your vital child

your vital child

A NATURAL HEALING GUIDE FOR CARING PARENTS

From the Natural Physician Team of
Mark Stengler, N.D.,
and Angela Stengler, N.D.

Foreword by William Sears, M.D.

RODALE

© 2001 by Mark Stengler, N.D., and Angela Stengler, N.D.

Illustrations © by Judy Newhouse
Cover photographs © by Corbis Stock Market (back), G&M David de Lossy/The Image Bank (top right), Mitch Mandel/Rodale Images, and Rosanne Olson/Stone (bottom left)

References in the Vaccinations chapter on page 483 were taken from ImmunoFacts® Facts and Comparisons, 2000; *Physicians' Desk Reference,* 1998 edition; and the U.S. Centers for Disease Control and Prevention Web site (www.cdc.gov).

Cover and interior design by Joanna Williams

Library of Congress Cataloging-in-Publication Data

Stengler, Mark.
    Your vital child : a natural healing guide for caring parents / from the natural physician team of Mark Stengler and Angela Stengler ; foreword by William Sears.
        p.   cm.
    Includes index.
    ISBN 1–57954–533–5 hardcover
    ISBN 1–57954–305–7 paperback
    1. Pediatrics—Popular works. 2. Children—Diseases—Alternative treatment—Popular works. 3. Naturopathy—Popular works. I. Stengler, Angela. II. Title.
RJ61 .S889 2001
618.92—dc21
                                                        2001004513

Distributed to the book trade by St. Martin's Press

2   4   6   8   10   9   7   5   3   1   hardcover

2   4   6   8   10   9   7   5   3   1   paperback

Visit us on the Web at www.rodalestore.com, or call us toll-free at (800) 848-4735.

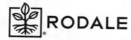

WE **INSPIRE** AND **ENABLE** PEOPLE TO IMPROVE
THEIR LIVES AND THE WORLD AROUND THEM

to you, the parent, for caring enough
about your child to read this book

contents

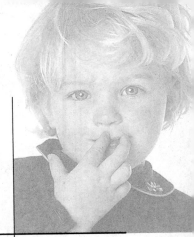

foreword

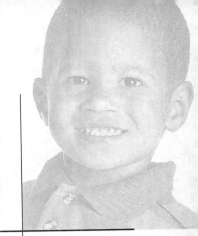

Pediatrics is a partnership between parents and doctor. This book will make you a more informed partner. Realistically, parents are their child's decision makers when it comes to medical treatment. The more informed you are about the available options—and the risks and benefits of treatment—the better able you are to make the wisest medical choices for your child.

In this book, you as parents will learn the meaning of natural medicine. You will learn how the body can heal itself given the proper tools. In fact, this may be considered a book of self-help tools to use as preventive medicine to keep your children healthy so that they need a doctor less. And when your children do need medical attention, you'll be an informed consumer who can work in partnership with your doctor to help heal your child.

More than 2,000 years ago, Hippocrates said, "Let food be your medicine." Little did the Greek father of medicine know that centuries later, the quality of our food would be so poor that we would have to take more medicine to treat the diseases caused by our nutritional deficiencies. But here you will learn the true meaning of the term *health foods*: foods that boost your child's immune system. In more than 30 years of pediatric practice, I have noticed that children whose parents feed them a nutritionally optimum diet are emotionally, intellectually, and physically healthier. Throughout this book, you will learn which foods are good medicine for your child. You will also learn how to raise a "pure child," one who is as free as possible from pollutants in his food and environment.

Parents are hungry for knowledge of herbal and other types of medicine. Which are safe? Which are effective? Throughout *Your Vital Child*, you'll find many sidebars with the title "Vital Fact" or "Vital Study," where the authors provide readers with as much research as possible about the most common health concerns affecting children today.

I was particularly impressed with the many self-help resources throughout this book. After reading *Your Vital Child,* parents will be able to put together their own medical plan for their individual child. This is a timely book. With the advent of managed care, many parents have less access to medical care and, by choice or necessity, have to formulate their own medical plan. This book will help you do exactly that.

William Sears, M.D.
Author, *The Baby Book*

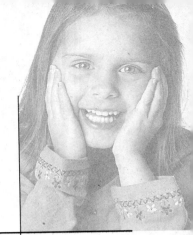

acknowledgments

The amount of work, time, and commitment needed to write such an important book could not have been managed without my husband, Mark. I love him more each day and admire him for his confidence in natural medicine. Our children are additional gifts from God, and I feel blessed to have such a loving family.

I encourage you to read this book and ask your health care provider questions. Never underestimate the importance of good nutrition, and always believe in your child's powerful natural healing abilities.

—Angela Stengler, N.D., La Jolla, California

First, I dedicate this book to our children: to our son, Mark Jr., and daughter, Hope, both of whom are truly vital children. Also, to all of our nieces and nephews in Canada.

I want to thank my wife, Angela, who coauthored this book with me. I have never met anyone as concerned about the health and well-being of children. You are an outstanding mother, wife, and doctor.

Thanks to Susan Clarey and Nancy Hancock for believing in this project; to Stephen George, Stephanie Tade, and Chris Potash of Rodale for their support and guidance; and to our book agent, Jeff Herman.

And thanks to those who helped review this book: Minh N Vu, M.Ac.O.M., L.Ac.; Ingrid Vu, M.Ac.O.M., L.Ac.; and Launa Boire, D.Ac., R.A.H.P.; to Prudence Broadwell, N.D., L.Ac., and Arden Moore for their contributions; and to those from whom I have learned, particularly at the National College of Naturopathic Medicine in Portland, Oregon.

—Mark Stengler, N.D., www.thenaturalphysician.com

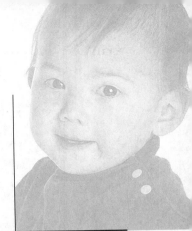

introduction

We titled this book *Your Vital Child* not just because we believe that natural therapies are vital to your child's health. The word *vital* means to be full of life and vigor, to be energetic. We feel that that's an excellent definition of children, too. We know that as parents or guardians, you want to see children full of health, in all areas of life. You want them to have maximum vitality. By augmenting a child's health and development with the natural healing traditions outlined in this book, parents will find the surest route to helping their children achieve a vitality that conventional medicine alone cannot.

We say this not just as parents and doctors but also as true believers who have seen the beneficial effects of natural healing. Dr. Mark has been studying various natural therapies since he was 10 years old. Dr. Angela became interested in natural and complementary therapies when she injured her foot in Europe. Soon after, in Britain, a health practitioner at a university clinic treated her with herbal medicine, which gave her tremendous relief from the bruising and swelling. We both spent 4 years at one of the top naturopathic medical schools in the world, and we did a great deal of internship with various doctors. Dr. Angela took extra training in natural childbirth and obstetrics and worked with many children. Dr. Mark received extra training in homeopathy, spinal manipulation, and oriental medicine. We both love to work with children in our clinic, and some parents travel long distances to receive consultation on the use of natural therapy for their children. We see the results firsthand when using natural medicine with children.

And we're not alone. Millions of people are healing themselves with the help of natural medicine. Seventy-five percent of Americans now take natural remedies on a regular basis, and a growing number are seeing naturopathic physicians, or natural health care practitioners. The dramatic increase in conventional doctors incorporating natural healing therapies into their practices is speeding the movement along. And with the popular shift toward preventive medicine, especially among modern parents, practitioners are increasingly prescribing natural therapies for children.

As doctors and as parents ourselves, we want the best for our children. We truly believe that a child cannot be vitally healthy without proper nutrition, regular exercise, unconditional love, and therapies that work in harmony with the healing systems of the body. Our training as naturopathic physicians includes a strong foundation in conventional medicine, and we respect what it can do. Drugs and surgery are appropriate for dealing with certain severe illnesses. But in many cases, such extreme treatments can cause more problems than they solve. For a child to achieve and maintain optimal health, we're convinced that parents must understand and take advantage of natural preventive and healing therapies.

It is our hope and our intention to raise the care of children to a higher level by giving parents and their family doctors the confidence to employ a wide range of natural health therapies safely and effectively.

How to Use This Book

Part 1 is designed to equip parents with everything they need to know about natural medicine. Here, we name the major healing modalities—nutrition, herbal therapy, vitamins and minerals, homeopathy, aromatherapy, and others—and explain how to use them to your child's best advantage. All the specifics about these modalities and how they relate to children are included. You'll learn how to make sure your child is getting the proper dosage, what therapies or supplements have potential side effects, and all the other essential things you need to know. We also provide an overview of the basic philosophy of natural medicine.

Breastfeeding gets an extended look as an important start to a healthy life, and factors that affect development—the environment, mental and physical exercise, and spiritual support—are also explored as they relate to health care. Research has shown that breastfeeding provides tremendous health advantages for children, such as improved immunity, better growth and development, and even benefits for the brain. We see the difference that it makes in children in our practice, and we felt compelled to share this knowledge with you.

Part 2 details more than 150 common childhood conditions and provides a convenient shortlist of proven natural remedies and preventive holistic treatments. After explaining the cause of the childhood condition and identifying its typical symptoms and typical conventional treatment, we provide two treatment options. The first is a Basic Plan that contains the most important and effective therapies or natural medicines to help treat your child for that specific problem. The supplements and therapies recommended in the Basic Plan are readily available at health food stores, pharmacies, online, and even in some grocery stores. This simple yet effective program is the perfect one to follow if you are new to natural therapies.

Following the Basic Plan is the Advanced Plan, which lists all the other natural therapies that are potentially helpful for a particular condition. For those who are experienced in natural therapies, or for those who want a more aggressive treatment program, the Advanced Plan provides an array of alternatives that are to be used *in addition to* what is suggested in the Basic Plan. This does not mean that all the Advanced Plan supplements and therapies given need to be followed. Instead, you should pick and choose the treatments that seem most indicated for and also most compatible with your child.

Part 3 presents a bonanza of quick-reference information about vaccination schedules, assembling a children's natural medicine kit, and how to deal confidently with common health care emergencies. Finally, we end with a resource guide that gives the names and addresses of organizations that can provide additional information on any of the natural healing modalities discussed in the book, and more.

The Philosophy of Natural Medicine

Learning the philosophical principles behind natural medicine is just as important as using the natural remedies themselves. They're the key to relieving symptoms in a safe and effective manner, and to identifying and treating the underlying causes of a child's health problems. The principles of naturopathic or natural medicine make a lot of sense, even to those who are new to natural healing. And, as you may be surprised to discover, all the great healing traditions of the world—including some aspects of conventional medicine—share most of the following principles in one way or another.

First, Do No Harm

This tenet, found in the Hippocratic oath that physicians take when they earn their M.D.'s, is a cornerstone of all responsible healing disciplines. Whatever treatment is chosen for a particular situation, it should not create more problems than it solves. It follows, then, that noninvasive treatments, whenever feasible, are preferred to minimize the risk of harmful side effects and to avoid creating a situation where the cure turns out to be worse than the disease. Thus, we might use massage or chiropractic for a child's muscular pain instead of using drugs that merely cover up the pain, increase the risk of further injury, or cause serious side effects. Or we may prescribe herbs, homeopathy, and supplements instead of frequently ineffective, side-effect-inducing antibiotics for a child who has reoccurring ear infections.

Find the *Real* Cause

Almost every illness has an identifiable underlying cause. In our experience, it often relates to a child's lifestyle, diet, or environment. For instance, many cases of colic are simply sensitivity to food ingredients that an infant ingests through formula or via the mother's breast milk. Identifying and removing the offending ingredient is often the most effective cure. Another good example is eczema. Creams that merely suppress the skin rash are not treating the cause. Identifying a cause—such as a nutritional deficiency or food sensitivity—allows you to treat the root problem, not just the symptoms.

Treat the Whole Person

For optimal health, healers need to focus on all the aspects that come into play in the life of a vital child. This is a complex set of factors, including physical, emotional, and even spiritual concerns. For example, we commonly find that children with asthma or irritable bowel syndrome have underlying emotional issues. When specific treatment is targeted toward these areas, the outcome is more successful than with physical treatment alone.

It's Better to Prevent Than to Treat

Most illnesses that children get are preventable, especially when parents learn to promote a healthy lifestyle in their children, which reduces overall susceptibility to disease. We are not just talking about colds and flu but also about more serious ailments, such as childhood type 2 diabetes. Many cases of this disease can be prevented through lifestyle habits (diet and exercise) and nutritional supplements. Another good example is childhood ear infections, which we find are also easily prevented with proper diet recommendations.

Trust in the Healing Power of Nature

The body has an inherent system to heal itself. The proper use of natural therapies helps to move the body in the direction of healing. Nature supplies powerful resources to activate the healing mechanisms of the body. The body, mind, and spirit are designed to be compatible with what nature has to offer: water, air, sunshine, and food.

Having said that, it's important to note that conventional treatments such as antibiotics and surgery are sometimes needed to allow the body to move in the direction of healing, and we will always note when such instances are necessary.

Part I

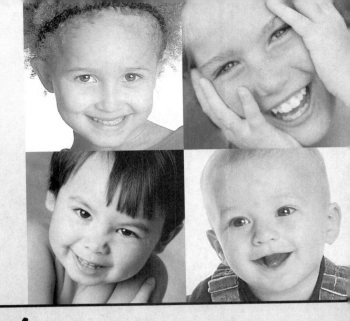

natural medicine
overview

children's building blocks of health

While it's important to treat the whole person, a person's whole health is the sum of individual components. Healers and parents need to consider each of those parts carefully in order to understand which natural or conventional therapies will work best to treat a child's illness and maintain their mental and physical well-being. Here, we'll examine each of the building blocks that comprise a child's health.

I. Genetics

To a certain extent, a child's health and healthy potential is laid out in the map of his or her genetic makeup. That's not to say that your children's vitality is "locked in" by their DNA. Research shows that through food, nutrients, and natural therapies we can change the way genetic information is expressed. Like most maps, genetics can provide you with a sense of direction, but it need not set you or your child on a course from which there is no deviation.

For example, a child may have a susceptibility to respiratory infections. If the child's diet is imbalanced or he is not getting enough sleep, he may be prone to repeated attacks of bronchitis. If his diet is healthy and he is getting plenty of rest, he is less likely to get sick. In addition, natural therapies such as homeopathy and supplements can minimize this genetic susceptibility. True, there are conditions where genetics are more of a controlling factor, such as cystic fibrosis, where mucus accumulation builds up in the lungs due to genetic abnormalities. In cases like this, there are natural treatments, such as nutritional supplements, that can at least reduce the symptoms and severity of the condition.

What's more, many of the illnesses that affect children when they get older—heart disease, osteoporosis, and cancer—take years to develop. And even if their genetic makeup puts them at greater risk for these diseases, a healthy lifestyle, good nutrition, emotional support, and all the benefits of the building blocks mentioned can reduce that risk of these and other diseases as they grow up.

II. Diet

One of the most important things you can do for your child's health is to surround her with nutritious and tasty foods. The quality of a child's diet can make a tremendous impact on her present health and vitality, and it sets the stage for her health as an adult. You may not be able to control whether your child gets hurt playing at school or whether an infectious epidemic hits your town, but you can control what your child eats and thereby optimize her health. Proper nutrition increases the enjoyment that children have in life because it positively affects their mood and energy levels. And it makes them more resistant to disease—especially to diet-related illnesses such as obesity, diabetes, cancer, fatigue, anemia, and most other chronic ailments. This section summarizes the most important things to focus on with regard to nutrition. Read it carefully and implement the recommendations in your child's diet.

The Five Basics of a Healthy Diet

1. Carbohydrates

These are individual sugar molecules joined together. There are two types of carbohydrates: simple and complex. Simple carbohydrates, such as sucrose and lactose, are composed of one or more monosaccharides, the simplest sugar molecules, which include glucose, fructose (fruit sugar), and galactose (a milk sugar). Most children consume far too many simple carbohydrates, which are abundant in candy, potato chips, and soft drinks as well as in white breads and other foods made with refined flours. When consumed in excess, especially on an empty stomach, the sugars in simple carbohydrates cause blood sugar levels to spike dramatically. This causes the pancreas to produce higher levels of insulin, the hormone responsible for transporting blood sugar to the cells where it is used for fuel. Over time, the pancreas becomes overtaxed, the body becomes more resistant to its own insulin, and all that excess blood sugar ultimately creates a host of problems, including immune system suppression, mood swings, attention problems, and weight gain. Too high a percentage of simple carbohydrates also predisposes children to diabetes, cavities, and heart disease.

Approximately 50 to 60 percent of your child's diet should come from complex carbohydrates. These provide a longer-lasting energy source than simple carbohydrates. They tend to make you feel fuller, they maintain blood sugar balance, and they contain more vitamins, minerals, and phytonutrients (nutrients found in whole plants that can have a range of health benefits) than simple carbohydrates. Examples of complex carbohydrates include whole grains (such as whole wheat pasta, whole wheat breads and cereals, and oatmeal), beans, brown rice, peas, and most root vegetables, such as carrots and yams.

Consuming carbohydrates with protein sources, fiber, and fat—that is, the good kinds of fat (see page 7)—also helps to smooth out the effect on blood sugar levels. This is another reason why a balance of all the nutrients is so important.

2. Proteins

Protein is found in plant and animal foods. The body uses protein as a fuel source and also to repair tissues, organs, and muscles. It com-

Animal versus Plant Proteins

	Positive	Negative
Animal Protein	Contains all of the essential amino acids; organic sources are available that do not contain hormones or antibiotics	Much higher in saturated fat, which can contribute to cancer and cardiovascular disease. May contain contaminants such as hormones, antibiotics, and microbes (parasites, bacteria, virus). Heavy metals can be found in fish (mercury in swordfish, tuna, and shark).
Plant Protein	Contains fiber and phytonutrients	Doesn't contain all essential amino acids
	Organic plants are free of the contaminants found in animal products	Nonorganic foods contain potentially harmful pesticides and herbicides

prises enzymes and hormones, and it is found in every cell in the body. Amino acids are the individual building blocks of protein. There are approximately 20 different amino acids. Ten of the amino acids are known as essential amino acids. Our bodies cannot manufacture these, so it is essential that we consume them in our diets. The remaining 10 nonessential amino acids can be manufactured in the body. Each has a positive and negative side. See the table above for a closer look at plant and animal proteins.

Quality protein sources include soy, eggs, poultry, legumes, fish, nuts, small amounts of dairy products (if a child is not sensitive to them), and limited amounts of meat. For infants, breast milk is the best source of protein.

Approximately 15 to 20 percent of your child's diet should consist of protein.

3. Fats

Most people fear fat because they associate it with obesity. But for a child to be healthy, fat is required in the diet. The key is to take in the right kind of fats and to reduce or avoid harmful fats. Children need fat in their diets for healthy brain development and function, for normal growth and development, and to help absorb certain nutrients. Fat is vital for healthy skin, nails, and hair, as well as for a healthy immune system and many other vital functions. All fats are composed of carbon, hydrogen, and oxygen molecules. The difference between the types of fats is the number of carbon atoms and the way in which they are arranged. There are three main categories of naturally occurring fats, plus a synthetic type that plays a large and unhealthy role in many people's diets.

Children who are vegan (eat plant foods only) can consume enough protein and get all the essential amino acids, provided that they get enough of a variety of complementary protein foods. It is best to consult with a nutritionist or doctor trained in nutrition to make sure that your vegan child is getting the right combinations of proteins.

Monounsaturated fats: These are fatty acids that have one double bond on the molecular level. The double bond affects the function of the fatty acid and makes it useful for certain cell functions. Monounsaturated fatty acids are healthy and are found in foods such as avocados and olive oil.

Polyunsaturated fats: All of the essential fatty acids are polyunsaturated fatty acids, meaning that they contain more than one double bond. Essential fatty acids must be taken in through the diet. Fish such as salmon and mackerel are examples, as are flaxseeds and flaxseed oil, walnuts, soybeans, and some other plant foods. See "Essential Fatty Acids" on page 8 for more information.

Saturated fats: In these fats, all the carbon molecules are filled (saturated) with hydrogen molecules. This makes fats solid to semi-solid at room temperature. Examples of foods high in saturated fats include red meat, pork, and dairy products. Lard is another example. Some oils, such as palm and coconut oil, contain large amounts of

Vital Study

A study published in the March 2000 issue of *Developmental Medicine and Child Neurology* shows that when infant formulas were supplemented with the fatty acids docosahexaenoic acid and arachadonic acid, it resulted in a mean increase of 7 points on the Mental Developmental Index of the Bayley Scales of Infant Development—a significant increase.

saturated fats. Saturated fats are associated with increased susceptibility to cancer, heart disease, and inflammatory conditions. Saturated fat is known to be a storehouse for many different types of toxins.

Hydrogenated and partially hydrogenated fats: Hydrogenation or partial hydrogenation is the commercial process of solidifying oils, a process that produces harmful trans fatty acids. These are "synthetic fats" that cause oxidation and damage of cells. Common food examples include margarine, cookies, crackers, many salad dressings, and many commercial baked goods. Alternative foods that do not contain these harmful fatty acids are available.

Approximately 25 to 30 percent of your child's diet should come from fats, with the majority of fats being polyunsaturated.

Essential Fatty Acids

Children need a proper balance of essential fatty acids, which are just that: essential nutrients that the body cannot manufacture and, in fact, cannot live without. Essential fatty acids are part of the cell membrane and necessary for cells to carry out their normal functions. They're involved with brain and retina development, balanced mood, hormone synthesis, pain and inflammation regulation, immune function, circulation, energy production, and skin, nail, and hair health, among other things. There are two essential fatty acids: alpha linolenic acid and linoleic acid.

Alpha linolenic acid (ALA): ALA is a member of the omega-3 fatty acid family. You have probably heard this term in regard to the health benefits of fish and flaxseeds. Other examples of foods that contain ALA include walnuts, green leafy vegetables, and canola oil.

Linoleic acid (LA): LA is a member of the omega-6 family. It's found in naturally occurring oils in foods such as corn, sesame, and borage, as well as in sunflower, safflower, and evening primrose oils.

Other Fatty Acids

While not essential (the body can manufacture them from essential fatty acids), these fatty acids are certainly beneficial.

Docosahexaenoic acid (DHA): This omega-3 fatty acid is found in high concentrations in breast milk and fish. Humans have the ability to make DHA from the essential fatty acid ALA, but the efficiency of this process varies depending on the individual. DHA plays a pivotal role in the development of a baby's brain and retinas. With the wealth of knowledge about the role of essential fatty acids, it is important that infant formulas be made to contain these critical fats. While we expect this to be mandatory at some point, you should look at adding sources of essential fatty acids to your infant's formula. DHA liquid pediatric formulas are readily available at health food stores and pharmacies. They can be given to the infant or added to formula.

The most common food sources of DHA are fish, especially cold-water fish such as salmon, mackerel, herring, and tuna. Other good sources include eggs and some types of algae.

Eicosapentaenoic acid (EPA): This omega-3 fatty acid helps to regulate inflammation, the immune system, blood clotting, and circulation (including to the brain). It is found in the same foods as DHA—fish.

Gamma linolenic acid (GLA): This member of the omega-6 family has a powerful effect on the functions of the brain. Some children require higher amounts of GLA for learning disorders, hyperactivity, and conditions such as eczema. Sources include borage oil, evening primrose oil, and black-currant seed oil.

Children who are on a vegetarian diet are at risk for deficiencies of essential fatty acids such as docosahexaenoic acid (DHA). Supplemental vegetarian sources of DHA are recommended for these children.

Vital Study

In a study published in *The Lancet* in 1995, researchers found that infants fed docosahexanoic acid (DHA) supplemented formula had better brain development and visual acuity than infants who did not receive DHA in their formula. They recommended that infants should receive DHA-enriched formulas. DHA is also used by nutrition-oriented doctors for the treatment of hyperactivity, mood disorders, and attention deficit disorder. Researchers in Europe have reported benefits in giving children with attention deficit disorder supplements combining fish oil and evening primrose oil.

Arachadonic acid (AA): This omega-6 acid is found in mothers' breast milk and helps with brain development. At approximately 1 year of age, an infant can make its own AA. Many animal products such as beef and turkey contain AA, so a deficiency is rare in our society. Too much AA can be a precursor to inflammatory conditions in the body. Linoleic acid can also be converted into AA. Sources of AA include animal fat, peanuts, and some algae.

The Importance of Fatty Acid Balance

Think of a scale with the omega-3 fatty acids on one side and the omega-6 fatty acids on the other. To maintain a balance, each side must be equal.

The problem with most children in our modern society is that this scale is tipped in favor of the omega-6 fatty acids. This imbalance can lead to a whole host of problems, including behavioral changes, decreased immunity, cardiovascular problems, joint problems, skin problems, and a variety of other medical conditions.

The physical signs of essential fatty acid deficiency or imbalance include:

- "Chicken skin" on the back of the arms
- Dandruff
- Dry eyes
- Dry or cracked skin
- Dry, listless hair
- Excessive thirst
- Frequent urination
- Irritability
- Poor wound healing
- Soft nails or nails that break easily

Conditions associated with fatty acid deficiency or imbalance include:

- Arthritis
- Asthma
- Attention deficit disorder
- Cardiovascular disease
  (heart attack, stroke)
- Cancer
- Depression
- Diabetes
- Dry skin

- Eczema
- Fatigue
- Hair loss
- Hypertension
  (high blood pressure)
- Lupus
- Memory problems
- Schizophrenia

Blood tests are available to determine fatty acid deficiencies or imbalances. These can be of value for attention deficit disorder, asthma, hyperactivity, and other childhood conditions.

4. Fiber

One of the keys of a healthy diet is to make sure that your child is getting enough fiber on a daily basis. Fiber gives your child a sense of fullness without empty calories. It may also reduce the risk of colon and other cancers, as well as of cardiovascular disease later in life. Constipation, straining to have a bowel movement, abdominal pain, or hard stools can all be signs that your child is not getting enough fiber.

Plant foods are the only source of fiber. There are two types of fiber, and most plant foods contain a mix of both.

Soluble fiber dissolves in water and is found in foods such as oat bran and beans and peas. This type of fiber helps to slow the absorption of glucose from the intestines into the bloodstream and thus improves blood sugar balance. It also helps to keep cholesterol levels in check.

Insoluble fiber does not dissolve in water, but instead helps to bind water and bulk up stool for efficient bowel movements. It also helps to bind excess fats and toxins in the digestive tract so that they can be excreted.

To calculate how many grams of fiber your child needs, take the age of your child (in years) and add 5. For instance, a 3-year-old would

Fiber Content of Common Foods

	Serving Size	Soluble Fiber (g)	Insoluble Fiber (g)	Total Fiber (g)
Fruits				
Apple	1	0.4	2.6	3
Banana	1	0.5	1.3	1.8
Blackberries	½ c	0.4	4.5	4.9
Blueberries	½ c	0.2	1.9	2.1
Grapefruit	½ grapefruit	0.1	0.3	0.4
Grapes	10 grapes	Trace	0.5	0.5
Honeydew melon	½ c chunks	0.1	0.4	0.5
Peach	1	0.6	1.1	1.7
Raisins	¼ c	0.2	1.4	1.6
Vegetables and Legumes				
Artichoke (fresh, cooked)	1 medium	3.5	2.9	6.4
Black beans (dry, cooked)	½ c	0.1	2.7	2.8
Broccoli	½ c florets	1.6	1.0	2.6
Brussel sprouts (frozen, cooked)	½ c	0.4	2.8	3.2
Green peas (canned or frozen)	½ c	0.3	2.8	3.1
Lentils (dry, cooked)	½ c	0.1	2.8	2.9
Lettuce	½ c torn	0.2	0.3	0.5
Spinach (cooked, canned, or raw)	½ c cooked or canned 2 c raw	0.3	2.0	2.3

require 8 grams of fiber a day. As a general rule, though, giving your child 5 or more servings of fruits and vegetables a day usually gives them all the fiber they need. Note that children with sensitive digestive systems, who are susceptible to bloating, gas, cramps, and so on, often do better with the steaming or cooking of fibrous vegetables such as broccoli, carrots, and cauliflower.

	Serving Size	Soluble Fiber (g)	Insoluble Fiber (g)	Total Fiber (g)
Vegetable soup, canned	1 c	0.6	1.6	2.2
Grains				
Bread, rye	1 slice	0.2	0.5	0.7
Bread, white or Italian	1 slice	0.2	0.6	0.8
Bread, whole wheat	1 slice	0.3	2.2	2.5
Cereal, Rice Krispies	1 c	0.1	0.4	0.5
Cereal, Special K	1 c	0.1	0.7	0.8
Cereal, Total cornflakes	1 c	0.1	0.8	0.9
Cookie, oatmeal	1 large	0.3	0.6	0.9
Cookie, plain sugar	1	0.1	0.1	0.2
Crackers, Ritz	4	0.1	0.2	0.3
Muffin, blueberry	1 small	0.2	0.6	0.8
Oats, whole (cooked)	½ c	0.5	1.1	1.6
Pancakes	2	0.2	0.7	0.9
Rice, medium grain (cooked)	½ c	0.1	0.3	0.4
Nuts				
Almonds, roasted	22	0.1	2.4	2.5
Peanuts	30 to 40	0.1	1.9	2
Walnuts	14 halves	0.1	1	1.1

5. Water

The majority of the human body is water, making it a critical substance for all of our cells, organs, and tissues to work properly. This includes the brain. Mild dehydration can interfere with concentration and cause headaches. Most children do not consume enough water on a daily basis. Infants who are exclusively breastfed do not need to drink water, as they get plenty in the breast milk. Children should consume an average of 40 ounces a day. Warm climate, exercise, and consumption of soft drinks and high-sodium foods lead to the loss of water in children. A child needs more water to help recover when he is sick.

Keeping Your Child on a Healthy Diet

Now that you know the essentials of a good diet, here are some guidelines for incorporating these essentials into what your child eats every day.

Think of yourself as your child's "food coach." A coach guides you in specific areas to improve your knowledge and skills. A good coach also provides support and helps to motivate you to make the best choices. This is a great approach to take with your children. Being parents ourselves, we know that a firm but caring and passionate approach works best when it comes to providing healthy meals and snacks for your child. Here are some tips to help you become an effective food coach for your children.

Do not rely on a child to tell you when he is thirsty. By the time a child feels the need for fluids, he is already somewhat dehydrated.

1. Learn as much as you can about nutrition. This book and many others are loaded with sound, effective advice on optimal nutrition for children.

2. Be a role model for nutritious eating. Kids learn more by watching than from listening to parents preaching.

3. Start young. While it's easiest to shape a child's eating preferences in the first 3 years of life, working with children of any age helps them develop good eating habits that will allow them to make smart choices as adults.

4. Be enthusiastic about eating healthfully. Enthusiasm begins with the belief that you really can make a difference in the quality of your child's health and vitality. The more enthusiasm you display, the more positively your kids will respond to the meal plans.

5. Be patient. In a society where junk food is the norm, it takes time to adapt to a healthful diet.

Avoid the SAD Diet. By examining the standard American diet (SAD), it's all too easy to get a picture of what should *not* be fed to kids on a regular basis. The standard child's diet is high in sugar, saturated fat, and animal protein. Many of the foods are loaded with artificial sweeteners, dyes, and preservatives. The SAD diet is deficient in plant foods such as fruits, vegetables, legumes, whole grains, and nuts, as well as in fish. Most children do not drink enough water on a daily basis, drinking soft drinks or sweetened fruit juice instead. Pesticides, herbicides, and other toxic chemicals are present in the food supply (including some leading-brand baby food). The short- and long-term effects of many of these pollutants are unknown, although we do know that a child's maturing immune and nervous systems are more susceptible to these chemicals.

Stick to whole foods. Your child's diet should be one that focuses on whole foods, which are unprocessed and as fresh as possible. A whole-foods diet will be much richer in nutrient and enzyme content than a diet made up of packaged and processed foods. Examples of whole foods include whole grain breads and cereals, fruits, vegetables, fresh fish and meats, and nuts and seeds.

Add the spice of variety. Every food has a different nutritional profile. By fitting as many different healthful foods as possible into your child's diet, you expand the amount and types of nutrients that your child will consume. In addition, a varied diet will expand your child's desire for a wider variety of foods. When it comes to fruits and vegetables, try to provide the whole spectrum of colors—green, yellow, red, and so on. They all contain different phytonutrients, or plant nutrients, that are valuable for your child's developing body and that can help prevent serious illnesses.

Go organic. More than 1 billion pounds of pesticides and herbi-

Vital Study

Researchers at the University of Tennessee, Knoxville studied preschool children and found that the foods most commonly consumed were fruit drinks, carbonated beverages, 2% milk, and french fries. Vegetables dominated children's "least favorite foods" lists. (Published in 1999 in the *Journal of the American Dietetic Association*.)

cides are sprayed on U.S. crops each year. Yes, it is realistic to assume that your child is ingesting these potential toxins. According to studies by the nonprofit, public interest Environmental Working Group (EWG), based in Washington, D.C., more than one-quarter million American children ages 1 through 5 ingest a combination of 20 different pesticides every day. More than 1 million preschoolers eat at least 15 pesticides on a given day. Overall, 20 million American children age 5 and under eat an average of 8 pesticides every day.

The long-term effect of pesticide and herbicide exposure on children is unclear. Population studies on adults suggest a link between these substances and certain types of cancers and neurological diseases. As parents and doctors, we do not want to wait until "absolute" scientific evidence links these chemicals to various diseases. Pesticides that have been considered safe and that have been used for decades are only now being banned. For example, in December 2000, the U.S. Environmental Protection Agency (EPA) stated that Diazinon, the second most commonly used home pesticide, was a risk to children. The agency is now restricting its consumer use.

The EPA admits that pesticides pose a risk to children's health. It has stated: "Children are at a greater risk from some pesticides for a number of reasons. Children's internal organs are still developing and maturing and their enzymatic, metabolic, and immune systems may provide less natural protection than those of an adult. There are 'critical periods' in human development when exposure to a toxin can permanently alter the way an individual's biological system operates." Children may be exposed more to certain pesticides because often they don't eat the same foods as adults.

Organic foods, on the other hand, have not been sprayed with

How Safe Are Your Fruits and Vegetables?

According to Mothers and Others, a New York City–based nonprofit group devoted to making the environment and our food supplies safer, the following 10 fruits and vegetables (nonorganic) contained the highest amounts of toxic pesticides:

1. Peaches
2. Apples
3. Pears
4. Winter squash
5. Green beans
6. Grapes
7. Strawberries
8. Raspberries
9. Spinach
10. Potatoes

synthetic chemicals and have been grown in safe soil. Look for foods that are labeled "certified organically grown." Or visit local farmers' markets and get to know the vendors. Learn who uses organic farming practices and who doesn't. As a general rule, though, you'll be exposing your child to fewer contaminants by going organic than not.

Clean your fruits and vegetables. All foods, whether they are organic or not, should be washed and cleaned thoroughly to rinse off bacteria as well as pesticides. The problem with soft foods such as pears is that the pesticides saturate into the core of the fruit. We recommend washing your fruits and vegetables with water or with special soaps available that rinse off pesticides.

Be finicky about fish. As we have mentioned, fish is an excellent source of protein and essential fatty acids. Unfortunately, certain species of fish are known to contain dangerous levels of mercury and other toxins. Below are lists of fish that are deemed to be safe from mercury and those that are considered borderline or unsafe. The quality and safety of fish depends on the area in which you live. You can check the status of fish contamination in your area by visiting the EPA's Web site (www.epa.gov)

or by checking with your state department of health. Safe fish include:

- Anchovy
- Catfish
- Clams (though bacterial and parasite contamination can be a problem)
- Cod, Pacific
- Crab
- Flatfish, Pacific
- Herring
- Mahi mahi
- Oysters (though bacterial contamination can be a problem)
- Pollack, Pacific
- Salmon, wild Alaskan
- Sardines
- Scallops, farmed
- Tilapia, farmed

Be cautious about eating the following fish; in general, they are not considered safe and shouldn't be eaten more than once a month. Check with the EPA or a local agency about the contamination levels of these fish in your area:

- Chilean seabass
- Cod, Atlantic
- Grouper
- Flatfish, Atlantic
- Halibut
- Lobster
- Mackerel
- Ocean perch
- Orange roughy
- Oreo dory
- Pollock, Atlantic
- Rockfish, Pacific
- Shark
- Snapper
- Striped bass
- Swordfish
- Tuna

Keep 'em regular. It is important that your child eat regular meals. This will help to maintain regular blood sugar levels. Regular meals improve concentration, mood, and energy levels. Snacks between meals are important for kids who are very active.

Pack a lunch. Many schools are infiltrated by well-known fast food chains. While fast foods pose no problem when eaten on occasion (once a week), they should not be what your child eats on a regular basis for lunch. They are loaded with harmful trans fatty and saturated acids, artificial preservatives and sweeteners, and sugars.

Eat out safely. You can enjoy eating out with your children and still get a relatively healthful meal. Here are some pointers:

- If your child cannot read yet, give him menu options that do not include fried foods.
- You don't have to order for your child from the kids' menu. Adult portions are often quite large, making it easy to share your meal with your child.
- Tell the waiter that you do not want a dessert menu or sample at the end of the meal.
- Choose fruit juice, milk, or water over soft drinks.
- Choose fruit or steamed vegetables instead of french fries as a side dish.

Introducing Food to Your Baby

There is no need to go out and purchase a lot of jars of baby food. It's a good idea, however, to have some jars of organic baby food on hand in your diaper bag and cupboard as backup. There are brands available that use non-GMO (non-genetically modified) organic baby foods.

What's the best way to feed your baby? Use your own food! For example, purchase fresh organic veggies, steam them, then puree them in a blender or food processor (add the water from steaming them—it contains valuable vitamins and minerals), cool, and serve. You can make homemade baby food as thin or thick as your baby

Vital Study

According to a 1993 study published in the *Journal of Applied Nutrition*, the following beneficial minerals are found in higher quantities in organic foods than in other foods:

Boron	Phosphorus
Calcium	Potassium
Chromium	Selenium
Copper	Silicon
Iodine	Sodium
Iron	Strontium
Lithium	Sulfur
Magnesium	Vanadium
Molybdenum	Zinc
Nickel	

Meanwhile, some toxic minerals are known to be higher in conventionally grown foods, including:

Aluminum	Lead
Cadmium	Mercury

can tolerate. You can mash and blend potatoes, fruits, beans, and meat. Your child does not need her own separate "menu" at mealtime. Just make sure that you are serving appropriate foods for her age.

You can prevent food reactions and health problems by systematically and correctly introducing solid foods to your baby. This section tells you how.

Introduce one new food every 4 or 5 days, and watch your child for any food sensitivity reactions. Symptoms such as runny nose, diarrhea, moodiness, or skin rashes can be associated with a food sensitivity. When you find that the food is not causing any problems, put it into rotation, serving it only every 3 to 5 days. For optimal health, avoid wheat, cow's milk, eggs, sugar, and citrus fruit until your child is at least 1 year old. Wheat-free, dairy-free, fruit juice–sweetened snacks are available.

Birth to 6 months

- Breast milk or iron-enriched formula

6 months

- Pureed, strained vegetables such as squash, carrots, and yams
- Pureed, strained fruits such as pears and peaches
- Enriched baby rice cereal

7 to 9 months

- Any of the following foods can be mashed or pureed with breast milk or water (don't combine foods, however): millet, barley cereal, mashed potatoes, lentils, avocados, apples, applesauce, and pear juice or apple juice (dilute juices with at least 50 percent water).

Your baby may be able to start drinking from a cup at this point. You can start giving "finger foods" around 9 months of age. ("O" cereals from the health food store are a good choice, since they contain no sugar or preservatives.)

Caution: Watch out for choking hazards, such as overly hard or large food items.

9 to 12 months

- Peas
- Cooked eggs (yolk first)
- Cheese
- Oatmeal
- Beans
- Broccoli and cauliflower

12 to18 months

- Whole yogurt with live cultures (plain or vanilla; do not use products with sugar)
- Wheat products
- Cow's milk, enriched-calcium soy milk, rice milk, and/or goat's milk
- Cooked whole eggs
- Poultry
- Beef
- Fish
- Increased variety of fruits, such as strawberries and melons

Some children may be able to start to use utensils at this age.

2 years

- Nut butters
- Oranges and other citrus fruits
- Tomatoes
- Deli meat (nitrate/nitrite free; avoid all cured and smoked meats since they contain nitrates)

Healthy Meal Ideas for Toddlers

Following are samples of foods you can feed a toddler for meals and snacks.

Breakfast: Oat pancakes, cultured yogurt (whole milk or low-fat preferred, not fat-free for children under 2), enriched baby rice cereal, eggs, sprouted grain toast with natural nut butter (almond or peanut) or jam, waffles, cut-up fruit

Snacks: Sliced apples or bananas, mangoes, cantaloupe, cheese, vitamin-enriched "O" cereal, puffed wheat, and veggie sticks are healthful choices. Your local health food store may sell toddler granola bars; look for brands such as Barbara's and Health Valley. You can also look for cookies that are free of hydrogenated fats, artificial colorings and flavorings, preservatives, and nuts. Or try wheat-free or whole wheat muffins with honey or fruit juice, not sugar, as the sweetener. Avoid artificial sugar substitutes.

Lunch: Nitrate-free chicken dogs or hot dogs, nitrate-free deli meat, rice pasta with cheese, steamed vegetables, sprouted grain toast, fish, homemade burritos

Dinner: Fish, brown or basmati rice, any rice mix without MSG, turkey loaf, tofu, steamed veggies, tacos made with chicken, lentils, navy beans, homemade soups, Tater Tots or french fries (baked, not fried), baked or broiled potatoes

III. Physical Exercise

Research has proved, time and time again, that exercise improves immunity and mood and prevents childhood diseases such as obesity and diabetes. It is the natural instinct of a child to get a lot of activity and movement. Television and the computer have been allowed to interfere with this vital building block. The best activities are the ones that get your child moving and active, and that she likes. These could be swimming, walking, biking, soccer, even playing hide and seek—whatever your child enjoys. Enroll your children in active programs at an early age so that they learn to enjoy participating. If there are no children's sports programs in your area, or if they are out of your price range, don't worry: There are numerous activities that are free and that will provide quality exercise for you and your kids.

Make it a point to set aside at least 30 minutes each day to focus on play with your child that involves movement. Things that we like to do with our oldest son include playing chase (in or out of the house), riding bikes, kicking or throwing balls around, playing in the sprinkler, jumping rope, and dancing or marching to music. Also, simple games such as Simon Says or singing "Ring around the Rosie" can leave you and your kids winded after 30 minutes of play. Going to the park is an excellent option, and it's good to get the kids out of the house at times. We always make an effort to play with our son outside for 30 minutes or more every day. This helps Mark Jr. burn off some energy, get some fresh air, and mingle with the neighborhood kids as well. In addition, outside play provides quality time for child and parents.

IV. Mental Exercise

A healthy body is not much good without a healthy mind. A child's brain develops at an incredible rate over the span of childhood. Think of the mind like a muscle; without exercise, it becomes weak and inefficient. It is important to keep a child's mind stimulated while allowing him time to play by himself or with friends. Reading together, playing board games, and doing crossword puzzles are all fun ways to exercise your child's mind. Turn off the TV and read to your children or sing the ABCs. You'll be amazed at how much your kids enjoy being with you. Here are some easy ways to ensure that your children get mental exercise every day.

1. Give your child a quiet time each day. Start with 5 minutes and move up to 20 minutes, depending on the age of the child. Designate a place in the house where she can sit and look at books or read quietly.

2. Do a craft each day with your child. For example, with our son, it may involve one of the following: coloring a picture, drawing a picture of the family, copying shapes, making macaroni necklaces, baking bread, pasting pictures onto cardboard, or finger painting. There are loads of craft ideas that range from easy to difficult. Even drawing on the sidewalk with chalk provides mental stimulation, especially when you combine it with learning about colors.

3. Play pretend and make-believe with your child. For example, use socks for puppets, or dress up in old clothes. Or imagine that you are wild animals. Or even reverse roles: Let your child play the parent, and you play the kid.

Have fun with imaginative play. This is the perfect time to use all those toys your kids have! Remember, making learning fun is a priority with children.

V. Emotional Support

The emotional state of a child has a direct effect on her physical and mental health. Spending time with your child, actively listening to her, being patient, and counseling her are essential for her to develop to her fullest potential.

It is important that your child knows that you are listening to her. Don't read the newspaper while your child is talking to you. And definitely turn off the TV. Look her in the eye and respond when she tells you about her day or asks you a question.

When asking a child about his day at school, be specific. Don't just ask, "How's school?" Ask pointed questions. Find out what the schedule is at school so that you can ask about his classes, story time, recess, and so on. Being a parent requires that you provide emotional support for your child. Don't expect a day care provider or teacher to do that job for you. Get involved with your children's activities. Volunteer when you can. It is important that your children feel that you are interested in them. Children need love and stability more than material possessions.

Discipline is invaluable in a child's life and an important step to providing them with emotional support. There are many forms of discipline, ranging from time-outs and restrictions to controlled spanking. You as a parent must find a form of discipline that works for you and your child. Kids crave boundaries, and they won't hate you for putting limits on them. Start discipline at a young age. By the time your child is 2 years old, you should already be explaining the consequences of bad decisions and actions. Follow through with your rules.

But most important, give your child constant love and affection. Don't wait for special occasions to give your child a hug. Rather, make it a regular habit to hug your child and tell him that you love him. This is the most powerful emotional expression that you can give to your child.

VI. Spiritual Support

The human spirit is most evident in children. Their need for love and acceptance is obvious. We believe that you cannot have a happy or healthy family without God. It is imperative to incorporate religion into your child's life starting at infancy. You, as parents, need to feel confident that your child is raised knowing the importance of prayer and the love that God has for him. Raising your child with a strong faith will give him more direction and guidance as he grows up.

VII. Environment

The physical environment to which a child is exposed plays an important role in her health. You can do many things right: feed your children a balanced diet, exercise with them, and give them unconditional love and proper medical care. But if they are exposed to too many harmful pollutants, children will not be able to reach their full potential of health and vitality. A child's immunity and other vital systems are still maturing and are more susceptible to the damaging effects of toxins. Also, we know that the body stores many of these environmental toxins (for example, lead in the bones and aluminum in the brain), so they can lead to health problems over a lifetime.

According to the EPA, between 1987 and 1994, an estimated 2.2

Vital Fact

Researchers at Children's Hospital Medical Center of Cincinnati found that blood levels of lead even well below commonly accepted toxic levels can affect cognitive skills in children. The team evaluated data for 4,853 American children between the ages of 6 and 16 and found that as blood lead levels rise, scores for reading and basic math skills drop significantly.

billion pounds of industrial environmental pollutants were released into the air, water, and land. These include pesticides and herbicides, heavy metals (lead, mercury, aluminum, arsenic, cadmium, and others), and industrial contaminants such as volatile organic compounds (VOCs) and dioxins. All have been linked to a variety of health problems, ranging from neurological and cognitive problems to increased risk of cardiovascular problems and even cancer. Even electromagnetic fields, created by high-tension lines and other electrical equipment, are suspected to affect health and may pose a risk. To minimize your exposure to these environmental factors, take the following precautions.

Keep your water pure. Have your water tested by a reputable lab for contaminants such as heavy metals. Filtered water systems (reverse osmosis) for drinking water are recommended. If you live in an older home, make sure that the pipes do not have a lead lining and that the paint on the walls does not contain lead. If you live in an apartment, there are inexpensive water purifiers that can be added to the tap, or water containers that contain a filter that removes lead.

Be a metal deflector. Avoid heavy metal exposure that you can control—for instance, secondhand smoke, which exposes kids to lead and cadmium; aluminum pots and pans; and mercury fillings, which many dentists recommend removing from adult teeth and replacing with safer alternatives. It is an excellent idea to have your child screened for lead toxicity. Your doctor can do this with a urine or blood test. A hair analysis is a good screening tool for most of the heavy metals; this is available from your doctor or natural health care practitioner.

Minimize VOC exposure. Volatile organic compounds, or VOCs, are carbon-containing compounds that evaporate very quickly. Health problems associated with VOCs include asthma, allergies, headaches, fatigue, and possibly even cancer. The compounds are found in cleaning products, paints, carpets, glues, and many other products used in the home. Plastics and pesticides can also contain VOCs. As you can see, these examples include a lot of things to which your child is exposed, and it's impractical to expect that you can avoid them all. But there are things you can do to minimize exposure. One of the most important things is to realize that new products containing VOCs can give off gas. To keep that gas from staying in your house, leave new furniture, rugs, and so on out in the open air for at least a day (or if that's not practical, open the windows in whatever room they're located) before your child is exposed to them.

You should also *maintain* good ventilation in your home by keeping windows open when possible, especially when you've put down new carpeting or bought new furniture, as we just mentioned. Good ventilation allows VOCs to go outside.

Of course, whenever you can, choose low-VOC or VOC-free products, which may be labeled as such. (See "VOC Information" on page 507 for companies that can provide more details.)

Deal with dioxins. Dioxins are a class of chemicals that are released into the air from the production of vinyl, the burning of waste, the manufacturing of herbicides and household cleaners, and the bleaching of paper. Dioxins end up in the water and, ultimately, in the food we eat. These substances are carcinogenic and hormone disrupters, and they can cause neurological problems. Dioxins are primarily released into the air during the production and incineration of polyvinyl chloride (PVC), also known as vinyl. PVC is also contained in home construction and decoration materials, water, gas, sewage pipes, window frames, doors, blinds, shower curtains, imitation leather, furniture, wallpaper, and some baby toys (including teething rings).

As much as possible, try not to purchase vinyl products. Pay attention to the toys that your kids play with. Many manufacturers are now producing teething rings and other plastic toys without PVC. If it does not say "PVC-free" on the label of the plastic toy you are buying, you should call the company and ask. If the toy does contain PVC, make sure that your child does not continuously bite or suck on it.

Be wary of electromagnetic fields and currents. In the computer age, where virtually every device generates some level of electromagnetic energy, it's nearly impossible to stay away from all electromagnetic fields (EMFs) and currents. But it is a good idea to stay away from the largest EMF generators, particularly electrical power generators and power lines. We also recommend avoiding prolonged, up-close contact with certain electrical devices, especially electric blankets, cellular phones, and even home computers.

herbal medicines
for children

Herbal medicines are plants or plant substances used for medicinal purposes. They can be used to prevent, maintain, or improve health. Eighty percent of the world's population relies on herbs as a primary form of medicine. Many cultures use herbal therapies as a first line of treatment for infants and children. For example, hospitals in China train doctors to specialize in herbal medicine for infants and children. As herbal therapy enters mainstream medicine, more doctors are becoming educated and willing to recommend these treatments to their patients.

We find that most children respond more quickly than adults to herbal medicines. By following the guidelines in this chapter, you can strengthen your child's immune system and optimize his health. Start with common herbs, such as echinacea for a cold, or peppermint for an upset stomach. Your confidence will grow with each successful use of the herbs.

There may be times when you'll want to combine herbal treatments with conventional therapies. For example, we've seen children with attention deficit problems who still have problems even though they are taking conventional medicine such as Ritalin. In these cases, we can use herbs as well as other natural therapies in combination with the conventional prescription. Eventually, the child can decrease or completely eliminate the need for Ritalin, relying solely on natural therapies. Another use of herbs has to do with antibiotic treatment. In cases where a child is on antibiotics, herbal medicine can be used to speed up recovery and strengthen the immune system. In part 2, we give specific recommendations regarding the use of herbs and other natural therapies in these and other situations.

We encourage you to discuss the integration of herbal medicine and conventional medicine with your family doctor. More doctors are learning to integrate herbal medicine into their practices. Try not to get frustrated if a doctor seems uninterested or skeptical. Nowadays, there are more and more practitioners willing to learn about natural therapies. It would benefit you and your family to find a health care provider knowledgeable in herbal medicine.

Safe Use

We prominently review the herbs that are safe to use with children. Be suspect of any herbs for children not mentioned in this book. There are herbs that are toxic and that should not be used on children. Most toxic herbs are not available in your typical health food store, drug store, or supermarket supplement section. If you are unfamiliar with an herb or combination of herbs and cannot find any valid literature, then simply do not use it. Please pay particular attention to how to calculate the specific dosage for your child. This is important to achieve a therapeutic effect with herbs.

Herbal Preparations

Herbal remedies come in variety of different forms, for a variety of reasons. Here's a primer on the different forms you'll find.

- **Tinctures and glycerite.** A tincture or liquid extract is the preservation of herbs in water and alcohol. Tinctures are one of the most common forms of herbal medicines, along with capsules and teas. Since they are in a liquid form, tinctures are easy to absorb and assimilate. Some herbs require an alcohol extraction process so that certain medicinal constituents are pulled out of the plant and made available to the user. Children may not like the taste of a tincture due to the alcohol, but the taste can be improved by adding the tincture to a small cup of hot water and letting it sit for a few minutes. This allows some of the alcohol to evaporate. Then, you can add it to juice.

Glycerin-based tinctures, also known as glycerite, have had the alcohol removed and are easier for children to take. Glycerin is made from soaps and oils. It preserves herbs and is great for kids. It has no toxicity and can be sweetened easily for a taste kids love.

- **Capsules.** These contain the dry powder of the herb. They are popular because they're convenient. They are easy to take, as there is no taste involved, and they are easy to store in containers. If the herb(s) you need are available only in capsule form and your child cannot swallow capsules, you can open the capsules up and mix the contents into water, juice, or food.
- **Tablets.** These contain powdered herbs that have been compressed with binders and substances that make the tablet smooth and easy to swallow. The advantage is that more material can be compressed into a tablet. The downside is that many children cannot swallow tablets. However, you can crush the tablet.
- **Lozenges.** Herbs can be made into a dissolvable lozenge. A common example is echinacea/zinc lozenges.
- **Teas (decoctions and infusions).** A tea involves an herb or herbal combination soaked in water. There are two main ways to make a tea.

A *decoction* is used for harder plant parts, such as the bark, root, and seeds. These tough parts require more time and heat to extract their medicinal ingredients. To make a tea, heat the herb (1 tablespoon of a dry herb or 3 tablespoons of a fresh herb) in 1 cup of water until it boils and then let it simmer, covered, for 15 to 25 minutes. Then, let the mixture sit for 10 minutes, strain, and serve.

The more common preparation for a tea is an *infusion*. This is used for the softer part of herbs, such as leaves and flowers. It is effective for herbs such as peppermint leaf. Commercial preparations of tea bags are available, or you can use dry or fresh herbs.

For a tea bag, add one bag to a cup of hot or boiling water and let it sit for 10 to 15 minutes. For dry or fresh herbs, bring 1 cup of water to boil in a kettle and add 1 tablespoon of a dry herb or 3 tablespoons of a fresh herb to the water. Cover with a lid and let it sit for 10 to 15 minutes. Strain and serve.

- **Syrups.** Syrups can be added to decoctions and infusions to sweeten them.
- **Creams.** To make a cream, the desired herb is blended with an emulsion of water in oil. This allows the oily mixture to blend with skin secretions and penetrate the skin for healing purposes.
- **Salves.** These are mixtures of herbal oils or extracts with beeswax.
- **Liniments.** These are topical herbal preparations in oil.
- **Compresses and fomentations.** A compress involves the application of a hot or cold herbal extract to the skin. The herb can be applied directly to the skin, or it can be applied to the skin using a cloth that has been saturated with a decoction or infusion of the herb (this second method is called a fomentation). Fomentations are good for skin rashes or local inflammation.
- **Poultices.** In a poultice, plant material is applied to the skin by mixing the herb into a paste and applying it to the affected area between two thin pieces of cloth.
- **Steams.** Herbs or herbal (essential) oils are added to water that is steaming hot. Steam therapy is useful for ailments of the upper respiratory tract.
- **Suppositories.** Certain herbs can be inserted into the rectum or vaginal opening for a local treatment. Suppositories also provide a good way to get some herbs into the bloodstream.
- **Baths.** Herbs can also be delivered through the skin. Adding herbal preparations to a warm bath and having the child exposed to the bath for 15 minutes or longer can be effective. An example is an oatmeal bath for itchy skin breakouts or rashes.
- **Standardized extracts.** These are herbal extracts that have been standardized to certain levels of active compounds. This can be important in duplicating the level of active compounds used in a study.

At this time, there are many herbs with unknown active constituents. Standardized extracts are generally found in capsule form, although they can be found in tinctures, tablets, and occasionally teas as well.

Herbal Terminology

These terms are used to describe the properties and actions of herbs. We have avoided these terms in this book and have instead used common terms. However, this list can be helpful when consulting other works on herbal medicine.

Abortifacient: A plant that causes miscarriage or expulsion of the fetus. It is important that a pregnant woman avoid these. An example is the herb pennyroyal.

Adaptogen: A substance that helps the body adapt to stress, whether it be physical, mental, or emotional. Often referred to as a tonic. Supports energy levels. Many of the adaptogen herbs work in part by supporting adrenal gland function. Siberian ginseng is a classic example.

Alterative: An herb that helps improve general health by balancing and tonifying body functions. Alteratives improve nutritional status through improved digestion and elimination. They are sometimes referred to as blood purifiers. Alteratives generally have a low potential for toxicity and can be used on a long-term basis. A good example is burdock root.

Analgesic: A pain reliever. Also called an anodyne. An example is white willow.

Anticatarrhal: Something that decreases mucus production. Herbal examples are goldenseal and mullein.

Antidepressant: A substance that relieves feelings of depression. One example is St. John's wort.

Antidote: This counteracts the effect of a poison. Licorice is one example.

Antiemetic: An herb that prevents vomiting—for instance, ginger.

Antifungal: This destroys or prevents fungal infections. Tea tree oil is an example.

Antigalactic: Something that reduces or stops breast milk secretion. One example is sage.

Antihelmintic: An herb that destroys parasites. Examples include garlic, wormwood, and black walnut.

Anti-inflammatory: This reduces inflammation in the body. Examples: licorice root, bromelain, boswellia, white willow, and black cohosh.

Antimicrobial: A substance that prevents or destroys microbe (virus, bacteria, fungus, and so on) growth. Examples are echinacea and lomatium.

Antioxidant: Something that prevents the damage of cells by free radicals. Examples are ginkgo, astragalus, hawthorn berry, milk thistle, thyme, and wild oregano.

Antiparasitic: This prevents the growth of or destroys parasites. Examples include black walnut, clove, garlic, and wormwood.

Antipyretic: An herb that reduces fever—for instance, yarrow.

Antiseptic: This prevents the growth of microbes on the skin. Examples are calendula and propolis.

Antispasmodic: Something that prevents or reduces muscle spasms. Examples are black cohosh, chamomile, kava, valerian, and wild yam.

Antitussive: This relieves or suppresses coughing. Examples are horehound and wild cherry bark.

Antitumor: This fights or suppresses tumor growth. Astragalus and echinacea are two examples.

Astringent: An herb that causes contraction of the tissues. Useful in conditions such as bleeding or diarrhea. Examples are geranium, sage, witch hazel, and yarrow.

Bitter: Bitter-tasting herbs stimulate the digestive organ secretions and actions—stomach, liver, gallbladder, and pancreas. They can also help to increase an abnormally low appetite. Examples are gentian root, burdock, goldenseal, and dandelion root.

Bronchodilator: An herb that causes relaxation and dilation of the bronchial tubes (respiratory passageways). Often used to treat coughs, bronchitis, and asthma. Examples are peppermint, ma huang, and yerba santa.

Calmative: An herb that gently calms the nerves. Chamomile, hops, kava, passionflower, and valerian are good examples.

Carminative: This prevents or reduces gas. Examples include ginger root, fennel, anise, and peppermint.

Cathartic: An herb that stimulates bowel evacuation (a laxative). Cascara sagrada, senna, and rhubarb are cathartics.

Cholagogue: Something that stimulates bile flow from the gall-bladder—for instance, dandelion root.

Choleretic: This stimulates bile production in the liver. Milk thistle, burdock, and dandelion root are examples.

Demulcent: An herb that has a soothing and healing effect on the mucous membranes of the body. Slippery elm is a demulcent for the digestive tract.

Diaphoretic: An herb that causes perspiration. This can be useful in cases of colds to help the immune system expel the virus. Examples are yarrow and boneset.

Diuretic: Something that promotes urination. Dandelion leaf and parsley are examples.

Emetic: An herb that causes vomiting. Ipecac is an example.

Expectorant: An herb that promotes the expulsion of mucus from the respiratory tract—for instance, horehound, lungwort, or yerba santa.

Febrifuge: An herb that reduces fever. White willow is one example (used with adults).

Galactagogue: This stimulates milk flow. Examples include blessed thistle, fennel, and fenugreek.

Hemostatic: An herb that stops bleeding—for instance, cinnamon and yarrow.

Hepatic: An herb that acts on the liver to stimulate bile flow. Examples include burdock, milk thistle, licorice, dandelion root, yellow dock, and artichoke leaves.

Hypnotic: An herb that induces sleep—for example, valerian.

Storing Herbs

Most of the medicinal herbs used today come in commercial packaging. Therefore, it's easy to store them. Here are some general guidelines to remember:

Tinctures: Store them in the cupboard so that they are not exposed to light.

Capsules and tablets: Make sure that lids are closed at all times, and do not store bottles in an area with high humidity.

Teas: Bagged teas should be kept in an area that is dry and out of the light.

Herbs bought in bulk should be stored in an airtight glass container. The temperature should be between 55° and 65°F. Make sure to keep bulk teas out of the light as well.

Safety note: As with pharmaceutical medications, make sure you store herbal products out of the reach of children.

Hypotensive: An herb that lowers blood pressure. Hawthorn berry and garlic are two examples.

Immunomodulator: An herb that supports the action of the immune system. Astragalus, echinacea, garlic, lomatium, Oregon grape root, and osha are examples.

Laxative: An herb that promotes fecal expulsion. Examples include cascara sagrada, senna, aloe, and rehmania.

Lymphagogue: This stimulates activity of the lymphatic system. Herbal examples are burdock, ceanothus, and pokeroot.

Mucolytic: An herb that thins mucus secretions—for instance, goldenseal.

Nervine: An herb that relaxes and calms the nerves. Chamomile, passionflower, valerian, skullcap, and lavender are examples.

Nutritive: An herb that is nourishing to the body, such as nettle.

Palliative: An herb that relieves symptoms but does not cure the disease. For example, a child might sleep well when taking passionflower before bedtime, but cannot sleep unless she uses passionflower.

Prophylactic: An herb used to prevent a disease or condition. For instance, you might use echinacea to prevent a cold.

Rubefacient: An herb that is irritating to the skin and mucous membranes. Used to increase bloodflow to the affected area. Horse-radish, for example, opens up the sinuses.

Sedative: A calming herb. Examples include valerian, passion-flower, and chamomile.

Stimulant: This increases energy or has an exciting action. Gin-seng is one example.

Synergist: An herb that acts to increase the effectiveness of an-other herb or herbs in a formula, so that the sum of the herbs is greater than its parts. Licorice root is an example.

Tonic: This nourishes and restores normal function. An example is Siberian ginseng.

Vermifuge: This promotes expulsion of intestinal worms. Worm-wood is a vermifuge.

Vulnerary: An herb that promotes tissue healing—for example, calendula applied topically to cuts and scrapes, or aloe applied to burned skin.

Helping Your Child with Herbs

This section provides creative ways to administer herbs to children. Medicine doesn't have to taste bad to be good. In fact, many herbal medicines not only work better than conventional medicines but also taste better!

For example, if a tincture that has an alcohol base is used, put the desired amount of herb in ¼ cup hot water for 5 minutes to let the alcohol evaporate out, let the mixture cool, and then add it to water or juice. One of our favorites is to mix herbal teas with juice and freeze them like Popsicles. Here are some other strategies you can try.

1. Mix herbal capsules or crushed tablets into foods such as oat-meal, applesauce, and jam.

Case History

Seven-year-old Jennifer came to our clinic with a sore throat and a mild fever. Her parents said that she had had these symptoms for a few days. Our medical exam indicated that her symptoms were caused by a viral infection, for which antibiotics are powerless. We prescribed an herbal formula in an alcohol tincture for Jennifer that consisted of echinacea (for its antiviral and immune-stimulating effects), licorice root (which is sweet-tasting and antiviral), and mullein (which is throat-soothing). Jennifer didn't like the taste of this herbal combination, so we had her mom put the recommended dosage in a highly diluted fruit juice smoothie. Jennifer felt better by the next day, and her symptoms were completely gone within 3 days.

2. Use a dropper to put the desired amount of tincture in the child's juice (dilute the juice with 50 percent water). Concord grape juice hides bad-tasting herbs well.

3. For children who are stubborn, who refuse to eat or drink anything with herbs, or who will not take any medicine, there is one aggressive solution left: Use a plastic dropper and squirt the desired amount in the side of the child's mouth. This way, he can't spit it out.

Precautions

As with any substance, whether it is a food, drug, or pollen, allergic reactions can occur with herbs. Although it's rare, your child could be allergic to an herb or herbal formula. When using a herb or herbal formula for the first time, give a small amount, such as 3 drops, and see if there is any adverse reaction for the next 2 hours. Chances are, there will not be a problem. If a severe allergic reaction does occur—such as wheezing, difficult breathing, or hives—seek medical attention immediately and discontinue any further use of the herb. If more mild reactions occur, such as itching or a mild rash, choose another herb that has a similar action.

Frequency of Use

For acute conditions: Give the recommended dosage every 2 to 3 waking hours to relieve symptoms and support the body's response. For infectious conditions, continue the herbal treatment for 3 to 5 days after the symptoms have resolved, to prevent a relapse.

For chronic conditions: Give the recommended dosage two to three times daily.

The Natural Physician's Top Herbs for Children

The following are 13 herbs every parent should know about. These are the herbs most commonly used with children.

Astragalus: Astragalus is a Chinese herb that has been used medicinally for more than 1,000 years. It is one of our favorite herbs for supporting the immune system. It is especially effective for preventing colds, bronchial infections, and shortness of breath. It can be used long-term if needed. An example of this type of use would be with children with asthma who are prone to respiratory tract infections in the winter. It is also one of the best herbs to use for children undergoing chemotherapy and/or radiation treatment for cancer; it supports their immune system and helps to prevent secondary infections. Hospitals in China prescribe astragalus on a routine basis for people undergoing conventional cancer treatment. In addition, astragalus works to strengthen the digestive system and can help with lack of appetite and diarrhea. It is best to avoid using astragalus when a fever is present (although it may be used in some herbal combinations).

Calendula: As you know, children are prone to all kinds of cuts and scrapes. It is important to have a bottle or salve of calendula at home. This is an incredible herb to help disinfect wounds and to speed up the healing process.

Wash minor cuts and scrapes with soap and water, and then apply calendula—preferably calendula succus, a thicker form of the tincture. We see children's wounds heal twice as fast when calendula is applied two to three times daily versus not using calendula.

Cascara sagrada: Many parents have called us up over the years concerned about an acute case of constipation with a child. A typical case is a child who has not had a bowel movement for 3 days or longer. Cascara sagrada is one of the better herbs to use to get the bowels moving.

Herbs can be taken with or between meals. If your child is prone to digestive upset, have him take the herbs with meals. If the herbs are being used to strengthen digestion, we recommend giving them 15 minutes before mealtime.

This herb works to stimulate movement of the muscles of the colon. We recommend it on a short-term basis only (an average of 1 to 3 days). Keep in mind that this herb does not treat the cause of constipation.

Chamomile: Chamomile tea has been used throughout the ages for children with upset tummies, restlessness, and fussiness. It has natural anti-inflammatory effects on the digestive tract to relieve abdominal pain and gas. This makes it helpful for stomachaches and colic.

Echinacea: Echinacea works to reduce the severity and length of an illness, such as a cold, once a child has caught the cold "bug." Keep in mind that most of the infections your child gets are viral. Antibiotics have no effects against viruses, only against bacterial infections. Herbs such as echinacea are effective against viruses and other types of microbes. Echinacea not only has a direct effect against microbes but also stimulates and supports the white blood cells of the immune system—the immune system's "army." One question always arises: "Is echinacea safe for kids to use?" The answer is yes, it's very safe. We, as well as thousands of other natural health care doctors and herbalists, prescribe echinacea to children on a routine basis. The other question that mothers always ask us, and justifiably so, is: "Is it safe to take echinacea if I am pregnant or am nursing?" The answer to this question is also yes. This is based on the fact that echinacea has been used by pregnant women for more than the past 100 years without reports of adverse effects. The "Vital Study" on page 52 also confirms its safety.

A concern parents often have is whether echinacea will affect fertility. This question is asked because of a 1999 study that suggested that common herbal supplements, such as St. John's wort, ginkgo, and echinacea, might adversely affect fertility. Researchers took hamster eggs, removed the outer coating, and exposed the eggs to the herbs. They then mixed in human sperm, which will usually penetrate the eggs. At higher dosages, the herbs either impaired or prevented the sperm's ability to penetrate the eggs. High concentrations of *Echinacea purpurea* interfered with sperm enzymes. Based on this,

The Natural Physician's Quick Dosage Guide for Children

Here are simplified calculations that parents can use to calculate the dosage for their children.

Note: Most children's dosages usually range between 5 and 30 drops per dose.

Acute Dosage: Use 1 drop of tincture for every 3 pounds of body weight, or 3 milligrams of the capsule extract for every pound of body weight. Give every 2 to 3 waking hours until the illness resolves.

Chronic Dosage: Use the same calculation as for the acute dosage, but give this dosage only two times daily.

some researchers have prematurely concluded that echinacea may interfere with fertility. Is this a valid conclusion? No. There are several problems with it. In the body, any herb is first broken down by the digestive system. In this study, the researchers used the whole herb in relatively high concentrations, which would never contact sperm in real life. Also, the experiment was done in a laboratory petri dish. To be valid, human studies would have to be done. We have no problem recommending echinacea for short-term use in pregnancy or as needed for infections in those trying to conceive.

Another question parents ask us is whether their children can take echinacea on a long-term basis. There are no definitive studies that show a problem with taking echinacea on a long-term basis. However, we generally prescribe it on a short-term basis. We have parents give it to children who have colds or infections. We also recommend it if the kids are around other sick children or adults, to prevent an infection. For children who are getting repeated colds and infections on a regular basis, we may have the parents give echinacea for the entire winter season. We also prescribe it for long-term use (2 weeks on and 1 week off) for children who have a junk food diet when, for one

(continued on page 52)

Common Herbs for Kids and Their Uses

Following is a handy reference guide to some common herbs and their medicinal uses for children. More uses may be indicated for adults.

Herb	Medicinal Uses	Parts Used
ALOE VERA (Aloe barbadensis)	Topically for burns and scrapes; juice used interally for ulcers and inflammatory bowel disease	Leaves
ANISE (Pimpinella anisum)	Internally to reduce intestinal gas, colic, bronchitis	Seeds
ASTRAGALUS (Astragalus membranaceus)	Internally to support immune system; adaptogen	Root
BLACK WALNUT (Juglans nigra)	Internally to prevent or treat infections from parasites worms, and yeast	Husk
BURDOCK (Arctium lappa)	Internally for skin conditions such as rashes and acne, to improve liver function, for detoxification; antimicrobial	Root
CALENDULA (Calendula officinalis)	Topically for cuts, scrapes, rashes, burns; antiseptic	Flowers
CASCARA SAGRADA (Rhamnus purshiana)	Internally as a laxative	Bark
CATNIP (Nepeta cataria)	Internally for colic, fevers, restlessness; as a digestive aid	Leaves and flowers
CAYENNE (Capsicum frutescens)	Internally to improve circulation, as antiseptic, to stimulate sweating in first stages of colds, sore throats; topically to relieve pain	Fruit
CHAMOMILE (Matricaria recutita)	Internally for indigestion, nervousness, colic	Flowers
CINNAMON (Cinnamomum spp.)	Internally for colds, diarrhea, digestive upset, bleeding	Inner bark
CLOVE (Syzygium aromaticum)	Topically as an anesthetic for teething	Clove
COMFREY (Symphytum officinale)	Externally for sprains, burns, wounds, fractures	Root

Forms Used	Side Effects/Cautions	Comments
Gel, cream, salve	Children should not take aloe vera juice internally except under the guidance of a practitioner.	One of nature's top healing herbs for the skin.
Tea, tincture	None	Sweet taste that children like; often blended with bad-tasting herbs
Tea, tincture, capsule	None known	Can be used on a long-term basis.
Tincture, capsule	Large doses can be sedating to circulatory system.	Use under the guidance of a health professional for the treatment of worms or parasites. For short-term use only.
Tincture, capsule	None known	Good general detoxifier, especially for skin conditions.
Tincture (applied topically), creams, salves	None	Excellent herb to promote healing and prevent infection of the skin.
Tincture, capsule	For short-term use only; long-term use can lead to electrolyte loss.	Best used under the guidance of a health care professional.
Tea, tincture	None	Only a few drops are needed for colic and restlessness for infants and children.
Tincture, capsule, topical ointment	Digestive upset	Topical ointment is used as a pain reliever.
Tea, tincture, capsule	Rare allergic reaction	Best used on a short-term basis.
Tea, tincture, or as a food	None in normal dosages	A warming herb, useful when a child is chilly.
Essential oil	Too high a dosage can be irritating to the mucous membranes.	Apply 1 to 2 drops of clove essential oil to gums during teething to reduce pain. Use only under the guidance of a health professional.
Poultice	Not to be taken internally due to toxic alkaloids.	Speeds healing of wounds and skin conditions.

(continued)

Common Herbs for Kids and Their Uses (cont.)

Herb	Medicinal Uses	Parts Used
CORNSILK (*Zea mays*)	Internally for bed-wetting, urinary tract infections	Golden silk of corn
CRANBERRY (*Vaccinium macrocarpon*)	Internally for prevention and treatment of urinary tract infections	Ripe fruit
DANDELION (*Taraxacum officinale*)	Internally to stimulate gallbladder and liver function and general digestion; leaf has diuretic effect	Root and leaf
ECHINACEA (*Echinacea purpurea* or *angustifolia*)	Internally for immune system enhancement; antiviral, antibacterial, antifungal	Roots and flowers
ELDERBERRY or elder flowers (*Sambucus nigra*)	Internally for colds, flus, coughs, sinusitis	Berries, flowers
ELECAMPANE (*Inula helenium*)	Internally for respiratory tract infections, digestive support	Root
EYEBRIGHT (*Euphrasia officinalis*)	Internally or externally for conjunctivitis (pinkeye), allergies affecting the eyes, sinus and nasal congestion	Whole herb
FENNEL (*Foeniculum vulgare*)	Internally for intestinal gas, colic, respiratory tract infections	Seed
FENUGREEK (*Trigonella foenum-graecum*)	Internally for digestive tract inflammation, colic, blood sugar imbalances	Seed
FEVERFEW (*Tanacetum parthenium*)	Internally for migraine headaches, arthritis	Leaves
FLAXSEED (*Linum usitatissimum*)	Internally for inflammatory skin conditions, dry skin, constipation, arthritis	Seeds
GARLIC (*Allium sativum*)	Internally and externally for immune system support, ear infections; antiviral, antibacterial, antifungal; reduces cholesterol levels	Cloves
GENTIAN (*Gentiana lutea*)	Internally for digestive stimulation	Root
GINGER (*Zingiber officinale*)	Internally to reduce intestinal gas and for sore throats and colds; anti-inflammatory; stimulates digestion	Root
GINKGO (*Ginkgo biloba*)	Internally for memory and attention deficit disorder; to improve circulation	Leaf

Forms Used	Side Effects/Cautions	Comments
Tea, tincture	None	Used as a tonic for the urinary tract.
Unsweetened juice, capsule	None	Dilute 50-50 in water and have child sip during the day to treat urinary tract infection.
Tea, tincture, capsule	Diarrhea. Do not use if gallstones are present.	Not generally used in younger children.
Tea, tincture, capsule, tablet	Caution for children allergic to the daisy family	Effective for colds, flus, sore throats, and respiratory tract infections. Nature's antibiotic.
Tea, tincture	None	One of the best herbal medicines for the flu.
Tea, tincture	None in normal doses. High doses can cause vomiting and digestive upset.	A lung tonic.
Tincture, capsule	None	Can be used as an eyewash or taken internally.
Tea, tincture, capsule	None in normal doses	Excellent digestive tonic. Sweet-tasting.
Tea, tincture	None	One of the better herbs for diabetes.
Capsule, tincture	Not recommended for children under 2 years of age.	Reduces inflammation.
Ground-up seeds (powder), oil	Too much oil can cause diarrhea.	Excellent for chronic skin conditions—supplies essential fatty acids.
Fresh cloves, tincture, capsule	Digestive upset	Commonly used as eardrops for ear infections. Also used for sore throats and upper respiratory tract infections.
Tincture, capsule	Can aggravate gastritis or ulcers.	Useful to treat malabsorption and low appetite after an illness.
Tea, tincture, capsule	None in normal doses	One of the best herbs for intestinal gas. A warming herb.
Tincture, capsule	Headache, digestive upset, blood thinning	Not commonly used in kids under 10 years of age.

(continued)

Common Herbs for Kids and Their Uses (cont.)

Herb	Medicinal Uses	Parts Used
GINSENG: American ginseng *(Panax quinquefolius),* Siberian ginseng *(Eleutherococcus senticosus),* and Chinese ginseng *(Panax ginseng)*	Internally to counteract physical, mental, emotional stress; also for immune system support and fatigue; American ginseng used for asthma	Root
GOLDENSEAL *(Hydrastis canadensis)*	Internally for colds, sore throats, flu, ear infections, digestive tract infections, fungal infections, sinusitis	Root
GOTU KOLA *(Centella asiatica)*	Internally for concentration, connective tissue healing	Whole plant
HAWTHORN *(Crataegus oxycantha)*	Internally for heart conditions	Berry
HOPS *(Humulus lupulus)*	Internally for stomachache due to anxiety, restlessness, insomnia, colic	Strobile (female flower)
HOREHOUND *(Marrubium vulgare)*	Internally for bronchitis, asthma, coughs	Flowering herb
HORSETAIL *(Equisetum arvense)*	Internally for urinary tract infections	Stems
KAVA *(Piper methysticum)*	Internally for anxiety, insomnia, hyperactivity, muscle spasms	Root
LAVENDER *(Lavandula angustifolia)*	Externally and internally for stress, anxiety, headache, muscle spasms, insomnia	Flowers
LEMON BALM *(Melissa officinalis)*	Internally for respiratory tract infections, fevers, depression, cold sores; antiviral; also used externally	Whole herb
LICORICE *(Glycyrrhiza glabra)*	Internally for immune system support, coughs, sore throats, digestive tract inflammation, heartburn, adrenal gland support, liver support; antiviral, anti-spasmodic, anti-inflammatory	Root
LOMATIUM *(Lomatium dissectum)*	Internally for immune system support, colds, urinary tract infections; antiviral, antibacterial	Root
MA HUANG *(Ephedra sinica)*	Internally for asthma, bronchitis, sinusitis	Stems of branches

Forms Used	Side Effects/Cautions	Comments
Tea, tincture, capsule	Chinese ginseng can cause overstimulation.	American and Siberian ginsengs are cooling; Chinese ginseng is warming.
Tincture, capsule	Digestive upset	Very bitter. One of the best herbs to use for infections of mucous membranes. Not to be used on a long-term basis.
Tincture, capsule	None in normal doses	Sometimes used for attention deficit disorder. Decreases scar tissue formation after an injury.
Tincture, capsule	Caution when combined with heart medications	Best when prescribed by a natural health care practitioner.
Tea, tincture, capsule	None	Helps calm the nerves.
Tincture	None	Helps discharge mucus from the respiratory tract.
Tea, tincture, capsule	None	Not to be used on a long-term basis. Good source of silica.
Tea, tincture, capsule	Skin rash rarely occurs.	Strong action on the nervous system. Best prescribed by a natural health care practitioner.
Tea, tincture, essential oil	None	Calming to the nervous system and mind.
Tincture, salve	Not to be used if the child has hypothyroidism.	A calming herb.
Tea, tincture, capsule, cream	Large amounts can lead to water retention and thus increase blood pressure.	Sweet-tasting. Reduces toxicity and increases effectiveness of other herbs. Topical cream or gel used for cold sores.
Tincture, capsule	Skin rash in a small percentage of users	An excellent antiviral herb for colds and flus.
Tea, tincture	Large doses can cause heart arrhythmias, high blood pressure, headaches, vomiting. Avoid if the child has a preexisting heart condition.	Use only under the supervision of a health practitioner.

(continued)

Common Herbs for Kids and Their Uses (cont.)

Herb	Medicinal Uses	Parts Used
MAITAKE (Grifola frondosa)	Internally for general immune support, HIV, diabetes; antiviral, antitumor	Fruiting body (mushroom)
MARSHMALLOW (Althaea officinalis)	Internally to soothe mucous membranes of respiratory tract, digestive tract, and urinary tract	Root
MILK THISTLE (Silybum marianum)	Internally for liver congestion, hepatitis	Seed
MULLEIN (Verbascum thapsus)	Internally for coughs, upper respiratory tract infections; externally for ear infections	Flowers, leaves
MYRRH (Commiphora myrrha)	Internally and externally for sore throats, urinary tract infections, gingivitis, mouth sores	Resin
NETTLE (Urtica dioica)	Internally for anemia, detoxification, rashes	Whole herb
OATSTRAW (Avena sativa)	Internally for stress, depression, restlessness, fatigue, itchy skin	Seeds
OREGON GRAPE (Mahonia aquifolium)	Internally for respiratory tract and urinary tract infections	Root and stem bark
PASSIONFLOWER (Passiflora incarnata)	Internally for insomnia, restlessness, heart palpitations	Flower
PEPPERMINT (Mentha piperita)	Internally for colic, indigestion, nausea, fevers	Leaf
PLANTAIN (Plantago spp.)	Internally for urinary and respiratory tract infections (antiseptic, anti-inflammatory); topically for wounds and bites	Leaf
RED RASPBERRY (Rubus idaeus)	Internally for diarrhea, nausea, vomiting	Leaf and berry
REISHI (Ganoderma lucidum)	Internally for allergies, bronchitis, tumors, HIV, viral infections, immune support during chemotherapy and radiation treatments	Fruiting body (mushroom)
ROSEMARY (Rosmarinus officinalis)	Internally to soothe nervous system, for memory, to treat lice; antioxidant	Leaf
SAGE (Salvia officinalis)	Internally as an antimicrobial, to reduce secretions, and for intestinal gas	Leaves
ST. JOHN'S WORT (Hypericum perforatum)	Internally for anxiety, depression, viral infections; topically for burns, scrapes, nerve pain	Flowers, whole herb

Forms Used	Side Effects/Cautions	Comments
Tincture, or as a food	None	Often used for long-term immune support.
Tincture, capsule	None	An anti-inflammatory herb.
Tincture, capsule	None	Best studied herb for hepatitis. Shown to regenerate liver cells.
Tincture, capsule; topical oil for ear infections	None	A soothing herb. Antimicrobial.
Tincture	Large doses internally may cause kidney irritation and diarrhea. Use small doses only (1 to 5 drops).	Commonly used for infections of the throat and mouth.
Tea, tincture, capsule, salve	None	Very nutritive, very high in minerals. Also called stinging nettle.
Tincture, capsule, seeds	None	Oatmeal baths are used for itchy skin.
Tincture, capsule	None	Often used as an alternative to goldenseal for infections of mucous membranes.
Tea, tincture, capsule	None	A gentle nerve relaxer for children.
Tea, tincture, oil	Heartburn in some individuals	Provides acute relief of digestive complaints.
Tea, tincture	None	Works well topically for insect bites.
Tea, tincture; as a food (berries)	None	Tastes good.
Tincture, or as a food	None	Often used for long-term immune support.
Tea, tincture	None	Generally used in a combination herbal formula.
Tea, tincture	None in normal dosages	Used by mothers who are not breastfeeding to dry up their milk.
Tincture, capsule, oil	Small percentage of users develop sensitivity to light. Should not be combined with pharmaceutical antidepressants.	If using as a natural antidepressant for children, use only under the supervision of a health care professional.

(continued)

Common Herbs for Kids and Their Uses (cont.)

Herb	Medicinal Uses	Parts Used
SHIITAKE (Lentinus edodes)	Internally for general immune system support, HIV, hepatitis, cancer, bronchitis	Fruiting body (mushroom)
SKULLCAP (Scutellaria lateriflora)	Internally for nervousness, insomnia, anxiety, hyperactivity	Whole herb
SLIPPERY ELM (Ulmus fulva, U. rubra)	Internally to soothe mucous membranes of the respiratory tract, digestive tract, urinary tract; also for bronchitis, colitis, ulcers, urinary tract infections	Inner bark
TEA TREE (Melaleuca alternifolia)	Topically for skin fungus, burns, acne	Leaves
THUJA (Thuja occidentalis)	Externally for warts	Branches, leaves, bark
THYME (Thymus vulgaris)	Internally for respiratory tract infections (bronchitis), urinary tract infections; topically for skin fungus	Leaves and flowers
TURMERIC (Curcuma longa)	Internally as an anti-inflammatory and anti-tumor treatment	Rhizome (part of plant above-ground)
UVA-URSI (Arctostaphylos uva-ursi)	Internally for urinary tract infections	Leaves
VALERIAN (Valeriana officinalis)	Internally for insomnia, restlessness; antispasmodic	Root
WHITE WILLOW (Salix alba and spp.)	Internally for headaches, pain	Bark
WILD CHERRY (Prunus serotina)	Internally for cough, bronchitis	Bark
WITCH HAZEL (Hamamelis virginiana)	Topically for gingivitis, eczema, inflamed veins	Bark
YARROW (Achillea millefolium)	Internally for fevers, toothaches, digestive upset; improves circulation	Flowers, leaves
YELLOW DOCK (Rumex crispus)	Internally for sore throat, iron deficiency anemia; liver tonic	Root
YERBA SANTA (Eriodictyon californicum)	Internally for bronchitis, laryngitis	Leaves

Forms Used	Side Effects/Cautions	Comments
Tincture, food	Rare digestive upset	Used for long-term immune support.
Tincture, capsule	None	One of the best herbs to use for insomnia with children.
Tea, tincture, capsule, lozenge	None	A soothing herb.
Tincture, oil	Too high of a concentration can be irritating to the skin.	Excellent for athlete's foot.
Tincture, oil	Not to be taken internally by children.	An excellent topical treatment for warts.
Tea, tincture, capsule, essential oil	Too much of the essential oil can cause abdominal pain.	Mainly used in respiratory tract infection formulas.
Tincture, capsule	None	One of the best anti-inflammatory herbs.
Tincture, capsule	None in normal doses	One of the best herbs for urinary tract infections.
Tincture, capsule	A small percentage of users feel drowsy in the morning if the herb is used as a sleep aid.	One of the stronger nerve-relaxing herbs.
Tea, tincture, capsule	Do not use if the child is on blood-thinning medications or has hemophilia, as it thins the blood. Not to be used with a fever or during viral infections.	A natural alternative to aspirin. Also called willow or willow bark.
Tincture	Not to be used in large amounts or for prolonged periods of time.	For irritating coughs.
Tincture	Best used topically with children. Use as a mouth rinse for gingivitis and then spit out.	Natural anti-inflammatory.
Tea, tincture	External application may result in a rash.	Mainly used for fevers with children.
Tincture, capsule	None	Great for iron deficiency anemia. Contains a small amount of iron and enhances absorption of iron.
Tea, tincture	None	Helps to expel respiratory mucus.

Vital Study

A study conducted by the Hospital for Sick Children in Toronto in conjunction with the Canadian College of Naturopathic Medicine looked at the safety of echinacea and pregnancy. The study analyzed 206 women who used echinacea during pregnancy for upper respiratory tract infections, along with a control group of 198 pregnant women who had upper respiratory tract infections but never used echinacea. The researchers found no association with the use of echinacea and birth defects. There were also no differences in the rate of live births or spontaneous abortions between the two groups.

reason or another, the parents cannot change the diet. We find that echinacea works well by itself or in combination with other immune-enhancing herbs such as astragalus.

Fennel: Fennel is an old-time favorite remedy for colic. It helps to relieve intestinal gas and cramping. One-half to 1 teaspoon of warm fennel tea can do wonders for an infant with colic or for a child with intestinal gas. It is one of the more pleasant tasting teas. It is also effective for respiratory tract ailments.

Garlic: Garlic is one of those herbs whose "old wives' tale" medicinal uses have been proved by science to be true. Garlic is an ally of the immune system. It has antimicrobial effects against bacteria, viruses, and fungal infections. It works well in sinus, throat, and lung infections. Warm garlic oil is an effective topical treatment for earaches caused by bacterial infections. We like the combination of garlic oil and mullein oil for ear infections. A couple of drops in the ear every few hours can help reduce the pain and fight the infection.

Garlic also helps to prevent and treat infections of the digestive tract. It is effective against yeast overgrowth in the colon. And it improves circulation throughout the body and helps to normalize cholesterol levels.

Use fresh garlic as a food, unless your child has a sensitivity to it. Older kids can usually tolerate the capsule form.

Ginger: This is another spice that has many medicinal benefits. It works well for colds and sore throats, especially when the child is chilly, as it has a warming and anti-inflammatory effect. It also is one of the best herbs to relieve intestinal gas, diarrhea, nausea, and digestive upset. Studies have shown it to be effective for motion sickness. Some of our patients have reported it to be helpful for their children who get carsick.

Goldenseal: Goldenseal has a pronounced effect on the mucous membranes of the body. This herb is used for sinus, respiratory, and digestive tract infections. Goldenseal is a well-known antibacterial herb for mucous membrane infections and helps to dry mucus.

Licorice: There is a reason why Chinese and Western herbalists include licorice root in so many formulas. It has many medicinal qualities. It is very soothing to the respiratory and digestive tract. As a matter of fact, it is one of the best herbs for the treatment of ulcers.

It is also supportive to the immune system and strengthens the adrenal glands (glands that respond to stress).

This herb is sweet in taste and improves the flavor of children's tinctures and teas.

Mullein: This is one of the best herbs for soothing the respiratory tract. It works well in formulas for coughs, bronchitis, and asthma. As we mentioned before, it works well when combined with garlic oil in eardrops for earaches.

Passionflower: We like this herb because of its gentle but effective relaxing effect on the nervous system. When children are having problems going to sleep, it is one of the first herbs we recommend. It can be used by itself or as part of a formula for hyperactivity.

Yarrow: No parent likes to see a child struggle through a fever. Yarrow has the action of inducing and breaking a sweat when children have fevers. Warm yarrow tea or the tincture form can be helpful in cases of high fevers that are not resolving.

Herbs to Avoid

Avoid any herb with which you are not familiar or for which you cannot find information showing its safety. The vast majority of herbs that can be used with children are listed in this chapter. A reputable herbalist or knowledgeable natural health care practitioner can help answer your questions on herbal therapies for children.

Purchasing Quality Herbal Products

Follow these rules whenever you shop for herbs.

1. Make sure that the label provides easy directions and recommended dosages.

2. The label should list all ingredients in order of potency.

3. Look to see whether the specific parts of plants used are identified. For example, some herbs work better when their leaves are used; other herbs house their medicinal ingredients in the roots, not the leaves.

4. Purchase products that are wrapped in safety seals to prevent tampering and preserve freshness.

5. Make sure that the label lists an expiration date and lot number.

6. Buy products that are certified to be organic. This ensures that no pesticides or herbicides were used in harvesting and preparation.

7. Cautions should be listed on the container.

8. The company should be known for high standards in quality control.

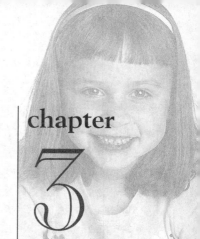

homeopathy
for children

Homeopathy is one of the fastest-growing alternative forms of medicine in North America. This form of medicine uses ultra-dilute amounts of plant, mineral, and animal substances to stimulate the healing systems of the body. Homeopathic remedies are effective for a wide range of conditions and are available in health food stores, pharmacies, and shopping centers; they cannot be made at home. Homeopathy can be used to strengthen the defense systems of the body and to stimulate healing of mental and emotional imbalances. These remedies are an excellent therapy to stimulate or help repair a damaged immune system. Since homeopathic medicines are ultra-diluted, they are extremely safe for children—no side effects or toxicity.

Homeopathic researchers are finding that each homeopathic remedy has its own "fingerprint" on the electromagnetic spectrum. It appears that homeopathic remedies work on a vibrational/energetic level. In some ways, each remedy has a different electromagnetic frequency and thus action, similar to the various actions of different acupuncture points.

The History of Homeopathy

The science of homeopathy is not a new development. Ancient Hindu literature describes the homeopathic effect in the 10th century B.C. In 400 B.C. Greece, Hippocrates wrote about the principles of homeopathy.

homeopathy for children   55

Case History

Soon after our son, Mark, learned to walk on his own, bam! His forehead collided with a coffee table. We were shocked by the huge bruise that quickly formed above his eye. After examining him, we immediately gave Arnica montana. Within minutes, the swelling went down. The next day, the color of his bruise was fading and the swelling had been reduced. For centuries, people have used Arnica to treat bruises and traumas. (And, yes, we did move that coffee table!)

The popularity of homeopathy spread in the early 1800s through the research and teachings of German medical doctor Samuel Hahnemann. Dr. Hahnemann was instrumental in developing the knowledge of the homeopathic remedies that are used today.

Homeopathy is a primary form of medicine all over the world. For example, in India, there are more than 120 homeopathic medical schools, tens of thousands of homeopathic practitioners, and millions of people who use homeopathy every year. More than half of all German medical doctors prescribe homeopathic medicines or refer patients to practitioners who use homeopathy.

The Law of Similars: Like Cures Like

The word *homeopathy* comes from the Greek root words *homoios,* which means "similar," and *pathos,* which means "suffering" or "disease." This relates to the fundamental law of homeopathy: "Like cures like." The "like cures like" principle means that a substance that can cause particular symptoms in healthy people can also stimulate healing in those who are ill with similar symptoms. A classic example is the homeopathic remedy Apis mellifica, a preparation of bee venom. When introduced to the body through a bee sting, bee venom results in stinging, burning, redness, and swelling. These same symptoms, no matter what the cause, can be improved or relieved by the Apis remedy. In fact, Apis stimulates a healing response whether a bee sting, arthritis, or a urinary tract infection is involved. In short, if the symptoms match those of the homeopathic agent, a cure can occur as the body's healing mechanisms are activated by the law of similars.

Homeopathic nosodes are an especially interesting example of the "like cures like" phenomenon. A nosode is a preparation made from the disease itself, similar to a vaccine. For instance, the Herpes simplex nosode can be given to help prevent recurrent cold sore outbreaks caused by the herpes simplex virus. As with other homeopathics, nosodes can also be given to help quicken recovery from a disease if the child is already sick.

Less Is More

One of the unique aspects of homeopathy is that the more dilute a remedy is made, the stronger the effect. Dr. Hahnemann and other homeopathic practitioners have found that homeopathy becomes more effective and powerful when prepared by a special process of dilution and succussion (shaking or pounding of the medicines). This process is referred to as potentization and indicates the strength of a homeopathic remedy (often simply called a homeopathic). Special laboratory equipment is used in homeopathic pharmacies and re-search centers throughout the world to produce homeopathics with this special technique.

Working with the Body's Systems

Homeopathy, like many of the natural therapies, works with the healing systems of the body. As you will see in the remedy chart on page 62, homeopathic medicines are prescribed based not only on the disease itself (such as the flu or anxiety) but also based on symp-toms that are expressed by the person. This allows for actual im-provement in chronic health conditions rather than merely suppressing symptoms. Symptoms are used to differentiate the homeopathic remedy for the individual, thus allowing the "whole" person to be treated.

Reasons for Using Homeopathy

There are five main reasons why we believe homeopathy is gaining popularity among doctors and parents for use with children.

1. Homeopathy is highly effective for chronic and acute diseases, including epidemics. It works to strengthen the immune and other healing systems of the body. It can be used to treat conditions for which conventional medicine has no effective treatment.

2. It is cost-effective. Compared with pharmaceutical medications, homeopathic remedies are quite inexpensive.

3. It is a preventive medicine. One does not have to have a disease to be treated with homeopathy. It can be used to optimize health.

4. It can be used to treat the whole person. Homeopathy takes into account all the factors of a child's health—the mental, emotional, and physical.

5. Side effects are not an issue. This is especially important when it comes to children, who are more prone to toxic side effects of medications than adults.

Prescribing Homeopathy

There are two basic ways parents can use homeopathy with their children.

Combination remedies: This refers to homeopathic formulas that contain two or more homeopathic remedies. If the remedy a child needs is in the formula, then it will be helpful. If the homeopathic remedy a child needs is not one of the ingredients, then usually nothing will happen, or only minor improvements will occur but will not last. Combination remedies are available in most health food stores or pharmacies. They are prepared for certain conditions, including colds, flu, teething, colic, diarrhea, rashes, and headaches.

Single remedies: This is the system used by trained homeopathic practitioners. The one remedy that matches up best to the patient's symptoms is prescribed. In general, this system is more effective than combination remedies, but it may require a knowledgeable practitioner to pick the correct homeopathic. If the single remedy choice is obvious, then go ahead and use single remedies for your child. This book lists the most common single remedies for each of many conditions.

Administering Homeopathics to Your Child

Homeopathic remedies are generally available in pellet, tablet, liquid, or cream form. For infants, pellets or tablets can be pulverized and mixed in an ounce of purified water, and then a few drops can be put in the child's mouth with a dropper or teaspoon. Children like the sweet taste of the pellets and tablets. Two pellets or tablets is a typical children's dosage. Homeopathic remedies are best taken 10 to 20 minutes between eating or drinking, and they should be taken away from strong-smelling odors such as eucalyptus or essential oils, which can interfere with their efficacy.

For severe acute conditions when the symptoms are intense (for instance, vomiting or severe headache), give the homeopathic remedy every 15 minutes for the first hour. If no improvements are noticed in that time, you should try a different remedy. If you find a remedy that improves the condition, it may not need to be taken again. If symptoms do return, give the remedy every 2 to 3 hours until you notice continued, consistent improvement. At that point, stop giving it.

For milder acute conditions (for instance, runny nose, mild bloating, or sore throat), give the remedy two or three times daily.

For chronic conditions, homeopathics are usually taken one or two times daily, or less frequently depending on the strength of the remedy prescribed. Improvements may be noticed in a few days or a couple of weeks. For long-standing conditions, it may take a month

Case History

Tyler, a 3-year-old, came to our clinic in tears because of pain from a severe ear infection. He had a high fever of 105°F. His face was flushed. He tugged at his right ear, and his pupils were slightly dilated. Based on Tyler's symptoms, we prescribed the homeopathic Belladonna. Within 10 minutes, Tyler fell asleep. In 20 minutes, his temperature had dropped to 100°F. By the next morning, Tyler was up and playing as if nothing had happened. Belladonna is one of the excellent homeopathic medicines for acute infections (viral or bacterial) when symptoms including fever and facial flushing are present.

or longer for improvements to occur. Professional consultation may be required for proper long-term use.

Which Potency to Use

Potency refers to the strength of the remedy. The number behind the name of the homeopathic indicates the dilution and strength of the medicine. The higher the number, the stronger the action of the remedy. For example, 30C is stronger than 12C, and 12X is stronger than 6X. There are two common scales of homeopathy available in the marketplace.

X: These are the lowest potencies used. *X* stands for a 1-in-9 dilution. So, 1X is equal to 1 part of the original substance diluted in 9 parts solvent. Many stores carry the 6X and 12X potencies for many of the remedies.

C: These are more dilute and stronger than the X potencies. The first dilution, that is, 1C, is equal to 1 part of the original substance in 99 parts solvent. Many stores carry the 12C and 30C potencies for many of the remedies.

Although the potency does matter, picking the right remedy is the most important aspect when it comes to success with homeopathy. Therefore, if you have access to only one potency (for instance, you wanted to use a 30C but only have a 6C), then use it—it will still work.

Storage

It's important to note that all homeopathic remedies should be stored away from strong odors (for instance, camphor or eucalyptus). If your child is using homeopathy, it is also best to keep him away from strong odors, such as eucalyptus or any essential oil, because homeopaths have found that these odors may nullify the effect of the homeopathic therapy.

Constitutional Homeopathic Remedies for Children

One of the fascinating areas of homeopathy is constitutional remedies, which are linked to physical, mental, and emotional characteristics. Based on a child's personality and physical symptoms, a homeopathic practitioner can accurately choose a constitutional homeopathic remedy to treat or prevent an imbalance by strengthening the child's overall healing and defense systems. This section describes common constitutional remedies for children as well as examples of success stories. If a remedy matches up closely to your child's constitution, you can try giving your child a 12C or 30C potency twice daily for a week or two and see if there are any changes. Once improvement has begun, stop the remedy unless progress halts, in which case you may give it again as needed. Otherwise, it is best to follow the advice of a qualified homeopathic practitioner.

Some acute remedies, such as Sulphur, are also useful as constitutional remedies. (See "Acute versus Constitutional Remedies: What's the Difference?" on page 68 for more information.)

Here are some of the more common constitutional remedies for children.

Calcarea carbonica

Physical symptoms: Children fitting this constitutional type tend to be plump or obese, tire easily, and are susceptible to infections, especially ear or upper respiratory infections. There can be a delay in development, such as a slow onset of walking, talking, or teething. Their nails may break or be brittle. They tend to sweat profusely on the back of the head when sleeping. Calcarea carbonica is also indicated for infants who spit up constantly and for children with chronic constipation. These children often crave eggs, sweets, and dairy products.

Mental and emotional symptoms: Independent, stubborn, and curious. The child is slow and meticulous.

Case history: At 1 month old, Josh weighed 10 pounds—big for his age. He was a big, plump, happy infant. His parents, aware of the benefits of homeopathy, brought Josh in for a checkup and to optimize his health. He had a mild case of cradle cap and would constantly spit up milk after almost every breastfeeding. Josh

(continued on page 66)

Common First-Aid Homeopathic Remedies for Children

Remedy	Used For
Aconitum napellus	Anxiety, bladder infections, colds, croup, ear infection, fever, flu, pneumonia, shock, urine retention
Antimonium tartaricum	Bronchitis, pertussis, pneumonia, respiratory tract infections
Apis mellifica	Allergic reactions, arthritis, bee stings, bladder infections, chicken pox, kidney disease, cold sores, hives, meningitis, sore throat, pneumonia
Arnica montana	Bruises, concussions, head injuries, nosebleed from trauma, postsurgery recovery (including dental work), sprains
Arsenicum album	Anxiety, asthma, bladder infections, bronchitis, cancer, colds, cold sores, colitis, diarrhea, eczema, fever, food poisoning, hepatitis, pneumonia, vaginitis
Belladonna	Appendicitis, arthritis, bladder infections, boils, convulsions, fever, flu, headaches, sore throats, tonsillitis
Bryonia alba	Appendicitis, arthritis, bronchitis, constipation, cough, flu, headache, lower back pain, pleurisy, pneumonia, tendinitis, toothache
Calendula	Cellulitis, postsurgery healing, wounds (scrapes, cuts, burns)
Cantharis	Bladder and urinary tract infections, skin burns
Chamomilla	Colic, ear infections, fever, teething pain and diarrhea from teething
Cina	Bruxism (tooth grinding), colic, convulsions, ear infection, worms (especially pinworms)
Coffea cruda	Insomnia
Colocynthis	Abdominal pain, colic, kidney stones, sciatica

Key Symptoms	Comments
Anxiety, fear of death, restlessness. One cheek red and the other pale. High thirst.	Mainly used in first stage of infectious diseases such as colds, flus, ear infections. Useful for shock and fear immediately after a physical or emotional trauma.
Sleepiness during a cough or bronchitis. Rattling cough in chest.	Specific for respiratory tract infections with lots of mucus that cannot be expelled.
Stinging pains that get better with cold applications. Swelling.	Excellent first-aid remedy for bee stings.
Bruised sensation	Given for physical trauma, especially where there has been bruising.
Anxiety, restlessness, panic. Chilliness. Burning pains that get better with heat. Worse from 12:00 to 2:00 A.M.	Good for many acute illnesses that match up to symptoms. Great acute remedy for asthma in children.
Fever, heat, redness, intense symptoms that come on in a hurry. Pupils may be dilated with fever. Cold hands and feet, but face is hot.	One of the most common first-stage remedies for infectious conditions in children. Commonly used for sore throats and right-sided ear infections.
Pain worse with any movement; child very irritable. Dryness of mucous membranes. Large thirst.	Commonly used for coughs and sprains/strains.
Cutting pain. Red, stinging pain. Pus formation.	Helps to speed the healing of cuts and scrapes, or to repair wounds that have been stitched after surgery.
Burning pain.	One of the most common remedies for urinary tract infections. Relieves pain and helps promote tissue healing after a burn.
Child irritable and inconsolable, averse to being touched during illness, capricious. High sensitivity to pain. One cheek red and the other pale during fevers.	The most common remedy for colic and teething. One of the top three most common remedies for ear infections.
Child angry, averse to being touched. Bluish discoloration around mouth. Constant boring of nose and rectum with fingers.	Specific for pinworms, which cause a child to pick at the nose and rectum.
Child wakes up from the slightest noise. Mind racing and cannot relax from overexcitement.	Mainly used for insomnia due to overexcitement.
Suppressed anger. Abdominal pain made better by applying pressure and bending double.	Excellent for abdominal cramps.

(continued)

Common First-Aid Homeopathic Remedies for Children (cont.)

Remedy	Used For
Drosera	Bronchitis, croup, pertussis, tuberculosis
Euphrasia	Allergy (hay fever), colds, eye inflammation (conjunctivitis, iritis), measles
Ferrum phosphoricum	Anemia, colds, ear infections, fever, flu, hemorrhage, nosebleed, pneumonia, sore throats, tonsillitis
Gelsemium	Chronic fatigue syndrome, fever, body aches, flu, headaches
Hepar sulphuris	Abscesses, acne, bronchitis, croup, ear infections, laryngitis, pneumonia, sinusitis, sore throats, tonsillitis
Hypericum perforatum	Injuries to nerves and spine, especially toes and fingers
Ignatia	Ailments from grief and stress; tight muscles
Ipecacuanha	Asthma, food poisoning, nausea, vomiting
Kali bichromicum	Asthma, bronchitis, sinusitis
Lachesis	Asthma, bleeding, cancer, diarrhea, ear infections, kidney stones, sore throats
Ledum	Abscesses, arthritis, bites, bleeding, bruises, puncture wounds, sprains, stings
Lycopodium	Appendicitis, asthma, bloating, bronchitis, colic, colitis, diabetes, ear infections, hepatitis, hernias, urinary tract infections
Magnesia phosphorica	Colic, muscle cramps, sciatica, toothaches
Mercurius solubilis or vivus	Abscesses, colds, colitis, conjunctivitis, ear infections, eczema, gastroenteritis, inflamed testicle, sore throats, tonsillitis

Key Symptoms	Comments
Violent coughing spells so severe that child has trouble catching breath and may turn blue.	Specific for severe coughs.
Red, irritated, burning eyes. Runny nose. Cough during the daytime.	Very specific remedy for hay fever where irritated eyes are the major symptom.
High fever without specific symptoms. Child has fever but does not act sick.	A common fever remedy when there are no other specific symptoms.
Drowsiness, dizziness, dullness. Chills up and down back. Muscles feel bruised. Headache that starts in back of head. Sensitivity to light.	Very common remedy for the flu.
Intolerant to cold and drafts. Child more irritable than usual. High sensitivity to pain. Thick, yellow discharge. High thirst.	Useful in the first stage of infectious conditions.
Nerve pain that is radiating, and sharp shooting pains.	Given immediately for puncture wounds that injure nerve tissue. Specific for when a child's fingers or toes get caught in a door or hit by a fallen object.
Child is crying, wants to be alone. Sighing. Changeable mood.	Useful after emotional traumas (such as the loss of a loved one or pet, or a sibling leaving for college) to help child recover.
Constant nausea not relieved by vomiting. Smell of food worsens nausea. Has a clean tongue despite vomiting.	Specific first-aid remedy for nausea. Do not confuse with syrup of ipecac, which induces vomiting.
Thick nasal discharge from the sinus or throat that is often yellow, green, and sticky.	One of the best remedies for sinusitis.
Fever, heat, left-sided symptoms, aversion to being touched on throat or wearing clothes that are tight around neck or waist	Commonly used for left-sided ear and throat infections.
Injury feels better with ice-cold applications.	Specific for puncture wounds.
Feels better with warm applications. Rightsided problems, stomachache in lower abdomen. Child gets full easily.	Relieves many digestive symptoms as well as right-sided ear infections and sore throats. Symptoms worsen between 4:00 and 8:00 P.M.
Better from heat and pressure.	Excellent for muscle cramps.
Sensitive to heat and cold. Sweating, alternating with chills. Symptoms worse at night. Excessive salivation. Bad breath with thick coating on tongue.	Commonly used for ear infections with discharge and raw, burning throat infections.

(continued)

Common First-Aid Homeopathic Remedies for Children (cont.)

Remedy	Used For
Natrum muriaticum	Allergies, colds, cold sores, depression, fever
Natrum sulphuricum	Asthma, concussions, diabetes, sinusitis, warts
Nux vomica	Asthma, colds, colic, constipation, flu, food poisoning, headaches, heartburn, sinusitis
Phosphorus	Anxiety, asthma, bronchitis, chronic fatigue, colds, croup, eczema, heartburn, nosebleeds, sore throat
Phytolacca	Mumps, inflamed testicle, sore throats, teething
Podophyllum	Diarrhea
Pulsatilla	Asthma, bladder infections, bronchitis, conjunctivitis, cough, ear infections, eczema, headaches, mumps, inflamed testicle, sinusitis
Rhus toxicodendron	Arthritis, eczema, flu, lower back pain, poison ivy rash, sprains, strains, tendinitis
Ruta graveolens	Arthritis, bursitis, muscle strains, tendinitis
Spongia tosta	Asthma, bronchitis, cough, croup, inflamed testicle
Sulphur	Abscesses, asthma, bronchitis, diarrhea, ear infections, rashes, sore throats, tonsillitis
Symphytum	Fractures, trauma to the eye

also displayed the classic Calcarea carbonica signs of sweaty feet and sweaty neck. We prescribed the Calcarea carbonica, and his parents reported that all of Josh's problems were gone within 5 weeks.

Lycopodium

Physical symptoms: These include problems with the digestive system—bloating, gas, burping that gets worse between 4:00 and 8:00 P.M. Children fitting the Lycopodium remedy picture often have large

Key Symptoms	Comments
Craves salt. Introverted (wants to be alone).	Excellent for reoccurring cold sores on the mouth.
Child is depressed.	Excellent remedy for problems after a head injury.
Chilly, nauseated, irritable, constipated. Pressure headaches in front of face, worse bending over.	Useful for digestive complaints of the upper abdomen.
Burning pains. High thirst for cold drinks. Bleeds easily.	Common remedy for respiratory tract infections and reoccurring nosebleeds.
Right-sided sore throat better with cold drinks.	Useful for right-sided sore throats and for teething that is relieved by teeth grinding.
Profuse, explosive diarrhea. Stool often contains yellow mucus.	Mainly used for diarrhea.
Fever with low thirst or no thirst. Child clingier than usual. Feels better with fresh air. Symptoms and mood very changeable.	Common remedy for many acute childhood illnesses that involve fever. One of the main remedies for ear infections and bronchitis.
Stiffness of joints worse from cold, wet weather, and movement. Better with warm applications. Child is restless.	Useful for arthritis and joint stiffness from overexertion. Specific for some cases of eczema.
Sprains and strains of tendons that result in stiffness and a bruised pain.	Useful for acute injuries of tendons.
Dry, barking cough that is worse with cold air.	A common cough and croup remedy.
Burning pains. Fever. Tremendous thirst for cold drinks.	The most common remedy for skin rashes.
Fracture pain.	Best remedy to be used for the healing of fractures.

appetites and crave sweets. However, some fill up very fast and can be poor eaters. They are also prone to respiratory problems and tend to have problems on the right sides of their bodies. They tend to be thinner-sized and chilly.

Mental and emotional symptoms: A "bullying" attitude to weaker, smaller children, demonstrating an underlying lack of self-confidence. The child is shy around adult strangers but rude and bossy to parents and siblings.

Acute versus Constitutional Remedies: What's the Difference?

An acute homeopathic remedy is the one most indicated and beneficial for an acute illness or trauma. For example, Arnica montana is an acute remedy for a child who falls down and suffers a bruise. In this case, to choose a remedy, all you need to know is that the child fell and became bruised. Arnica can be given to reduce the pain and quicken the healing of the bruised skin. Another example would be a child who is chilled with sore muscles from the flu. In this case, Gelsemium could be used as an acute remedy to help the child recover from this short-term viral illness.

A constitutional remedy is not generally used for an acute illness but is given to strengthen a person's resistance to disease, treat chronic disease, and optimize general health and vitality. In effect, you take the whole person into account when choosing a constitutional remedy, since the right remedy will be based on the person's constitution. This requires information about a child's personality traits, moods, mental and emotional state, and susceptibility to different illnesses. It also includes factors such as body type, body temperature, sleep patterns, food cravings, and fears. A constitutional remedy is more focused on long-term health benefits.

Case history: Jeff's parents brought him to our office for help with his digestive complaints. This 6-year-old suffered from chronic bouts of abdominal cramps and bloating. His flatulence buildup and release every evening at the dinner table was not appreciated. Diet changes did not seem to help. His parents described him as an active kid at school but said that he really lacked confidence in what he did. We prescribed Lycopodium, and within the first month, his digestive problems were greatly improved. Five months later, his parents reported on a follow-up visit that his digestive problems were still much improved and that his teachers felt that he was displaying a more confident attitude in his activities at school.

Natrum muriaticum

Physical symptoms: Children requiring this remedy often complain of headaches, some of which can be severe. Symptoms are usually worse between 10:00 A.M. and 3:00 P.M. The child craves salty foods. Cold sores break out from sun exposure. The child's eyes are extremely sensitive to the sun.

Mental and emotional symptoms: The child tends to be depressed and wants to be by himself. Children requiring Natrum muriaticum often have a history of emotional grief, such as the death of a loved one or the divorce of parents. They do not like to cry in front of others. It is important to them to be very neat and tidy in appearance.

Case history: Melanie's mother described her 3-year-old as a happy, outgoing child before her father was killed in a car accident a year ago. After the loss of her father, Melanie became withdrawn and was not interested in playing with kids anymore. Her mother also noticed that she craved salty foods and wanted to stay indoors all the time. In addition to recommending a children's counselor, we prescribed Natrum muriaticum. Melanie's mother reported an immediate improvement in her mood over the next month. She seemed happier and began to socialize more. She had not yet received counseling, which we still recommend.

Phosphorus

Physical symptoms: Children fitting this constitutional type often have reoccurring nosebleeds for no apparent reason. They also have a tendency for colds to turn into respiratory tract infections. Many children with asthma benefit from the Phosphorus remedy. Digestive upset such as tummyaches can be common. These children have a high thirst for cold drinks. They crave sweets and ice cream. They tend to be tall and lean, and they feel worse when they miss a meal.

Mental and emotional symptoms: The personality is usually of a child who is outgoing and very sociable. These children like attention. They have sympathy for others and do not like to be alone, especially in the dark.

Case history: Paul, a 4-year-old, was described by his parents as an extrovert, always seeking someone's attention. He was brought to our clinic because of reoccurring chest infections. Every winter, he would get bronchitis that would develop into pneumonia. His parents were concerned about all the antibiotics he had been on. He also suffered from reoccurring nosebleeds, which seemed to happen in both dry and moist environments. In addition to dietary changes, we prescribed Phosphorus. During his treatment with Phosphorus, and up to this day, Paul has not had pneumonia or required a prescription of antibiotics. And he no longer experiences nosebleeds.

Pulsatilla

Physical symptoms: A child who fits this profile tends to warm easily (she often sticks her feet out of the covers) and loves being in the open air. She is prone to ear and respiratory infections and to sinusitis, which often has a greenish yellow discharge. She craves sweets, especially pastries, and has low thirst. She often sleeps on her abdomen or back with her arms raised over her head. Infections cause yellow or green discharges.

Mental and emotional symptoms: The child is shy and clings to parents, yet craves attention and loves to be around people. She tends to stay in her parents' bedroom at night for fear of being alone. She has a very changeable mood; she can be sweet one moment and irritable the next.

Case history: Jordan, age 2, was a very cute and active boy. At age 14 months, he developed a severe infection that required hospitalization. Since then, he had become extremely clingy to his mother and insisted on sleeping in his parents' bed at night. He would not allow anyone to hold him but his mother. His actions persisted long after his hospitalization. After reviewing his case, we prescribed Pulsatilla. Within weeks, Jordan started interacting more with people, was less clingy with his mom, and finally started sleeping in his own bed. He was also less susceptible to bronchitis. Jordan illustrates how well constitutional homeopathic medicines can treat emotional imbalances.

Silica

Physical symptoms: The child has very low resistance to infections such as ear infections, colds, sinusitis, sore throats, and bronchitis. He is always coming down with something and has poor stamina. Children requiring Silica (sometimes also called Silicea) are often very thin and underweight, and may have brittle skin, nails, and hair. They are chilly and cannot stand drafts of cold air.

Mental and emotional symptoms: The child is usually stubborn and irritable, yet very sensitive to criticism and shy.

Case history: Sherry was worried about her 6-year-old son, Tony. Her pediatrician was concerned that Tony was extremely underweight for his age and height. She also stated that he was slow in school and very susceptible to respiratory tract infections. Sherry had been giving him vitamins and other supplements with no improvements.

Silica was an obvious choice by looking at Tony's thin frame and disproportionately large head. While sitting in our office, Tony would not take off his coat and scarf. His mother commented that he had a hard time staying warm. We prescribed Silica, and over the next 8 months, Tony made some incredible improvements. His memory began to improve, as did his resistance to colds and other respiratory infections. He began to put on weight at a more rapid pace, and his weight percentile increased from the 5th to the 40th percentile.

Sulphur

Physical symptoms: Children requiring this remedy tend to be prone to skin rashes and bad body odor. They have a large thirst (for

Vital Study

Acute diarrhea is the leading cause of death in children worldwide. A study published in *Pediatrics* in 1994 compared the effectiveness of homeopathic medicines with that of a placebo in the treatment of acute childhood diarrhea. Eighty-one children ages 6 months to 5 years were given various homeopathic medicines. The results demonstrated a statistically significant decrease in the duration of diarrhea and the number of stools per day in the group prescribed homeopathic medicines.

cold drinks) and appetite. They often crave sweets and spicy foods. They are almost always on the warm side and sweat easily (they usually kick their covers off at night).

Mental and emotional symptoms: These children tend to be very curious, always asking why and how something works, and they are very sociable. They like to be the leaders in groups of kids. They also tend to be messy and unorganized compared with other kids their own age.

Case history: Victor's parents stated that he has had eczema as long as they can remember. This 4-year-old was constantly scratching his skin, often to the point that it bled. He was a very active boy who liked to organize games with other children.

He was very warm, always throwing his covers off at night, even in the cold of winter. Victor loved spicy foods such as pizza. We had Victor's parents stop the use of cortisone cream, which his previous doctors had prescribed to suppress the eczema. We prescribed Sulphur based on all his symptoms. At first, his eczema got worse. We had Victor take oatmeal baths to reduce the itching. After a month on Sulphur, the eczema all over his arms and legs began to recede. Within 2 months, it was 60 percent improved. Five months after starting treatment, Victor was clear of his eczema. His parents were astonished, as it never came back. Sulphur has a detoxifying effect on the body and is one of the top skin remedies.

Tuberculinum

Physical symptoms: Children fitting the Tuberculinum remedy picture have problems with reoccurring bronchitis, pneumonia, and ear infections. Colds always turn into chest infections.

Mental and emotional symptoms: These children are hyperactive and aggressive and can be malicious.

Case history: Four-year-old Jeff had always been a healthy child. But for 4 months, he had had reoccurring chest colds that wore him down with coughs and fever. Even more troubling to his parents was the fact that Jeff was becoming very aggressive toward kids and adults. He started kicking, biting, and not listening to his parents. He would bang his head on the floor for no apparent reason. Knowing that Jeff had a very stable family life and excellent nutrition, we prescribed the homeopathic Tuberculinum. This homeopathic medicine is excellent for kids who are overly aggressive and hyperactive, crave milk products, have reoccurring respiratory infections, and even bang their heads on surfaces. After 1 week of taking the remedy, Jeff stopped banging his head. Over the next 3 weeks, his parents reported that his biting and kicking had calmed down. Over the next 2 months, he had times of aggression, but they were less frequent. His reoccurring chest colds also disappeared. Jeff's story illustrates how a constitutional remedy can treat the whole person—mentally, emotionally, and physically.

A Guide to the 12 Cell Salts

Cell salts are simplified forms of homeopathy that quickly and simply alleviate many childhood health problems. The German doctor Wilhelm Heinrich Schuessler discovered that 12 inorganic minerals were key constituents of cells. His theory was that a deficiency or imbalance of these cell salts led to disease. By supplementing these naturally occurring biochemical cell salts, one can stimulate the cells to assimilate nutrients more efficiently. Replenishing and balancing of these minerals restores the proper structure and function of each cell, tissue, and organ. Ferrum phosphoricum cell salt, for example, is a homeopathic dilution of iron, making it an excellent treatment for anemia because it bolsters iron assimilation in the cells, increasing the oxygen-carrying capacity of red blood cells.

How to Use Cell Salts

Cell salts are used similarly to other homeopathics. Just like other homeopathics, they are available in pellet, tablet, or liquid form. The most common potencies available are the 6X. They are best taken 10 to 20 minutes between eating or drinking. For infants, cell salt tablets

Cell Salts for Children

Name	Good For	Used For
Calcarea fluorica	Connective tissue	Ligament and tendon sprains/weakness, brittle teeth and gums, abnormal spine curvature
Calcarea phosphorica	Bone health	Fractures, teething, growing pains
Calcarea sulphurica	Wound healer	Abscesses, boils, acne
Ferrum phosphoricum	Iron metabolism, bleeding, fever	Anemia, to stop bleeding, fever
Kali muriaticum	Mucus	Fluid in ears, sore throat
Kali phosphoricum	Nerves	Nerve injuries, brain tonic, concentration, attention deficit disorder
Kali sulphuricum	Skin	Discharges
Magnesia phosphorica	Muscles	Muscle spasms, cramps, stomach cramps, relaxes nervous system, seizures, hyperactivity
Natrum muriaticum	Water balancer	Skin dryness, hay fever, grief, cold sores
Natrum phosphoricum	Acid-base balancer	Heartburn
Natrum sulphuricum	Detoxifier	Jaundice in newborns, hepatitis, head injuries
Silica (or Silicea)	Tissue cleanser	Acne, boils with pus discharge, sinusitis

can be crushed and given, or they can be mixed in an ounce of purified water and then a few drops put in the child's mouth with a dropper or teaspoon. Children like the sweet taste of the pellets and tablets.

For acute conditions, cell salts are often taken every 15 minutes or 2 hours, depending on the severity of the condition. For chronic conditions, cell salts are usually taken one to three times daily. Since they are of a low potency, cell salts are often used on a long-term basis. As with other homeopathics, they have no side effects or toxicity. They are the simplest remedies to use.

Note that all homeopathic remedies—including cell salts—should be stored away from strong-smelling odors (such as camphor or eucalyptus). The odor can cancel out the remedy's effects.

Bach Flower Remedies: An Introduction

In the early 1900s, British doctor Edward Bach (pronounced "batch") developed Bach Flower Remedies from flower and plant extracts. He believed that physical problems were a result of emotional imbalances. By relieving emotional blockages with the flower remedies, he theorized that physical ailments would improve. This is another simple system of homeopathy that parents can use safely on their children. Bach's 38 flower remedies focused on emotional problems, greatly addressing stresses faced by children. One of the beauties of this system

The Rescue Remedy

This common Bach Flower Remedy, easily found in health food stores and pharmacies, is a mixture of cherry plum, clematis, impatiens, rock rose, and star of Bethlehem. Rescue Remedy, as its name implies, is excellent during a crisis or acute situation. It helps to calm fear and anxiety and acts as a first-aid remedy. We often recommend Rescue Remedy after accidents, stresses in a relationship, and deaths in families. It even works for people (and their pets) who are anxious about flying.

It certainly worked for Shelly, a 9-year-old patient of ours who had to have blood drawn at our clinic. She was fearful and anxious about seeing needles. Her mother told us that the last time Shelly had had blood drawn, she had fainted. After reassuring Shelly, we gave her 5 drops of Rescue Remedy. Two minutes later, she had her blood drawn. She cried, but according to her mother, she was remarkably calmer than previous times. We also gave her 5 more drops after her blood was drawn to relieve any lasting anxiety. We now make it standard procedure to give Rescue Remedy before blood draws, injections, and any procedure in our clinic during which patients display fear or anxiety.

Bach Flower Remedies and Themes

Flower Remedy	Emotional Theme
Agrimony	Suppressed grief
Aspen	Fear and anxiety
Beech	Critical and intolerant
Centaury	Weak-willed and seeks praise of others
Cerato	Lack of confidence
Cherry plum	Fear of losing control
Chestnut bud	Repeating of old patterns
Chicory	Controlling of others
Clematis	Lack of motivation and concentration
Crab apple	Poor self-image
Elm	Feelings of inadequacy, being overwhelmed
Gentian	Self-doubt and discouragement
Gorse	Hopelessness
Heather	Loneliness
Holly	Negative feelings
Honeysuckle	Dwelling in the past
Hornbeam	Fatigue of mind and body
Impatiens	Impatience
Larch	Lack of self-confidence

is the lack of harmful side effects because of the microdilutions of the medicines. Bach Flower Remedies are gaining popularity in the health food arena because they are simple and easy to use. They are available in most health food stores and some pharmacies.

How to Use Bach Flower Remedies

Pick the Bach Flower Remedy or Remedies that match your child's emotional theme. It is common to mix two or more remedies together to fit your child's emotional makeup or imbalance. One

Flower Remedy	Emotional Theme
Mimulus	Fear
Mustard	Unexplainable sadness that comes and goes
Oak	Struggles against the odds and does not give up
Olive	Mental and physical exhaustion
Pine	Lack of satisfaction
Red chestnut	Overly fearful for others
Rock rose	States of terror, such as nightmares
Rock water	Too strict with self
Scleranthus	Indecisive
Star of Bethlehem	Emotional trauma
Sweet chestnut	Despair
Vervain	Argumentative
Vine	Strong-willed to the point of being dictatorial
Walnut	Emotional stress
Water violet	Independent
White chestnut	Persistent worry
Wild oat	Unfulfilled ambitions
Wild rose	Indifferent
Willow	Bitterness

remedy also can be used by itself. The correct Bach Flower Remedy or mixture will help move your child in the direction of mental and emotional healing.

Bach Flower Remedies can be dropped directly in the mouth or added to ¼ cup of water and sipped by a child. Up to six remedies can be combined in ¼ cup of water and sipped. For infants, ¼ teaspoon of the water can be given.

For acute conditions, give your child 2 drops of the indicated Bach Flower Remedy (or combination of Remedies) every 30 minutes, for up to three doses. If there is no improvement within 2 hours, try another remedy.

For chronic conditions, give your child 2 drops of the indicated Remedy (or combination of Remedies) twice daily. If there is no improvement within 2 weeks, try another Bach Flower Remedy or consult with a practitioner.

For more serious cases, it is prudent to consult a homeopathic practitioner. This increases the chance that your child will receive the right remedy. Chronic cases may require many different remedies in a proper sequence for optimal results to be attained. (To find a qualified practitioner near you, see "Homeopathy" on page 504.)

vitamins and minerals for children

A vitamin is an organic substance that is essential for life. Most vitamins cannot be synthesized in the body and so must be attained through the diet or from supplements. Vitamins fall into two main groups. Fat-soluble vitamins are those that require some amount of fat in order to be absorbed. They are also stored longer in the body. Common examples of fat-soluble vitamins include vitamins A, D, K, and E. The second major group of vitamins is termed water-soluble. This group does not need fat in order to be absorbed and is excreted out of the body much more readily than fat-soluble vitamins. Vitamin C and the B vitamins are water-soluble.

Minerals are inorganic substances that are important components of tissues and fluids. They are necessary for the proper functioning of vitamins, enzymes, and hormones, and for other metabolic activities in the body. Minerals compose 4 percent of the body's weight. Most of the minerals, such as calcium, phosphorus, and magnesium, are found in the bones. Some minerals are required in minute amounts; these are referred to as trace minerals. Chromium is an example of a trace mineral, as it is required in micrograms (one one-thousandth of a milligram) as opposed to minerals such as calcium, which are required in milligrams.

The Need for Vitamins and Minerals

Food is unquestionably the best source of vitamins and minerals for children. Fresh, organic foods from nature supply vitamins and minerals in the correct form and in ratios that are most compatible with a child's system. As described in the "Diet" section on page 4, this should be the focus of a child's vitamin and mineral supply. But in an age of refined and fast foods, many developing children do not take in sufficient levels of these nutrients. We know from the children we see, and from speaking to a wide variety of doctors and practitioners who work with children, that multiple nutritional deficiencies are very common in kids. The old adage that you can get all the vitamins and minerals you need from diet alone is just that: an old adage that is detrimental to the health of our children. Nutritional supplements, such as children's multivitamins, are necessary for most kids. This type of insurance policy against nutritional deficiencies can help to prevent many health problems and optimize a child's growth, development, and vitality. We are big advocates of food-based supplements that contain naturally occurring vitamins, minerals, and phytochemicals. Our experience also tells us that vitamin and mineral supplements make a difference in most kids' health.

Recommended Daily Allowances

The Recommended Daily Allowance, or RDA, is the average daily dietary intake level that is sufficient to meet the nutrient requirements of nearly all (97 to 98 percent) healthy individuals in a group. RDAs for different nutrients have been set by the U.S. National Academy of Sciences since 1941. Many health professionals feel that they are still too low to promote optimal health. The RDAs are currently being revised to what are termed Dietary Reference Intakes (DRIs). On the pages that follow, you'll find basic information for many essential vitamins, minerals, and other nutrients, including their RDAs where applicable.

Vitamins

Biotin

Function: Biotin plays an important role in the metabolism of fats, proteins, and carbohydrates. It also aids nail and hair growth.

Sources: Gut bacterial synthesis, organ meats, cheese, soybeans, eggs, mushrooms, whole wheat, and peanuts

RDA: None given, but the following are safe and adequate ranges:

Birth to 6 months: 10 micrograms (mcg)

6 months to 1 year: 15 mcg

1 to 3 years: 20 mcg

4 to 6 years: 25 mcg

7 to 10 years: 30 mcg

Deficiency signs: Seborrheic dermatitis (cradle cap) and hair loss in infants; brittle nails and hair

Toxicity: None reported

Vital Studies

According to studies published in the *Journal of the American Medical Association* and the *Annals of the New York Academy of Sciences,* the risk of bearing a child with a common birth defect known as a neural tube defect is reduced by 60 percent if a 400-microgram folic acid supplement is taken by the mother 1 month prior to conception and through the first trimester. Folic acid also decreases the risk of limb and urinary defects.

Carotenoids (carotenes)

Function: Carotenoids are potent antioxidants and help with immune function, growth and repair of tissues, and vision. There are more than 600 identified carotenoids. Some examples include beta-carotene, alpha carotene, gamma carotene, beta zeacarotene, cryptoxanthin, lycopene, zeaxanthin, lutein, canthaxanthin, crocetin, and capsanthin. Approximately 50 carotenoids act as precursors to vitamin A.

Sources: Yellow vegetables such as carrots, pumpkins, squash, and sweet potatoes; green vegetables such as broccoli, peas, collard greens, endive, kale, lettuce, peppers, spinach, and turnip greens; and certain fruits, including apricots, cantaloupe, papaya, peaches, watermelon, cherries, and tomatoes

RDA: None established

Deficiency signs: Increased susceptibility to developing certain cancers and cardiovascular disease

Toxicity: Relatively nontoxic. Too high of an intake can lead to carotenemia (yellowing of the skin), which disappears once intake is reduced.

Vital Fact

Even though folic acid is added to many foods, folic acid deficiency is the most common vitamin deficiency in the world.

Folic acid (folacin, folate)

Function: Folic acid helps to prevent neural tube defects and must be taken by mothers in early pregnancy. It is required for many processes in the body.

Sources: Dark green vegetables (spinach, kale, broccoli, and asparagus), as well as organ meats, kidney beans, beets, yeast, orange juice, and whole grains

RDA: Birth to 6 months: 25 micrograms (mcg)
6 months to 1 year: 35 mcg
1 to 3 years: 50 mcg
4 to 6 years: 75 mcg
7 to 10 years: 100 mcg

Deficiency signs: Macrocytic anemia (abnormally large red blood cells), irritability, weakness, weight loss, loss of appetite, shortness of breath or difficulty breathing, sore tongue, palpitations, forgetfulness, digestive upset, and diarrhea

Vitamin A (retinol, retinal)

Function: An antioxidant that aids in vision, growth, and development; strengthens the immune system; and fights respiratory tract infections.

Sources: Liver, chile peppers, carrots, vitamin A–fortified milk, butter, sweet potatoes, parsley, kale, spinach, mangoes, broccoli, squash

RDA: Infants under 1 year: 1,875 international units, or IU (375 retinol equivalents, or RE)
1 to 3 years: 2,000 IU (400 RE)
4 to 6 years: 2,500 IU (500 RE)
7 to 10 years: 3,500 IU (700 RE)
11 years to adult: males, 5,000 IU (1,000 RE); females, 4,000 IU (800 RE)

Caution: Higher dosages of vitamin A may be used only under a doctor's supervision.

Deficiency signs: Night blindness, susceptibility to infectious disease, follicular hyperkeratosis (bumps on the skin—mainly on the backs of the upper arms, shoulders, neck, buttocks, and lower abdomen), faulty tooth and bone formation, impaired growth

Toxicity: Overdoses of vitamin A can produce vomiting; joint pain; abdominal pain; bone abnormalities; cracking, dry skin; headache; irritability; and fatigue. Symptoms disappear after supplementation is discontinued.

Vital Study

A Harvard School of Public Health study looked at the effects of vitamin A supplements on 28,753 children and the effect on childhood mortality. Vitamin A supplementation reduced childhood mortality by 65 percent. This protective effect was the most significant in children who had growth problems or who had diarrhea.

Vitamin B₁ (thiamin)

Function: Vitamin B_1 aids in energy metabolism and neurological activity.

Sources: Pork, beef, liver, yeast, whole grains, and legumes

RDA: Birth to 6 months: 0.3 milligram (mg)
6 months to 1 year: 0.4 mg
1 to 3 years: 0.7 mg
4 to 6 years: 0.9 mg
7 to 10 years: 1 mg

Deficiency signs: Beriberi—a condition characterized by fatigue, loss of appetite, weight loss, gastrointestinal disorders, fluid retention, weakness, heart abnormalities, stunted growth, cyanosis (bluish skin), and convulsions.

Note: Children on the seizure medication Dilantin require extra B_1. See a doctor if your child is on this medication.

Toxicity: None reported

Vitamin B₂ (riboflavin)

Function: Vitamin B_2 helps with energy production and fatty acid and amino acid synthesis.

Sources: Organ meats such as liver, milk products, whole grains, green leafy vegetables, eggs, mushrooms, broccoli, asparagus, and fish

Vital Study

A study published in the *British Medical Journal* looked at the vitamin A levels of 180 children with rubeola (also known as 9-day measles). Ninety-one percent of the children were found to have levels below normal. They were given vitamin A (200,000 international units, or IU) supplements for 2 consecutive days. Results indicated an 87 percent decrease in death rate for the children under 2 years of age. *Note:* High doses of vitamin A should be used only under a doctor's supervision.

RDA: Birth to 6 months: 0.4 milligram (mg)
6 months to 1 year: 0.5 mg
1 to 3 years: 0.8 mg
4 to 6 years: 1 mg
7 to 10 years: 1.2 mg

Deficiency signs: Cracking at the corners of the mouth, inflamed tongue, reddening of eyes, vision problems, dermatitis, nerve damage, decreased neurotransmitter production, malformations and retarded growth in children and infants

Toxicity: None reported

Vitamin B_3 (niacin)

Function: Vitamin B_3 aids in energy production, the formation of steroid compounds, and red blood cell formation.

Sources: Organ meats, peanuts, fish, yeast, poultry, legumes, milk, eggs, whole grains, and orange juice

RDA: Birth to 6 months: 5 milligrams (mg)
6 months to 1 year: 6 mg
1 to 3 years: 9 mg
4 to 6 years: 12 mg
7 to 10 years: 13 mg

Deficiency signs: Pellagra—a condition characterized by dermatitis, diarrhea, dementia, weakness, lassitude, and loss of appetite

Toxicity: Large doses can cause dilation of the blood vessels and flushing of the skin. Time-released niacin products may result in liver damage.

Vitamin B_5 (pantothenic acid)

Function: Vitamin B_5 helps with the metabolism of carbohydrates, proteins, and fats for energy production. It also aids the production of adrenal hormones and red blood cells.

Sources: Organ meats, fish, chicken, eggs, cheese, whole grains, avocados, cauliflower, sweet potatoes, oranges, strawberries, yeast, and legumes

RDA: None given, but the following are safe and adequate dosages:

Birth to 6 months: 2 milligrams (mg)

6 months to 3 years: 3 mg

4 to 6 years: 3 to 4 mg

7 to 10 years: 4 to 5 mg

Deficiency signs: Numbness and shooting pains in the feet; fatigue

Toxicity: None reported

Vitamin B₆ (pyridoxine)

Function: Vitamin B_6 is important for the formation of body proteins, neurotransmitters, and red blood cells, and for immunity.

Sources: Meats, poultry, egg yolks, soy, peanuts, bananas, potatoes, whole grains, and cauliflower

RDA: Birth to 6 months: 0.3 milligram (mg)

6 months to 1 year: 0.6 mg

1 to 3 years: 1 mg

4 to 6 years: 1.1 mg

7 to 10 years: 1.4 mg

Deficiency signs: Mood abnormalities, sleep problems, anemia, impairment of nerve function, eczema, and cracking of the lips and tongue

Toxicity: Very high dosages can cause nerve symptoms—numbness and tingling. To our knowledge, this has been studied only in adults.

Vitamin B₁₂ (cobalamin)

Function: Vitamin B_{12} is important for the synthesis of DNA, the formation of red blood cells, and nerve development.

Vital Study

In a study published in *Schizophrenia*, 33 schizophrenic children under the age of 13 were placed on nicotinamide (a form of vitamin B_3), with doses from 1.5 to 6 grams daily, along with 3 grams of vitamin C. All recovered and then had their nicotinamide tablets switched to placebo tablets. Only 1 out of 33 kids failed to respond to B_3 therapy. All of the kids who responded to the B_3 therapy relapsed upon substitution with the placebo, and then improved again upon restarting the B_3.

Vital Study

A 1999 study in the *Journal of the American College of Nutrition* reported on the vitamin C intake among American schoolchildren. Among the 1,350 children ages 7 to 12 studied, 12 percent of the boys and 13 percent of the girls had mean vitamin C intakes that were less than 30 milligrams per day. Health care professionals should continue to promote at least five daily servings of vegetables and fruits, at least one of which should be rich in vitamin C.

Sources: Gut bacteria synthesis, organ meats, clams, oysters, soy, milk products, cheese, chlorella, and spirulina

RDA: Birth to 6 months: 0.3 microgram (mcg)

　6 months to 1 year: 0.5 mcg

　1 to 3 years: 0.7 mcg

　4 to 6 years: 1 mcg

　7 to 10 years: 1.4 mcg

Deficiency signs: Macrocytic anemia (abnormally large red blood cells), inflammation of the tongue, spinal cord degeneration, digestive upset, fatigue, and mental abnormalities

Toxicity: None reported

Vitamin C (ascorbic acid)

Function: Vitamin C is an antioxidant that bolsters immunity and helps with collagen formation, bone development, cancer prevention and treatment, gum health, and hormone and amino acid synthesis.

Sources: Citrus fruits, tomatoes, green peppers, dark green leafy vegetables, broccoli, cantaloupe, strawberries, brussels sprouts, potatoes, and asparagus

RDA: Birth to 6 months: 30 milligrams (mg)

　6 months to 1 year: 35 mg

　1 to 3 years: 40 mg

　4 to 10 years: 45 mg

Deficiency signs: Scurvy—a disease that is rare in North America but that is characterized by bleeding gums, poor wound healing, joint tenderness and swelling, and profuse bruising

Toxicity: The first symptom of too much vitamin C is generally diarrhea, which disappears when the dosage is reduced.

Vitamin D (D₂, or ergocalciferol; D₃, or cholecalciferol)

Function: Promotes calcium and phosphorus absorption from the intestines and increases calcium deposition into bones. Vitamin D_2 is derived from plant sources; vitamin D_3 is derived from animal sources.

Sources: Cod liver oil, coldwater fish (salmon, herring, sardines, mackerel), vitamin D–fortified milk, egg yolks. Small amounts are found in dark green leafy vegetables and mushrooms. Sunlight stimulates the body's production of vitamin D.

RDA: Birth to 6 months: 300 international units (IU)
6 months to 10 years: 400 IU

Deficiency signs: Rickets—softening of the skull bones, bowing of legs, spinal curvature, contracted pelvis, abnormal enlargement of the head, and increased joint space. Delayed tooth eruption.

Toxicity: Too high of an intake can cause nausea, loss of appetite, weakness, headache, digestive disturbance, kidney damage, calcification of soft tissues, and hypercalcemia (too much calcium in the blood).

Vital Study

A 1999 study published in the *Journal of Clinical Endocrinology and Metabolism* found that vitamin D supplementation of breastfed infants during the first year of life was associated with greater bone density in later childhood.

Vitamin E (tocopherol, tocotrienols)

Function: Vitamin E is an antioxidant that aids immunity. It includes alpha, beta, and gamma tocopherol as well as tocotrienols. Most supplements refer to alpha-tocopherol, although newer ones are including a blend. Make sure to look for natural forms of vitamin E, listed as d-alpha-tocopherol, as opposed to synthetic, which is listed as dl-alpha-tocopherol.

Sources: Vegetable oils, seeds, nuts, and whole grains

RDA: Infants under 1 year: 4.5 to 6 international units (IU)
1 to 10 years: 9 to 10.5 IU

Deficiency signs: Severe deficiency is rare. Hemolytic anemia (de-

Vital Fact

Inadequate intake of calcium (and other minerals) during childhood is a major risk factor for developing osteoporosis as an adult. According to the National Academy of Sciences, the most nutritional approach for reducing osteoporosis in our society is to ensure a calcium intake that allows children to reach their genetic potential for building bone mass. This is important, as 90 to 95 percent of the total bone mass you will ever reach is built by the time you reach your late teens.

struction of red blood cells) can occur in newborns. Muscle and neurological disorders are also symptoms.

Toxicity: Excess vitamin E can lead to muscle weakness, fatigue, nausea, diarrhea, and thinning of the blood.

Vitamin K (K_1, or phylloquinone; K_2, or menaquinone)

Function: Vitamin K is an antioxidant that aids in blood clotting and bone formation. Vitamin K_1 is derived from plants; K_2 is synthesized by intestinal bacteria; and K_3, or menadione, is derived synthetically.

Sources: Dark green leafy vegetables, parsley, broccoli, cabbage, spinach, soy, egg yolks, liver, and legumes; K_2 is synthesized by gut bacteria

RDA: Birth to 6 months: 5 micrograms (mcg)
6 months to 1 year: 10 mcg
1 to 3 years: 15 mcg
4 to 6 years: 20 mcg
7 to 10 years: 30 mcg

Deficiency signs: Deficiency is uncommon. Vitamin K is given to newborns to prevent internal bleeding. It is available through injection or supplemental drops, or found in multivitamins.

Toxicity: Excess vitamin K_2 or K_3 can cause hemolytic anemia (destruction of red blood cells). No toxicity is found with vitamin K_1, which is the type of vitamin K used in supplements.

Minerals

Calcium

Function: Calcium aids in bone and tooth formation, muscle contraction, heartbeat, blood clotting, and nerve impulses. We recommend calcium citrate or calcium citrate malate as the primary sources of calcium supplementation for children due to their high absorbability.

Sources: Kelp, cheese, collards, kale, turnip greens, almonds, yogurt, milk, broccoli, and soy

RDA: Birth to 6 months: 400 milligrams (mg)

6 months to 1 year: 600 mg

1 to 10 years: 800 mg

Deficiency signs: Bone deformity (rickets), growth retardation, muscle and leg cramps.

Toxicity: Normally, there are no toxic effects with large doses. Some researchers feel that those with a tendency to develop kidney stones should avoid high doses of calcium, although this has not been proved.

Chromium

Function: Chromium helps with blood sugar control.

Sources: Whole grains, meats, potatoes, liver, and brewer's yeast

RDA: None given, but the following are estimated safe and adequate daily intakes:

Birth to 6 months: 10 to 40 micrograms (mcg)

6 months to 1 year: 20 to 60 mcg

1 to 3 years: 20 to 80 mcg

4 to 6 years: 30 to 120 mcg

7 years and older: 50 to 200 mcg

Deficiency signs: Elevated blood sugar levels

Toxicity: Chromium is safe when taken in the recommended dosages. No toxicity is reported, but it has not been studied in children either.

Copper

Function: Copper is involved in collagen formation, red blood cell formation, energy production, and many other enzyme systems.

Vital Study

A joint research study by Indiana University School of Medicine in Indianapolis and Purdue University in West Lafayette, Indiana, looked at the absorption difference between two supplemental sources of calcium: calcium carbonate and calcium citrate malate. The calcium absorption from calcium citrate malate exceeded calcium carbonate by 55 percent.

Vital Fact

Chromium is an essential nutrient required for sugar and fat metabolism. Most people don't get as much chromium as they should. Insufficient dietary intake of chromium leads to signs and symptoms that are similar to those observed for diabetes and cardiovascular diseases. Supplemental chromium given to people with impaired glucose tolerance or diabetes leads to improved blood glucose, insulin, and lipid levels.

Sources: Whole grains, shellfish, nuts, eggs, poultry, organ meats, peas, dark green leafy vegetables, and legumes

RDA: None given, but the following are estimated safe and adequate daily intakes.

Birth to 6 months: 0.4 to 0.6 milligram (mg)

6 months to 1 year: 0.6 to 0.7 mg

1 to 3 years: 0.7 to 1 mg

4 to 6 years: 1 to 1.5 mg

7 to 10 years: 1 to 2 mg

Supplementation is generally not recommended except a small amount in a children's multivitamin (0.1 to 1 mg). Higher doses may be necessary with high doses of zinc supplementation.

Deficiency signs: Deficiency is rare, but symptoms could include low immune function, poor collagen and connective tissue strength, bone and joint abnormalities, and anemia.

Toxicity: Too much copper can cause nausea, vomiting, and dizziness.

Caution: Use only as part of a children's multivitamin.

Iodine

Function: Iodine is required to manufacture thyroid hormones.

Sources: Iodized salt and water; seafood, seaweeds such as kelp

RDA: Birth to 6 months: 40 micrograms (mcg)

6 months to 1 year: 50 mcg

1 to 3 years: 70 mcg

4 to 6 years: 90 mcg

7 to 10 years: 120 mcg

Since iodine deficiency is rare, amounts more than what is present in a children's multivitamin (for example, 0.15 to 0.25 milligrams) should be supplemented only under the guidance of a physician.

Deficiency signs: Iodine deficiency is rare in North America. Infants deprived of iodine during pregnancy can develop a condition known as cretinism. This condition is characterized by physical and mental impairment. Severe mental retardation can occur. Another condition known as goiter—an enlargement of the thyroid gland—can occur, as can general hypothyroidism.

Toxicity: Too much iodine can interfere with thyroid activity (hypothyroidism) and may cause acne eruptions and goiter.

Iron

Function: Iron is important for oxygen supply to cells, collagen synthesis, and normal immune function.

Sources: Liver and organ meats, beef, legumes, dark green leafy vegetables, kelp, and blackstrap molasses

RDA: Birth to 6 months: 6 milligrams (mg)

6 months to 10 years: 10 mg

For iron deficiency anemia, dosages of up to 60 mg daily are used under a doctor's supervision.

Deficiency signs: Iron deficiency is characterized by fatigue, paleness, poor memory and concentration, developmental delays and behavioral disturbances, chronic colds, and weakened immunity.

Toxicity: Too much iron is associated with an increased risk of heart disease and cancer. Acute iron poisoning in children can result in damage to the intestinal tract, liver failure, nausea and vomiting, shock, and death.

Caution: Never give iron in excess of the amounts prescribed by a doctor.

Magnesium

Function: Magnesium is important for bone and teeth formation, energy production, and muscle and nerve impulses.

Sources: Whole grains, nuts, legumes, soy, and green leafy vegetables

Vital Study

Data from the third National Health and Nutrition Examination Survey (NHANES III), which was conducted from 1988 to 1994, indicated that 9 percent of children ages 12 to 36 months in the United States had iron deficiency and that 3 percent also had iron deficiency anemia. The prevalence of iron deficiency is higher among children living at or below the poverty level than among those living above the poverty level, and it is higher among black or Mexican-American children than among white children.

RDA: Birth to 6 months: 40 milligrams (mg)
6 months to 1 year: 60 mg
1 to 3 years: 80 mg
4 to 6 years: 120 mg
7 to 10 years: 170 mg

Deficiency signs: Weakness, confusion, mood changes, muscle spasms/tremors, nausea, poor coordination, heart disturbances, insomnia, and susceptibility to kidney stones

Toxicity: Children who have kidney disease or who are on heart medications should not supplement magnesium unless instructed to do so by their doctors. Diarrhea is usually the first symptom of too much magnesium.

Manganese

Function: Manganese is required for enzyme systems involved with energy production and also for blood sugar control, fatty acid synthesis, thyroid hormone function, connective tissue and bone formation, and healing of sprains and strains.

Sources: Liver, kidney, whole grains, nuts, spinach, and green leafy vegetables

RDA: None given, but the following are estimated safe and adequate daily intakes:
Birth to 6 months: 0.3 to 0.6 milligram (mg)
6 months to 1 year: 0.6 to 1 mg
1 to 3 years: 1 to 1.5 mg
4 to 6 years: 1.5 to 2 mg
7 to 10 years: 2 to 3 mg

Deficiency signs: No symptoms have been observed in humans. Animal studies show growth problems.

Toxicity: Too much manganese can interfere with iron absorption and cause iron deficiency.

Molybdenum

Function: Molybdenum is active in enzyme systems involved with the metabolism of alcohol, uric acid, and sulfur.

Sources: Meats, whole grain breads, legumes, leafy vegetables, organ meats, and brewer's yeast

RDA: None given, but the following are estimated safe and adequate daily intakes:

Birth to 6 months: 15 to 30 micrograms (mcg)

6 months to 1 year: 20 to 40 mcg

1 to 3 years: 25 to 50 mcg

4 to 6 years: 30 to 75 mcg

7 to 10 years: 50 to 150 mcg

Deficiency signs: None known, but the inability to detoxify sulfites is reported.

Toxicity: None reported

Phosphorus

Function: Phosphorus aids in growth, bone production, and energy production.

Sources: Meats, fish, eggs, poultry, and milk products

RDA: Birth to 6 months: 300 milligrams (mg)

6 months to 1 year: 500 mg

1 to 10 years: 800 mg

Note: Phosphorus supplementation should be done only under the recommendation of a physician.

Deficiency signs: Deficiency is very rare.

Toxicity: Too much phosphorus in the form of phosphoric acid (a common ingredient of soft drinks) can cause the body to lose calcium.

Potassium

Function: Potassium helps with nerve transmission, water balance, acid-base balance, heart function, kidney function, and adrenal function.

Vital Study

Many doctors have observed a correlation between the ingestion of cow's milk and iron deficiency anemia. One Swedish study examined 367 healthy 2½-year-olds. The amounts of cow's milk and formula consumed were recorded. Researchers found that 10 percent of the children were iron-deficient. They also found that the intake of cow's milk was significantly higher in the children with iron deficiency.

Vital Fact

An 8-ounce glass of cow's milk contains approximately 300 milligrams of calcium. The absorption of calcium from milk is 25 to 30 percent. Therefore, about 75 milligrams of calcium are actually absorbed.

Sources: Fruits and vegetables, especially apples, bananas, carrots, oranges, potatoes, tomatoes, cantaloupe, peaches, plums, and strawberries; meat, milk, and fish are also sources

RDA: Birth to 6 months: 500 milligrams (mg)

6 months to 1 year: 700 mg

1 year: 1,000 mg

2 to 5 years: 1,400 mg

6 to 9 years: 1,600 mg

Caution: Potassium is generally not taken as an individual supplement by children. Extra supplementation should be under the guidance of a physician.

Deficiency signs: Muscle wasting, weakness, and spasm; fatigue; mood changes; heart disturbances; nerve problems

Toxicity: Impaired heart and kidney function. Children with heart or kidney conditions should not take potassium unless instructed to do so by a physician.

Selenium

Function: Selenium is an antioxidant that aids in cancer prevention, immunity, thyroid function, and development of the fetus during pregnancy.

Sources: Liver, kidney, meats, and seafood. Grains and vegetables are good sources, but selenium content depends on the level in the soil where they are grown.

RDA: Birth to 6 months: 10 micrograms (mcg)

6 months to 1 year: 15 mcg

1 to 6 years: 20 mcg

7 to 10 years: 30 mcg

Deficiency signs: In China, severe selenium deficiency in children is associated with a severe heart disorder known as Keshan disease. Selenium deficiency is associated with an increased risk of heart disease, cancer, and poor immune function.

Toxicity: Overdosing on selenium can lead to nausea, depression, teeth abnormalities, and vomiting.

Silicon

Function: Silicon is important for bone, cartilage, and ligament formation.

Sources: Unrefined grains, cereals, and root vegetables

RDA: None given, and little information exists about dosages for silicon. Five to 20 milligrams is an estimated safe dosage for children.

Deficiency signs: None known, but brittle hair and nails are suspected.

Toxicity: Miners who have inhaled large dosages of silicon over a prolonged period of time have developed silicosis, fibrotic formation of the lungs. The amounts found in foods and in children's multivitamins appear to be very safe.

Sodium

Function: Sodium contributes to acid-base balance, muscle contraction, nerve impulses, and amino acid absorption

Sources: Naturally occurring in meats, milk products, water, eggs, poultry, and fish. Abundant in canned foods and other commercially processed foods.

RDA: None given, but the following are established minimum requirements for healthy persons:

    Birth to 6 months: 120 milligrams (mg)
    6 months to 1 year: 200 mg
    1 year: 225 mg
    2 to 5 years: 300 mg
    6 to 9 years: 400 mg

Vital Fact

Compared with 25 years ago, children ages 5 and younger consume 8 percent less calcium, children ages 6 to 11 consume 15 to 20 percent less, and calcium consumption by teenagers is down 7 to 15 percent.

Vital Fact

Iron sulfate or ferrous sulfate, the most widely prescribed form of supplemental iron, can be constipating and irritating to the digestive tract. We recommend other forms such as iron citrate or iron glycinate, which are much better absorbed and do not cause the digestive irritation and constipation found with iron sulfate.

Supplementation is not generally recommended, as deficiency is rare.

Deficiency signs: Deficiency is very uncommon except in the case of dehydration through profuse sweating or diarrhea. Symptoms can include muscle weakness and cramping, low blood pressure, muscle twitching, mental confusion, and loss of appetite.

Toxicity: High blood pressure, especially when potassium intake is low

Vanadium

Function: Vanadium helps with blood sugar balance and bone and teeth development.

Sources: Shellfish, mushrooms, black pepper, and buckwheat

RDA: None given, but a safe children's dosage would be 5 to 20 micrograms.

Deficiency signs: None known, but blood sugar imbalances are suspected.

Toxicity: Little is known, but very high amounts may lead to cramps and diarrhea.

Zinc

Function: Zinc is involved in more than 200 enzymatic reactions. It is required to manufacture many hormones and for immunity, skin healing, growth, vision, and blood sugar metabolism. It is also an antioxidant.

Sources: Oysters, herring, shellfish, red meat, whole grains, legumes, and nuts

RDA: Birth to 1 year: 5 milligrams (mg)

1 to 10 years: 15 mg

Deficiency signs: Too little zinc can cause hair loss, poor wound healing, poor immune function, diarrhea, skin conditions (acne), and mental disturbance. White spots on the nails are another symptom.

Toxicity: Zinc toxicity is rare. Very high dosages can lead to immune system suppression, digestive upset, and anemia.

Other Nutrients

Alpha Lipoic Acid

Function: Alpha lipoic acid is an antioxidant involved in energy production.

Sources: Liver, yeast, potatoes, spinach, and red meat

RDA: None given. An estimated safe dose is 5 to 25 milligrams.

Deficiency signs: No specific symptoms given, but children with diabetes may benefit from supplementation.

Toxicity: None known

Carnitine

Function: Carnitine helps with energy production and heart function.

Sources: Meat, dairy products

RDA: None given, but 25 to 100 milligrams is a safe range for children.

Deficiency signs: Symptoms of deficiency include loss of muscle tone, recurrent infections, brain swelling, heart irregularities, and failure to thrive.

Toxicity: None

Choline

Function: Choline is required to manufacture the neurotransmitter acetylcholine. It also helps with the metabolism of fats.

Sources: Legumes, egg yolks, whole grains, and soy

RDA: None given, but 10 milligrams is a safe dosage for children.

Vital Fact

Zinc is a major mineral involved in cell division (similar to folic acid and B_{12}). It is very important for fetal development. Low levels are linked to low birth weight, growth retardation, and premature births. Women should take it as part of a multivitamin before, during, and after pregnancy (especially if they are breastfeeding).

Vital Study

In a 1998 study, researchers around the world interviewed mothers of children with primary brain tumors (tumors that originated in the brain) as well as mothers of kids without brain tumors (the control group). The researchers found that children of mothers who had supplemented multivitamins for two trimesters of pregnancy had a decreased risk of brain tumors. The greatest risk reduction was among children diagnosed under 5 years of age whose mothers had used supplements during all three trimesters. The study's researchers also noted that mothers who took multivitamins also often used other supplements (such as vitamin C), which could have played a role in the positive outcome.

Deficiency signs: Potential liver and kidney dysfunction

Toxicity: Rare

Coenzyme Q$_{10}$

Function: Coenzyme Q$_{10}$ is an antioxidant involved in heart activity and energy production.

Sources: Meat, seafood

RDA: None given, but 5 to 15 milligrams is a safe dosage for children.

Deficiency signs: Gum disease, heart failure, fatigue

Toxicity: None known

Inositol

Function: Inositol is a component of cell membranes. It is used to treat depression and to prevent complications of diabetes.

Sources: Citrus fruit, whole grains, nuts, seeds, and legumes

RDA: None given, but 5 to 10 milligrams for children is safe.

Deficiency signs: None known

Toxicity: None known

Selecting Vitamins for Your Child

Make sure to purchase vitamins that are free of artificial sweeteners and preservatives. We recommend that all parents give their children a multivitamin to prevent nutritional deficiencies. (See "Storing and Administering Supplements" on next page for important information on storing multivitamins.) Liquid and powdered multivitamins are available for children and infants who cannot swallow capsules or chew tablets. They can be mixed with juice and water. Multivitamins should be taken with a meal for optimal absorption and to prevent digestive upset. An optimal vitamin/mineral program for children would include:

- A children's multivitamin. This provides a base for most vitamins and minerals.
- A calcium and magnesium supplement, for an extra 500 to 1,000 milligrams of calcium and 250 to 500 milligrams of magnesium daily. Studies show that most children do not get enough calcium, even if they drink milk. It is even more important for children with a dairy sensitivity to supplement extra calcium. Calcium and magnesium supplements are available in a liquid form. They are almost always bought as a formula but can be given separately.
- Vitamin C. An extra 100 to 250 milligrams is beneficial for children who do not eat fruits and vegetables on a regular basis, or who are in day care regularly (because they are exposed to more germs). Vitamin C is available in liquid, powder, and chewable tablet forms for children. If chewable tablets are used, make sure to have your child rinse with some water after chewing, as the acidity can be hard on the gums and tooth enamel. Children sensitive to citrus fruits will tolerate a nonacidic vitamin C such as calcium ascorbate or Ester C.

Storing and Administering Supplements

Keep vitamin and mineral containers away from heat and dampness, out of the light, and make sure that the lids are tightly closed. Most liquid vitamins require refrigeration. Check the expiration date on all supplements before giving them to your child.

It is best to give vitamin and mineral supplements with meals. This is especially true for fat-soluble vitamins, to ensure optimal absorption and utilization. Water-soluble vitamins can be taken between meals but may cause digestive upset in some children.

Vital Study

In a double-blind placebo study published in *The Lancet,* 60 children ages 12 to 13 were examined for the effect of a multivitamin on intelligence. Each child was given either a multivitamin or placebo for 8 months. Only the group receiving a multivitamin showed improvement in nonverbal intelligence.

phytochemicals and other supplements for children

A major area of interest for nutritional science is the therapeutic benefits of phytochemicals (plant chemicals), also known as phytonutrients. These naturally occurring substances give plants their characteristic flavor, color, aroma, and resistance to disease. Thousands of phytochemicals have been identified in fruits, vegetables, grains, and nuts. They have tremendous benefits to people because they help prevent diseases such as cancer and cardiovascular disease. For example, two phytochemicals found in cruciferous vegetables (such as broccoli and cauliflower), known as indole 3 carbinol and sulforaphane, help the body metabolize toxins and are associated with preventing certain types of cancers. And flavonoids found in citrus fruits protect against heart disease, stroke, and cancer.

Many phytochemicals are powerful antioxidants that protect against cell damage and environmental pollutants. Many also help cells detoxify more efficiently. For example, green vegetables are high in chlorophyll, which is a potent detoxifying phytochemical. Our children need all the support nature has to offer in our modern but toxic world.

The bottom line: You are what you eat. Children who grow up eating whole-food diets that include abundant amounts of plant foods stand better chances of avoiding cancer, heart disease, and other maladies. And there are many health benefits of phytochemicals that are yet to be discovered.

Good Food Sources of Phytochemicals

Foods	Phytochemical(s)	Health Benefits
Almonds and cashews	Saponins	Cardiovascular protection
Broccoli, cauliflower, kale, Brussels sprouts	Indoles, sulforaphane	Detoxification, cancer fighting
Carrots, cantaloupe, bell peppers, yellow squash, oranges, lemons, yams, sweet potatoes	Carotenoids, antioxidants	Cardiovascular protection
Flaxseed	Lignans	Cancer and cardiovascular protection
Oranges, lemons, limes, grapefruit	Carotenoids, flavonoids, d-limonene	Immune support, cancer fighting, cardiovascular protection, circulation, detoxification
Red grapes	Resveratrol, flavonoids	Cardiovascular protection
Soy products	Genistein, diadzein	Hormone balancing, cardiovascular protection
Tomatoes	Lycopene	Cancer and cardiovascular protection

Green Drinks: A Supplemental Source

Whole food supplements known as green drinks (so named because they contain a lot of green vegetables and herbs such as alfalfa, wheat grass, barley grass, chlorella, and spirulina) are emerging as popular sources of phytochemicals. These supplements fortify but do not replace the benefits of fruits, vegetables, and other plant foods in one's diet. Depending on the formulation, green drinks or whole-food supplements that are specifically designed for young children can be safely given to children over 2 years of age. The powdered forms can be mixed with a fruit juice such as apple or grape and help to keep children gently detoxified on a daily basis. There are whole-food formulas composed of fruits and vegetable extracts that are designed specifically for kids. Again, they are not intended to replace a proper diet. Check with your natural health care practitioner if you have questions about using a specific product with your child.

Other Nutritional Supplements

Walk into any health food store or your local grocery store and you can quickly be overwhelmed by the many shelves of nutritional supplements. In this section, we clear up the confusion and give you a description of the common supplements used with children. This section includes supplements that have not been covered in other chapters such as Herbal Medicines for Children and Homeopathy for Children.

- *Amino acids* are the building blocks of protein. When taken individually, they can influence the body's biochemistry. For example, GABA is an amino acid that has a calming effect on the body. Lysine is helpful to suppress herpes (cold sore) outbreaks. L-glutamine helps with tissue repair after surgery. Amino acids are best used under the guidance of a health care professional.
- *Bee pollen* is a powderous substance gathered from flowering plants by bees. It provides the essential proteins necessary for the rearing of young bees. It is a rich source of nutrients such as B vitamins, vitamin C, enzymes, trace minerals, amino acids, essential fatty acids, and sterols. Bee pollen is used for a variety of health reasons, including treatment of allergies (hay fever), arthritis, and fatigue, and immune system support. Allergic reactions to bee pollen are very rare but possible. It is important to use only bee pollen products that have been tested for heavy metals and other contaminants.
- *Bovine and shark cartilage,* derived from bovine (cow) and shark sources, are used for various medicinal effects. Bovine cartilage has been shown to enhance wound healing. Both types of cartilage are used to inhibit tumor growth. It is hypothesized that this type of cartilage cuts off blood supply to tumors. There are better clinical

data for bovine cartilage than for shark cartilage, but nothing definitive for either exists in research. Both types of cartilage are also used for the treatment of arthritis, and shark cartilage is also used for psoriasis.

   Caution: Only a doctor should prescribe bovine and shark cartilage to a child.

- *Brewer's yeast* is the dried cells of a type of fungus known as *Saccharomyces cerevisiae.* It is different from baker's yeast. It is grown specifically for health food use and termed *nutritional brewer's yeast.* It is a rich source of B-complex vitamins, amino acids, and trace minerals such as chromium. It is available in a powder or in capsule and tablet form. Brewer's yeast can cause digestive upset in young children. Start with a small amount (¼ teaspoon) and build up to 1 to 2 teaspoons daily.
- *Chlorella* is a type of edible marine algae. It is a rich source of chlorophyll, B vitamins, minerals, carotenoids, and vitamin E, as well as RNA and DNA that are thought to help with human cell repair. The high chlorophyll content makes chlorella an excellent detoxifier, even for heavy metal toxicity. It is a natural source of vitamin B_{12} and protein for vegetarians. Supplemental sources are generally available in tablet, capsule, or powder form.
- *Chlorophyll* is the phytochemical responsible for the green color in plants. It has antioxidant effects, which may help prevent cancer. Chlorophyll helps to build red blood cells, improve cellular detoxification, relieve constipation, improve wound healing, and ameliorate bad breath and foul-smelling stools. It is available in liquid form or as an ingredient in chlorella, spirulina, and other green foods.
- *DHA,* or docosahexaenoic acid, is a type of long-chain fatty acid found in high concentrations in the brain. Infants and children have a very high demand for this substance for brain and retina development. Fish such as salmon are an excellent source, as is breast milk. (For a more thorough description, see "Essential Fatty

Acids" on page 8.) It is available in liquid and capsule form. Vegetarian sources are available.

- *Enzymes* as supplemental sources exist in two forms: plant- and animal-derived. We generally recommend plant-derived enzymes, also called microbial-derived enzymes, as they are more stable when exposed to stomach acid. Enzymes are often used to help break foods down more efficiently. This makes them useful for digestive problems such as irritable bowel syndrome and gas. Enzymes can also be added to baby formula to help with colic. Proteolytic enzymes (which break down proteins) such as bromelain can be found in whole foods as well as supplements. They provide a natural anti-inflammatory action.

> *Caution:* Fiber supplements should be prescribed to children only under the guidance of a health care professional. If they are used, it is important that plenty of water be consumed—at least 8 ounces—with the supplement, followed by at least eight 8-ounce glasses of water throughout the day to prevent the bowels from plugging up.

- *Fiber supplements* are easy to find at grocery and health food stores. Fiber is found in many foods such as fruits, vegetables, legumes, and grains. Fiber is the indigestible portion of plants. It has many functions, such as helping to absorb toxins and fats and balancing blood sugar levels. Fiber, along with enough water, is important to prevent constipation. The most common fiber supplements contain psyllium seeds and psyllium husks in a capsule.

- *Fish oils* such as salmon oil and tuna oil are a rich source of omega-3 fatty acids that promote cardiovascular health. They are also a good source of DHA. (To learn more about DHA, see "Essential Fatty Acids" on page 8.)

- *Flaxseed oil* is a rich source of omega-3 fatty acids, especially alpha linolenic acid (ALA). It is commonly used to improve skin health and treat constipation in children. Caution must be used so that diarrhea does not occur.

- *Glandulars* are concentrated extracts from bovine or pork sources. The concept is to take the same glandular as the gland in which you want to stimulate or improve function. For example, thymus glandular can be used to support the thymus gland in order to improve immune system function. Glandulars are generally available in tablet form and need to be crushed up for children to use. They are best taken between meals.

Caution: Honey should never be given to children under 1 year of age, as it may contain bacteria that can cause botulism.

• *Honey* is made from the mixture of the nectar from flowers and the enzymes from bees. It contains carbohydrates, minerals, and a variety of vitamins. It acts as a natural antiseptic and is sweet-tasting.

• *Kelp* is a type of seaweed that is a rich source of iodine, which is needed for thyroid hormone production. It also contains magnesium, iron, and potassium. It is available in powder or capsule form. It is generally used for its helpful effects on a low-functioning thyroid.

• *Lactobacillus acidophilus* and *L. bifidus* are two types of bacteria found throughout the digestive tract and other areas of the body. These "friendly bacteria" help to prevent the overgrowth of bad bugs. They also help to synthesize certain vitamins such as vitamin K and biotin, and help to break down fiber in the colon. Antibiotics, especially broad-spectrum antibiotics, deplete these friendly bacteria, which can lead to conditions such as diarrhea, yeast overgrowth, digestive problems, and fatigue. A children's probiotic supplement (a supplement containing beneficial bacteria) containing acidophilus and bifidus is recommended while the child is taking antibiotics and for 2 months after antibiotic use. *Lactobacillus rhamnosus* is another good strain to use to replace the good bacteria. This type of supplement is best taken between meals. It is available in liquid and capsule form. Yogurt with live cultures also contains these good bacteria.

• *Propolis* is a type of glue that bees make from the resins of certain tree barks. It is used by the bees to sterilize the hive and protect it from invaders. Humans use propolis for its antimicrobial effects. It has been shown to have antiviral, antibacterial, and antifungal effects. It also stimulates the immune system. It is a rich source of bioflavonoids, which exert natural anti-inflammatory effects on the body. Propolis works well as a topical application for cuts and scrapes, to accelerate healing and to prevent infection. This would be the most common use with children. It is also available in capsule form.

- *Spirulina* is a type of blue-green algae found in warm, sunny climates. It has a high protein content as well as B vitamins, including B_{12}. It is a source of the fatty acid gamma linolenic acid and also contains chlorophyll, carotenoids, and other phytochemicals.
- *Wheat germ* is the tiny embryo of the wheat kernel. It is a good source of vitamin E and B vitamins. It should be used with caution in children under 2 years of age, as digestive upset may occur. Fresh wheat germ should be refrigerated after it is made.

aromatherapy
for children

An increasingly popular method for helping children's ailments is aromatherapy. The essential oils from plants, leaves, bark, roots, seeds, and flowers are used to treat a wide range of conditions. Aromatherapy can help provide relief from many childhood conditions, from insomnia to hyperactivity. It is effective for physical, psychological, and emotional symptoms.

Aromatherapy is nothing new. Ancient Egyptians and Greeks used aromatic substances as medicine to heal wounds and preserve mummies. A French cosmetic scientist, Professor Rene-Maurice Gattefoss, coined the term *aromatherapy.* After accidentally burning his hand, he applied lavender oil, which quickly relieved the pain and healed his skin. Being a scientist, he purposely burned his hand again and dipped it in lavender and found that it healed his skin in a remarkable way again.

More than 1,000 essential oils exist. Most are not actually oils as one would think of vegetable oils. They received the name *oils* because the majority of them will float on top of water. Each oil may contain 300 or more compounds. Unlike vegetable oils, most essential oils do not go rancid or stain clothes (as long as they are high-grade quality). Plants actually contain very small amounts of the essential oils. For example, 12 pounds of lavender flowers are needed to produce an ounce of lavender essential oil, and 30 roses are required to make a single drop of rose essential oil.

Most essential oils are extracted by manufacturers using steam distillation. Delicate flowers such as jasmine undergo solvent extraction.

It is important that pure sources are used to obtain the full range of aromatic compounds.

The recommended aromatherapy treatments for the conditions in this book were chosen for their effectiveness, high-grade quality, and accessibility.

Ways to Use Aromatherapy

There are three methods you can use to harness the power of aromatherapy for your child: inhalation, baths, and topical application. Here we will discuss each in detail, along with any necessary precautions associated with each method.

Inhalation

This is the most common and safest way to use aromatherapy. For children, put 1 to 2 drops onto a tissue and slip it under the bottom sheet in a crib or bed. This works especially well when using oils such as lavender for insomnia. Do not allow inhalation directly from the essential oil bottle, as it can be too strong for the child and may contaminate the oil. For colds, inhalation using hot, steaming water and adding essential oils works well. Careful adult supervision is, of course, necessary to prevent burns. Adding essential oils to a vaporizer is a way to provide fragrance to a room while benefiting from the aroma. Vaporizers require occasional cleaning and sterilization.

Caution: Do not use the steam inhalation technique with a child who has asthma.

Baths

After running a warm bath, add the desired aromatherapy oil(s). Swish the water briskly around to disperse the essential oil or oils. Have the child bathe for a minimum of 10 minutes. For children between the ages of 2 and 12, use 2 to 3 drops of essential oil(s). For those over the age of 12, use 4 to 6 drops.

Caution: Never use essential oils in a bath with infants under 2 years of age. Their skin is too sensitive. Topical or inhalation methods should be used instead.

Topical Application

Dilution is very important when using essential oils topically. More is not better when it comes to aromatherapy. The oil needs to be diluted in a carrier such as grape seed oil, olive oil, or sweet almond oil, available at health food stores or wherever aromatherapy oils are sold.

The general rule of thumb is to use 1 drop of essential oil for each year of the child's age, up to a maximum of 12 drops in 20 millileters of carrier oil. For newborns to 6-month-olds, use 1 drop of essential oil in 40 millileters of carrier oil. For infants 6 months to 1 year old, use 1 drop of essential oil in 30 millileters of carrier oil.

Note: Apply the aromatherapy blend under clothing to keep young children from getting it on their hands and transferring the oil to their mouths and eyes.

Massage is one of the most soothing and effective ways to apply the essential oils. Compresses are another good method. To make a compress, add 3 drops of essential oil to 5 cups of water (warm or cool). Dip in a facecloth or cotton cloth, wring it out so that it is not dripping, and lay it on the desired area for 5 to 10 minutes. Make sure to check the skin after the first 2 minutes to ensure that it has not become irritated.

Skin test: To see whether your child is sensitive or allergic to the essential oil(s) you want to use, simply dab a small amount of the oil (diluted in the carrier oil) on the back of your child's arm. Look for any signs of allergic reaction, such as redness or itching, over the next 12 hours. If there is a reaction, use a more dilute mixture or try a different essential oil.

Cautions with Aromatherapy

1. Never use essential oils undiluted on the skin unless otherwise guided by a professional aromatherapist, as most concentrated oils can be too caustic and cause burning or irritation.

Emergency Situations with Aromatherapy

Skin becomes irritated:	To relieve irritated skin from essential oils, wash with soap and water or a mild detergent. If the rash does not clear up in a few days, seek medical attention. If there is blistering, seek medical attention right away.
Essential oil gets in the eyes:	Place a small drop of plain carrier oil (such as olive oil) into the affected eye or eyes. The oil helps to absorb the essential oil. Rinse with water and pat with a cloth. Seek medical attention immediately to have the eyes examined.
Child becomes sick and nauseated:	If a child becomes sick, nauseated, or confused or gets a headache from the essential oils, get him to breathe some fresh air. Symptoms should improve immediately and should continue to improve over the next couple of hours. If there is no improvement, seek medical attention.
Child swallows essential oil:	Call the Poison Control Center or 911 immediately. Do not try to induce vomiting.

2. Never let your child swallow aromatherapy essential oils, as they can be toxic. Also, keep essential oils away from the genitals, ears, mouth, and nose.

3. Never put aromatherapy products into the bath of an infant under 2 years.

4. Never apply essential oils before going out in the sun. Oils such as bergamot, cold-pressed lime, neroli, lemon, grapefruit, angelica root, cumin, lovage, and verbena can cause sun sensitivity.

5. Do not use essential oils at the same time as taking homeopathic remedies. Some essential oils may counteract the homeopathic treatment. If both are used, spread the time between each as long as possible. Essential oils such as eucalyptus, peppermint, rosemary, and

spearmint should be avoided completely when using homeopathy.

6. Store essential oils out of the reach of children. They should be stored in a cool, dark, dry place.

Common Essential Oils for Children

Roman Chamomile

An excellent anti-inflammatory for the skin, muscles, and joints. A good nerve tonic. One of the most common oils used for allergies.

Eucalyptus

A powerful antiseptic oil against viruses and bacteria. Helpful for colds, sore muscles, and headaches. Avoid with a child who has high blood pressure or epilepsy.

Geranium

Rejuvenating to the nervous and immune system. Avoid using at nighttime with children, as it may keep them awake.

Lavender

The most popular essential oil. Used on cuts and burns, and for general tissue healing. Works well for headaches and insomnia. Calming.

Neroli

A good antidepressant. Reduces muscle spasms.

Niaouli (or Niauli)

This essential oil from Australia is good for skin healing. Powerful antibacterial effect.

Orange

A relaxing, soothing oil that helps depression, anxiety, and other nervous conditions. The "sweet" type is best to use with children as opposed to the stronger "bitter" orange oil. Avoid using when exposed to sunlight.

Case History

Philip, a rambunctious 8-year-old boy, had problems sleeping at night. His father said that Philip would resist going to bed, try to stay up all night, and fidget in bed. We recommended giving Philip a bath each night with 3 drops of lavender oil placed in the bathwater. We explained to Philip's father that lavender is a nontoxic essential oil that helps people to relax. The lavender bath is a nightly routine for Philip, who now sleeps soundly.

Patchouli

Useful for skin problems such as acne and eczema.

Peppermint

Helps calm upset stomachs, headaches, and sore muscles, and improves mental alertness. Do not use before bedtime, as it can be stimulating. Avoid if child has high blood pressure.

Tea Tree (Ti Tree)

A strong antiseptic with antifungal, antibacterial, and antiviral effects. Great for athlete's foot. Helps to combat a fever and promotes sweating. Make sure it is well-diluted for use on children's skin.

Thyme

Supports the immune system and has strong antiseptic properties. Use "sweet thyme" with children.

Purchasing Quality Aromatherapy Oils

As with most products, the better-quality aromatherapy products produce better results.

1. If possible, ask a reputable aromatherapist in your area what products he or she recommends that are of high quality.

2. The oils should be guaranteed to be pure, not diluted. Talk with aromatherapy practitioners to find out which brands they recommend. Reputable companies can provide records proving the purity.

3. The label should contain both the English and Latin names of the oil(s).

4. The bottle must be of tinted glass, not just dipped in dye. Dark blue and amber are common.

5. Purchase only essential oils that have been kept out of light and direct sunlight.

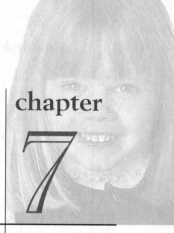

hydrotherapy for children

A simple but effective therapy that works well on children is hydrotherapy. The term *hydrotherapy* refers to water therapy that can be applied in many different forms. Manipulation of circulation with hydrotherapy can help many children's ailments, including fevers, colds and chest colds, headaches, sinusitis, insomnia, and various other conditions. Although it is a gentle treatment, hydrotherapy can have profound health benefits. In addition, hydrotherapy is an effective way to stimulate the immune system, optimize circulation, and promote detoxification.

Constitutional Hydrotherapy

The most powerful of the hydrotherapy treatments is constitutional hydrotherapy, so called because it has benefits for the entire constitution of a person. Naturopathic doctors have been using this technique for more than 60 years, and its origins go back hundreds of years. Hydrotherapy has five main effects:

1. It optimizes circulation.
2. It detoxifies and purifies the blood.
3. It enhances digestive function and elimination.
4. It tonifies and balances the nervous system.
5. It stimulates and enhances the immune system.

Hydrotherapy is particularly helpful for children who have digestive problems, respiratory problems such as sore throats and bronchitis, and infections such as colds or flu.

Caution: If a child has asthma, this procedure should be used only under the guidance of a physician.

Frequency of treatment: For acute conditions, one or two times daily; for chronic conditions, once daily.

Directions: Only an adult should apply this treatment.

1. Have the child lie in bed on his back.

2. Cover the child's bared chest and abdomen with two thicknesses of toweling that have been placed in hot water and wrung out. (Wet towels can also be heated in a microwave oven.) The towels should be hot but tolerable for the child. Place a small section of the toweling on the child first to make sure that it is not too hot.

3. Cover the hot towels with a dry towel.

4. Cover the child with blankets to avoid a chill. Leave the towels on for 5 minutes. After 5 minutes, remove the hot towels and replace them with a single thickness of a thin towel that has been run under cold water and then wrung out (some moisture should be left in the towel).

5. Place the cold towel on the bared chest and abdomen. Cover it with a dry towel and blankets. Leave these on for 10 minutes. The towel should be warm after 10 minutes. If not, leave it on longer, or prepare a new towel that isn't as cold and wet.

6. Take the cold towel off and have the child turn over and lie on his stomach. Repeat the same procedure on the back: 5 minutes of hot towels, followed by 10 minutes of a thin, cold towel.

Note: For young babies and toddlers, use a washcloth instead of towels to apply the hot and cold therapy. Hold the baby during the treatment.

Comment: The alternation in hot and cold increases white blood cells to help fight off infections. It also increases circulation to the digestive organs and to other organs of elimination.

Case history: Jason was a 5-year-old who came into our office with a nasty case of bronchitis. In addition to prescribing an herbal formula, we had his mother give Jason a constitutional hydrotherapy treatment every day for 3 days. It helped tremendously. Jason's mother told us that it helped relieve the congestion in his chest and also helped him sleep better.

Foot Hydrotherapy

A simpler treatment than constitutional hydrotherapy, foot hydrotherapy helps to relieve respiratory congestion, headaches, and insomnia.

Frequency of treatment: For acute conditions, one or two times daily; for chronic conditions, once daily.

Directions:

1. Have the child sit on a chair or couch and place both feet in a bucket of comfortably warm water for 5 to 10 minutes. (This step and the next step can be skipped with infants.)

2. Remove the child's feet from the water and dry them.

3. Put on a pair of cotton socks that have been placed in cold water and wrung out.

4. Cover with a pair of dry wool socks (or cotton, if wool is not available).

5. Leave the socks on for 30 minutes or longer. The child should rest; she can go to sleep with the socks on.

Comment: Foot hydrotherapy works by diverting bloodflow to the feet and away from the upper body, thus reducing congestion.

Hydrotherapy Headache Treatment

You can help alleviate a child's headache simply by putting his feet in warm water and placing an ice pack around his neck. This treatment works best at the onset of a headache; do it for 10 to 15 minutes. The hot and cold water strategy causes blood to move away from the head and toward the feet, relieving the child of head congestion and pain.

Case History

Dr. Angela knew about the value of foot hydrotherapy for children with colds, sore throats, and fevers before Dr. Mark did. At first, he teased her about prescribing such a simple treatment, but after seeing her success in 12 straight cases, he, too, started recommending it. Most parents tell us that foot hydrotherapy also helps relax their children and is great for relieving congestion of the sinus and upper respiratory tract.

massage and acupressure for children

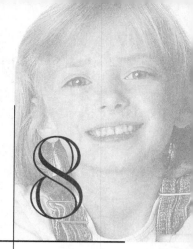

Your child can be safely massaged at home. Massage is a great way to help your child relax and improve her overall health. It improves circulation, detoxification, and elimination. It is therapeutic for a child to be touched by her parent. You can use your bare hands or an oil such as olive oil or almond oil (make sure to avoid the area around the eyes). Gently stroke the skin in the direction of the heart. For example, if you are massaging the legs, stroke upward. If you are working on the neck, stroke downward. The abdomen is best massaged in a clockwise manner. Massage therapists are available who specialize in pediatric massage.

Acupressure has likely been used since the beginning of human existence. People have always had the instinct to push on "sore spots" to relieve pain. This was also done by parents to relieve discomfort for their children, as pain relief is one of the many benefits of acupressure. For more than 4,000 years, traditional Chinese medicine has relied on a system of medicine that establishes harmony and balance in the body. Its theory is based on the concept of energy channels. It is believed that energy circulates through the different channels of the body, known as meridians. When there is a blockage of this energy, pain and disease can occur. The use of acupressure releases this blockage so that balance is restored. Although the mechanisms are not completely understood, modern scientific explanation of the benefits of acupressure/acupuncture is that it restores normal electrical flow through the cells and tissues. Also, different acupressure points have reflexes or connections to different organs in the body and can help normalize their function. In addition, it has been shown that acupressure causes the release of the body's natural painkillers and the release of immune factors that promote healing. Although acupressure relieves physical problems, it also can have benefits for the emotional and mental health of a child. The obvious benefit of acupressure as compared with acupuncture is that there are no needles involved—a major plus for children.

Acupressure Channels

There are 12 major meridians on the body. Six flow on the front of the body, and six are located on the back. The channels are identical on each side of the body. Each is connected to a specific organ, such as the heart or stomach. Aside from the 12 meridians, there are two extra channels, known as the governing and conception channels, that also have acupressure points. Each point has a corresponding organ name, such as Large Intestine 4, which is the fourth point on the Large Intestine channel. Different points are used for different disorders.

Administering an Acupressure Treatment to Your Child

1. Make sure that your child is relaxed. The room should be free of noise. If possible, the child should be wearing light clothing. Acupressure is best done by having the child lie down on a bed or comfortable surface. Make sure that she is warm. Talk to your child and let her know that you will be touching her to make her feel better.

2. Locate the desired point to which you will apply pressure. Press on the point using your thumb or fingers. The pressure should not cause the child pain. Some points may be very tender, indicating a blockage. Start with very light pressure, see how the child feels, and adjust the pressure accordingly. Press the acupressure point and hold for 10 to 15 seconds. This can be repeated 5 to 10 times to see if it helps with the relief of symptoms. Chronic conditions will need

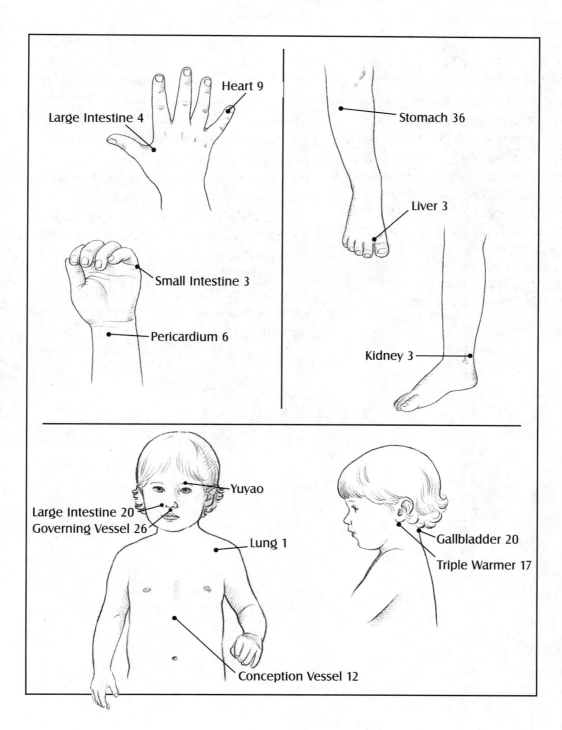

Heart 9

Large Intestine 4

Stomach 36

Liver 3

Small Intestine 3

Pericardium 6

Kidney 3

Yuyao

Large Intestine 20

Governing Vessel 26

Lung 1

Gallbladder 20

Triple Warmer 17

Conception Vessel 12

Case History

Tiffany, age 12, came to our clinic with her mother. Tiffany had a clogged sinus. In addition to giving her homeopathic and herbal remedies, we had Tiffany push on two acupressure points located on the outer-lower corner of each nostril, known as Large Intestine 20. Tiffany tried this technique under our supervision, and she immediately noticed that her sinus and head pain dramatically subsided. For the next 2 days, she noticed considerable sinus pain relief whenever she pushed on these points.

more treatments to see whether the acupressure is working. Some children may prefer a rubbing or massage over the acupressure points; this is fine to do as well. Since the same channel runs on both sides of the body, try to stimulate both points simultaneously. For example, Large Intestine 4 is located on the web of tissue between the thumb and index finger. You can grab both of your child's hands and stimulate Large Intestine 4 with your thumbs on each hand at the same time.

3. After the treatment, let your child relax in a quiet atmosphere, and give her a glass of water to drink to help her body detoxify.

the importance
of breastfeeding

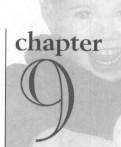

It's hard to believe, but for decades, many doctors maintained (and some still do) that there was no difference in the health benefits between breastfeeding and bottlefeeding. Thankfully, today, more enlightened health professionals—including the American Academy of Pediatrics—agree that breastfeeding provides the optimal food for babies.

Obviously, we feel the same way. That's why we've devoted this extended section to helping parents understand just what an amazing source of vitality breast milk can be. Indeed, breast milk contains everything newborns need—in the amounts in which they need it—for their physical and mental development. Nutritionists cannot devise a better formula (although they keep trying) than this milk, custom-made by a mother for her child.

Our message to mothers is clear: If you can breastfeed, you should make every effort to do so. Even if you work, you can provide breast milk to your baby, since milk can be pumped and stored in bottles or even frozen for your baby's use when you are not available. With practice and experience, you can overcome any societal pressures you may have about nursing your child either in public or in private. And if you need help and support, we have included several resources to turn to for information on breastfeeding, as well as ways to meet other nursing mothers who are sharing your experiences.

If you cannot breastfeed, then of course you should not. (See "What If You Are Not Breastfeeding?" on page 131 for other options.) If you choose not to breastfeed, that is, of course, your decision, and it does not mean that you're a bad mom. But bear in mind that breastfeeding confers many nutritional and psychological benefits to your baby, as we'll discuss here. Breastfeeding also help moms, too. It can help you to recover faster from the ordeal of pregnancy. There are even some studies that suggest that breastfeeding can reduce your risk of diseases (including cancer) later in life. Most important, breastfeeding helps cement a bond between you and your child that will last a lifetime.

You may seem hesitant at first—it may seem like an embarrassing or complicated task—but in many ways, nothing could be more natural than providing your child with milk that your own body has made for your baby's exclusive use.

The Makeup of Milk

Human milk contains fat, carbohydrates, protein, minerals, vitamins, essential fatty acids, immune factors, and many other nutrients. And it constantly changes, adapting to a baby's needs as it grows. For example, foremilk (the milk at the beginning of a feeding) is different from hindmilk (the milk at the end of a feeding). Colostrum (the milk present right after birth) is different from transitional and mature milk.

In fact, there are even normal variations in breast milk depending upon the time of day, the stage of lactation, the mother's nutritional status, and the genetics of each individual mother. But to keep things simple, let's look at the three major phases of breast milk.

Phase 1: Colostrum

For the first week postpartum (after birth), the breasts secrete a yellowish, thick fluid known as colostrum. The yellow color of colostrum is due to the presence of beta-carotene. Sodium, potassium, and chloride concentrations are higher than in mature milk, and the ash content is high. In addition, protein, fat-soluble vitamins, and minerals are present in greater percentages when compared with transitional or mature milk.

Colostrum's high protein and low fat content are just what nature ordered. Colostrum is also rich in potent antioxidants, such as vitamin A, carotenoids, and vitamin E, which protect the baby's cells and immune system from oxidative damage.

Colostrum is responsible for establishing bifidus flora, the good gut bacteria essential for proper digestion. Colostrum also helps the passing of meconium (the first bowel movement a newborn has). Also included in the colostrum are important antibodies, which provide protection against viruses and bacteria.

Vital Fact

Studies have shown that breastfed infants have fewer cavities and better dental health than bottlefed infants. This may be due to fluorine, and to other factors such as selenium, found in human milk.

In all, colostrum is extremely valuable not only for the initial development of the baby but also for reducing the susceptibility to various health problems later in life. The maturing effect colostrum has on the immune, digestive, and other systems of the body can never be received again after that first week of breastfeeding. We often refer to colostrum as the gold of breast milk.

In the first 3 days of life, the volume of milk the baby will get is between 2 and 20 millileters per feeding. Women who have had other pregnancies, especially if they have previously nursed, have colostrum more readily available at delivery, and the volume increases more rapidly.

Phase 2: Transitional Milk

The transitional phase from colostrum to mature milk starts from 1 to 2 weeks postpartum. The concentration of immunoglobulins (immune factors) and total protein decreases and the lactose, fat, and total caloric content increases to match the baby's growing needs. The water-soluble vitamins increase, whereas the fat-soluble vitamins decrease to the levels in mature milk. Studies on transitional breast milk have shown that changes in the composition of the milk are rapid at first and then taper off until the composition of the breast milk is relatively stable by day 36.

Vital Fact

The role of essential fatty acids in nerve cell development may have a bigger impact on the quality of nerve health than researchers originally thought. Studies have shown that multiple sclerosis, a nerve-related disorder, is rarer in countries where breastfeeding is common.

Phase 3: Mature Milk

By the first month's of a baby's life, the breast milk has matured and contains more than 200 constituents whose descriptions are still being defined. Let's examine the major components of mature human milk to see why it is so valuable.

Water is the most plentiful constituent and is especially important since it contributes to the temperature-regulating mechanism of the newborn (25 percent of newborn heat loss is due to evaporation of water from the lungs and skin). That means that a breastfeeding woman must drink water—at least eight 8-ounce glasses of water per day. Studies have shown that the water requirements of infants in hot, humid climates can be provided entirely by the water in human milk.

Lipids or fats are required for many of the essential functions in growth and development. They provide a well-tolerated energy source, as well as cholesterol and essential fatty acids. Breast milk contains the fat-digesting enzyme lipase, which allows maximum intestinal absorption of fatty acids. Fats contribute approximately 50 percent of the baby's calories.

Fats are the most variable part of human milk. The concentration increases during nursing (meaning that there is more fat in the breast milk at the end of feeding than at the beginning), but it can change depending on the mother's diet. The type of fat a mother eats will cause an increase in that type of fat in her milk. For example, a diet high in polyunsaturated fats will cause an increased percentage of polyunsaturated fats in the milk, without changing the total fat content.

There is increasing interest in breast milk fats due to long-range studies of breastfed infants that show more advanced development at 1 year, 8 to 10 years, and 18 years compared with formula-fed infants. There is also increasing interest in supplementing infant and baby formulas with missing ingredients such as the essential fatty acid docosahexaenoic acid, or DHA, which is found naturally in breast milk. And there is recent interest in supplementing mothers' diets during pregnancy and lactation, because dietary DHA levels have declined in the last half-century as women have avoided animal products (fish, eggs, and animal organs). Studies have shown that full-term, breastfed infants have greater concentrations of DHA in their brains compared with formula-fed infants. Essential fatty acids are essential to life, as they are involved with normal biochemical and functional development.

> ## Vital Fact
>
> The iron absorbed from human milk is 49 percent of the iron available. Only 10 percent of cow's milk iron and 4 percent of iron from formulas is absorbed. In addition, breastfed infants have higher iron storage levels.

Cholesterol, which most people think of only as a harmful substance associated with heart disease, is in fact a nutrient required for life. Cholesterol is essential for all membrane health. Breastfed infants have higher plasma cholesterol levels than formula-fed infants, and some animal studies suggest that an infant diet high in cholesterol (such as in human milk) may actually protect against high cholesterol problems later. Presently, though, commercial formulas contain little or no cholesterol compared with human milk.

Proteins are made up of amino acids, which are found in breast milk. (Taurine, for example, is an important amino acid for brain and eye development.) Important proteins in breast milk include immune-enhancing immunoglobulins; lactoferrin, which protects against gastrointestinal infections; whey; and human casein, which is vastly different from the cow casein in cow's milk. Cow casein, it's worth noting, is the protein mostly commonly associated with cow's milk allergies.

Carbohydrate is also present in breast milk—particularly lactose, which is also referred to as milk sugar. This component is especially important for newborn growth. It has been shown to enhance calcium absorption and is thought to be critical to the prevention of rickets (bone deformity). Lactose is also a component of galactose,

Vital Fact

Additional factors that influence iron absorption include higher amounts of vitamin C and lactose. Lactose is in higher concentration in breast milk than in commercial formulas. In fact, commercial formulas may not even include lactose.

which is needed for the production of other sugars that are essential to central nervous system development.

A number of carbohydrates in breast milk have bifidus factor activity, which helps to establish the important gut bacteria *Lactobacillus bifidus.*

Fluorine is a somewhat controversial component of breast milk. It's been held by some experts that fluorine levels in human milk are insufficient, requiring supplementation. Since fluorine has been accepted as a significant dietary factor in decreasing cavities, it is important that we look at the research surrounding this.

The amount of fluorine in human milk reflects to some degree the level in the water supply. The American Academy of Pediatrics Committee on Nutrition has stated, "It may not be necessary to give fluoride supplements to breastfed infants who are living in an area where water is fluoridated," which is often the case in most of the United States. The Academy also states that fluoride supplements should not be given to infants during the first 6 months after birth, whether they are breastfed or formula-fed, since excess fluoride intake can cause dental problems.

Iron is another controversial nutrient, and many new parents—as well as many of our patients—worry about whether their breastfed infants are getting enough iron from human milk. The fact is, they are. According to studies, an infant who is exclusively breastfed for the first 6 months is not at risk for iron deficiency anemia. Historically, breastfed infants have not been anemic (the exception is preterm infants; we'll discuss that under "Anemia" on page 153).

You should supplement iron to your baby only if he is iron-deficient. Giving iron to newborns inactivates lactoferrin by saturating it with iron. Lactoferrin is an iron-binding protein in human milk that does not allow the growth of certain bacteria in the gut. Experts think that it protects against certain gastrointestinal infections in breastfed infants.

Zinc is another mineral essential to human life. Zinc deficiency has been associated with failure to thrive and skin lesions. Zinc absorption from human milk is 41 percent, whereas cow's milk is 28 percent, standard infant formula is 31 percent, and soy formula is 14 percent.

While we cannot list every component of breast milk and its comparison with formula and cow's milk, it is important to point out more of the crucial substances found in human milk. These include but are not limited to vitamins A, C, D, E, and K; the B vitamins; enzymes; hormones; prostaglandins; growth factors; and iodide, copper, selenium, chromium, manganese, magnesium, calcium chloride, and potassium.

Human Milk and the Prevention of Allergies

The American Academy of Allergy, Asthma, and Immunology describes food allergy as an adverse reaction to food caused by one or more immune hypersensitivity mechanisms. Symptoms associated with food allergy include asthma, eczema, hives, and runny nose, as well as colic, failure to thrive, chronic respiratory disease, and chronic gastrointestinal disease. Research has shown that children whose parents both have allergies have a 47 percent chance of developing some allergic condition. If only one parent has allergies, then the child has a 29 percent chance of allergies. If neither parent has allergies, the child still has a 13 percent risk. Heredity obviously plays a role in the development of allergies. But can human milk prevent allergies?

According to many studies, the evidence shows that 6 months or longer of exclusive breastfeeding makes a difference in atopic (allergic) diseases. Human milk contains antibodies to major food proteins, which are helpful for the breastfeeding infant. These antibodies also provide protection against bacterial, viral, and toxic exposures.

One study of 500 babies born to families that were at high risk for

Vital Study

For a study published in the journal *Clinical Allergy*, 120 women who had previously had children with allergic conditions were told to avoid all milk, dairy products, eggs, fish, beef, and peanuts throughout pregnancy and lactation with a subsequent child. The control group had no restrictions. The mothers' avoidance of these foods was associated with less and milder eczema in their children, in particular for the children who were breastfed.

developing allergies clearly showed that breastfeeding for even a short period of time leads to a lower incidence of wheezing, prolonged colds, diarrhea, and vomiting. The babies in this study were divided into groups. No benefit was shown when soy milk was given instead of cow's milk. However, breastfeeding prevented allergic symptoms.

Prospective studies have determined that infants at high risk for atopic illness (determined by family history) had significantly less disease when breastfed, especially when solid foods were delayed.

What can a mom do during pregnancy and lactation to further prevent her infant from developing allergies? Researchers have concluded that avoiding common dietary allergens during pregnancy and lactation increases the protective beneficial effect of exclusive breastfeeding on the incidence of eczema in high-risk infants.

What about the long-term effects of breastfeeding? Once again, researchers have concluded that breastfeeding is protective against atopic eczema, food allergy, and respiratory asthma throughout childhood and adolescence.

If either parent in your family has a family history of atopic disease, the following guidelines must be followed to help prevent your child from developing allergies.

1. Reduce the number of highly allergenic foods that the mom eats during her last trimester of pregnancy. (See "Food Allergies and Food Sensitivities" on page 298 for common problem foods.)

2. Continue to avoid these foods during lactation.

3. Do *not* introduce solid foods until the baby is 6 months of age. If you are unable to breastfeed this long, a hypoallergenic commercial formula can be introduced.

What If You Are Not Breastfeeding?

If you have chosen not to breastfeed or can't for whatever reason, commercial formulas are available for your child that are healthful and that can provide adequate nutrition.

Some nonbreastfeeding moms make up their own formula devised by their midwives or natural health care practitioners. Since these can be time-consuming, we find that most mothers choose commercial formulas. We recommend starting out with a hypoallergenic formula, or with a dairy-free formula for infants who cannot tolerate dairy products. If you are breastfeeding part-time and giving formula part-time, we recommend that you use a low-iron formula. This is to avoid providing excessive iron that could bind with lactoferrin and interfere with its protective activity.

No matter what formula you are using, we recommend adding essential fatty acids to your child's bottle daily. Your natural health care practitioner or local health food store may provide quality sources of docosahexaenoic acid (DHA), an important fatty acid, in forms specifically for babies. DHA for babies usually comes in a liquid, which should be added to the formula-fed infant's diet when the baby is 4 to 6 weeks old. We also suggest adding a baby probiotic formula to your infant's bottle daily.

4. Breastfeed for at least the first 6 months of the child's life.

5. Avoid all environmental allergens as best as possible (animal dander, dust, pollen, cigarette smoke, and so on).

6. Talk to your natural health care provider about prescribing a constitutional homeopathic remedy for your child to take to strengthen her immune system.

7. Talk to your natural health care provider about adding essential fatty acids such as DHA to the breastfeeding mom's diet, which may reduce the risk of allergy development.

Should You Take Supplements while Breastfeeding?

Since exclusive breastfeeding is preferred for the first 4 to 6 months of life, what can we do to ensure quality breast milk? All over the world, women produce adequate and even abundant milk on very in-

Cow's Milk versus Mother's Milk

	Cow's Milk	Mother's Milk
Protein	80% casein, 20% whey;* no immuno-globulins (for the immune system)	40% casein, 60% whey; contains immunoglobulins
Fats	Higher in saturated fats; no significant amount of essential fatty acids	Rich in essential fatty acids
Carbohydrates	Hard for nonbreastfed babies to digest	Twice as much lactose for energy and growth; colostrum increases good bacteria, which help to digest lactose
Vitamins and minerals	Lower amounts of A, E, C, and B vitamins	Much higher amounts of A, E, C, and B vitamins
Good bacteria	None	Colostrum fuels the growth of good bacteria
Processing	Pasteurization and homogenization, which cause loss of enzymes and change protein structures†	None

*Whey is much easier to digest and less allergenic than casein.
†We do not recommend raw or nonpasteurized milk as a substitute.

adequate diets. Women in primitive cultures with modest diets produce milk without any problems to speak of. They do not complain of any fatigue or loss of well-being that some well-fed Western mothers experience.

It is important to add 500 calories daily to your diet when breastfeeding, unless you have a high metabolic rate (in which case, you should add more). The protein content and calcium content of the milk are independent of what the mother eats. Amino acids, certain fatty acids, and water-soluble vitamins can vary depending on a mom's diet. However, calcium, minerals, and fat-soluble vitamins need to be replaced. It is not necessary to take a vitamin when you are breastfeeding, but it does guard against deficiencies. It is necessary, though, to have a balanced diet. Since most women do not have a balanced diet, we recommend to all our breastfeeding moms that they take a multivitamin for the first 6 months of lactation (unless the baby gets fussy from the mom's multivitamin). We also recommend the following:

- Avoid diets and medications that promise rapid weight loss.
- Eat a whole grain diet, and avoid processed foods and cereals.
- Eat hormone- and chemical-free lean poultry, plenty of coldwater fish, and eggs. Add DHA as a supplement (for the mom) if you do not regularly eat fish and eggs.
- Protein is very important and should not be minimized during lactation.
- If you are unable to tolerate dairy products, make sure to take an additional 1,000 milligrams daily of calcium and 500 milligrams of magnesium.
- Eat as many vegetables as possible—especially those rich in vitamin A, such as carrots and spinach.
- Drink when you are thirsty. Filtered or spring water is the best choice.
- Keep in mind that caffeine passes into the breast milk. Two cups of coffee or tea daily will probably not hurt your baby.
- Avoid trans fatty acids, which are found in margarine and many fried foods. These also pass through the breast milk.
- Avoid artificial sweeteners.
- Keep in mind that dyes found in sodas may change the color of your milk. Reports of pink-orange milk have been traced to orange soda, and green milk has been traced to vitamins, seaweed, and Gatorade. Your baby's urine may also change color.
- Just as in pregnancy, what you eat goes to your baby, so pay attention to the quality of your foods. For example, one glass of orange juice is much better for you than an orange soda. If you must have carbonation, add some carbonated water to the juice.

Vital Fact

Developmental psychologists have found that infants with a strong attachment to the mother through breastfeeding are psychologically independent at 2 years old and have the most mastery of themselves at age 5. Breastfed children also have less anxiety entering school than bottlefed children.

Cow's Milk: Is It a Problem?

Cow's milk and formulas derived from cow's milk can be hard on babies. Nutrition-oriented doctors will tell you that cow's milk is the most common food sensitivity/allergy that they see in both children and adults. Our experience has shown the same. This is not to say that all children have problems with cow's milk. However, if your child suffers from or has a susceptibility to one or more of the following conditions, work with a nutrition-oriented doctor to go on a cow's milk–free diet to see whether the condition improves. In the case of infants, the breast-feeding mother typically goes off of milk products; bottlefed infants switch to a formula that is free of cow's milk protein.

Conditions linked to cow's milk sensitivity may include but are not limited to iron deficiency anemia, intestinal bleeding, sinusitis, ear infections, runny nose, constipation, arthritis, a weakened immune system, bronchitis, colic, eczema, allergic shiners (dark circles under the eyes), fatigue, mood swings, and attention problems.

Cow's milk alternatives include soy milk, rice milk, oat milk, and almond milk. These alternative milks are available calcium-enriched to ensure that your child gets enough of this valuable mineral.

When to Wean

Changing from one method of feeding to another is the process called weaning. As the mother starts to wean her child, the child becomes more dependent on other food sources, such as solid foods. This does not mean that solid food replaces breast milk; it supplements it. As soon as solid food is started, however, the process of eliminating the need for breast milk is the next step.

Weaning is a very complex time of adjustment for the mom and the baby. Boys tend to be weaned earlier than girls. This may be due to the fact that boys' energy intakes at all ages are greater and that the male rate of growth is faster than females'. Psychosocial pressures may also lead to the earlier weaning of the boy infant.

When is the proper time to start the weaning process? How long should a baby (or toddler) breastfeed? In primitive cultures, the age of weaning is between 2 and 5 years old. There are many formulations (based on birth weight, length of gestation, and so on) that researchers into breastfeeding have used to determine the proper age of weaning, but ages range from 2.3 years to 6 years. Interestingly, before the availability of baby food and artificial formulas, infants were traditionally breastfed for 3 to 4 years. Presently, most traditional societies do not wean until the baby is at least 1 to 2 years of age.

Vital Fact

In developing areas, breastfeeding continues for at least 1 to 2 years after the introduction of solid foods. The benefits for babies include protective effects on the digestive system and reduced risk and severity of infections.

No nutritional advantage results from introducing solid foods before the infant is 4 to 6 months old. It is important to begin iron-containing foods at 6 months because that is when the stores of iron from birth are starting to decrease. Protein becomes increasingly important toward the end of the first year, because the protein content of breast milk decreases as the infant grows heavier. The content of protein in breast milk begins to drop after 9 months of lactation. Developmentally, the infant is ready to learn to chew solids at about 6 months and can even start to learn to use a cup. (See "Introducing Food to Your Baby" on page 19.)

Many of our patients breastfeed their children until at least 1 year of age. More and more mothers are beginning to decrease the number of breastfeedings by the time their children are 1½ and have completely weaned their children by the age of 2. We prefer that moms breastfeed until the child is at least 1 year, double the amount of time that most conventional doctors typically recommend.

Part 2

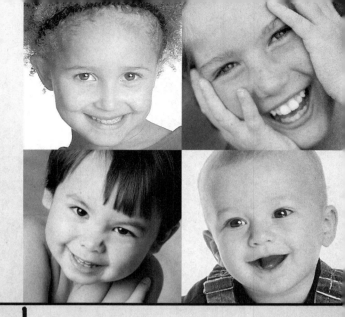

conditions from abscesses to warts

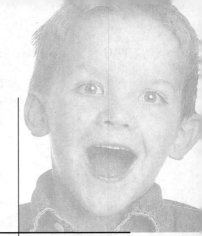

how to use
this section

In this section, you'll find 151 of the most common problems affecting children, and the natural therapies that treat them most effectively. In order to use these natural therapies properly, you'll need to have some basic information. This brief introduction tells you what you need to know. To learn more about the treatments discussed below, consult the relevant chapters in part 1.

A Note about Nutritional Supplements

For many of the conditions in part 2, we recommend nutritional supplements that fight illness and help restore vitality. Unless otherwise indicated, the dosages listed for these supplements are the maximum daily dosages your child should take.

For instance, if your child already takes a 250- to 500-milligram magnesium supplement daily as part of a program for optimal health, and she experiences growing pains, you still would not give her more than the maximum daily dosage (500 milligrams) listed in "Growing Pains" on page 316.

Dosages for Herbal Remedies

The following are acute and chronic dosages for herbal remedies.

Acute dosage: Use 1 drop of tincture for every 3 pounds of body weight, or 3 milligrams of the capsule extract for every pound of body weight. Give this dosage every 2 to 3 waking hours until the illness resolves.

Chronic dosage: Use 1 drop of tincture for every 3 pounds of body weight, or 3 milligrams of the capsule extract for every pound of body weight, but give this dosage only two times daily.

Choosing the Right Homeopathic Remedy

In many cases, there are several homeopathic remedies from which to choose for a particular condition. You should choose the one that best matches your child's symptoms. This does not mean that your child has to have all the symptoms listed. If you see a couple of symptoms listed that match up well, that's enough to pick the remedy—especially as you compare it with the other remedies listed. It is rare that a child will exhibit *all* of the symptoms listed under the description of a homeopathic remedy.

Aromatherapy Treatments and Dosages

There are three main methods of aromatherapy.

Baths: After running a warm bath, add the desired aromatherapy oil(s). Swish the water briskly around to disperse the essential oils. Have the child bathe for a minimum of 10 minutes. For children under the age of 12, use 2 or 3 drops of essential oil(s). For those over the age of 12, use 4 to 6 drops.

CAUTION: Never use essential oils in a bath with infants under 2 years of age. Their skin is too sensitive. Topical or inhalation methods should be used instead.

Topical application: Dilution is very important when using essential oils topically. More is not better when it comes to aromatherapy. The essential oil needs to be diluted in a carrier such as grape seed, olive, or sweet almond oil. *Never* use undiluted essential oils on your child's skin. The general rule of thumb is to use 1 drop of essential oil for each year of the child's age, up to a maximum of 12 drops in 20 millileters of carrier oil. For newborns to 6 months of age, use 1 drop of essential oil in 40 millileters of carrier oil. For infants 6 months to 1 year, use 1 drop of essential oil in 30 millileters of carrier oil.

Massage is one of the most soothing and effective ways to apply the essential oils.

To make a compress, add 3 drops of essential oil to 5 cups of warm or cool water. Dip in a facecloth or cotton cloth, wring it out so that it is not dripping, and lay it on the desired area for 5 to 10 minutes. Make sure to check the skin after the first 2 minutes to ensure that the child's skin is not irritated.

Inhalation: This common form of aromatherapy works well for most children. We describe it in detail whenever it is recommended. When using a vaporizer for inhalation, add one or two drops of essential oil to the vaporizer and let the fragrance fill the room.

CAUTION: Inhalation techniques should *not* be used with a child who has asthma.

A note about aromatherapy interactions: Do not give homeopathic remedies at the same time that you administer aromatherapy remedies. There's no harmful interaction, but the strong scents associated with aromatherapy can negate the effect of homeopathic remedies.

How to Find
Acupressure Points

When performing a recommended acupressure treatment on your child, you may find it helpful to consult diagrams of the acupressure points we discuss. You'll find acupressure diagrams on page 121. Also note that throughout part 2, when locations of acupressure points are measured in finger-widths, they are based on a child's finger-widths.

Abscesses and Boils

An abscess is an accumulation of pus that can occur anywhere, inside or outside of the body, including the skin, organs, and interior tissues. When an abscess forms around a hair follicle, it is known as a boil. Boils often surface on the buttocks, underarms, neck, and face. They begin as small, firm and tender nodules that become red and swollen. Within 2 to 4 days, a pustule usually forms in the center of the infected area. Some days later, the abscess will tend to rupture and drain the white- or yellow-colored pus.

If the abscess forms an elevated lump and the skin is red, painful, swollen, and warm but has no pustule, it's known as a carbuncle.

Abscesses can occur on anyone at any age. They are generally triggered as the result of an impaired immune system, trauma, improper drainage of tissues, bacterial invasion, or poor nutrition. Skin abscesses tend to develop in places where tight clothing rubs against the skin and around small puncture wounds or cuts. The infected area becomes tender, red, and swollen, and fever may be present. Delayed or improper treatment of the abscess can lead to a spreading of the infection.

Depending on the severity and location of the infection, antibiotics may be required. In some cases, the abscess may need to be drained by a doctor. Check with your doctor for any skin abscess that appears on the face, contains red streaks, or is filled with fluids. Consult your child's dentist or pediatrician for any mouth abscesses. If antibiotics are re-quired, ensure a quicker recovery by simultaneously using natural treatments. Never squeeze a boil or carbuncle: Not only is this extremely painful but it can also prolong and worsen the infection.

■ BASIC PLAN

Diet
Avoid sugar and dairy products as they can impair the immune system.

Keep the child well-hydrated with purified water, diluted fruit juice, herbal teas, and soups and broths.

Nutritional Supplement
Vitamin C—Supports the immune system and has mild anti-inflammatory effects. A supplement with bioflavonoids is preferable. Dosage: the child's age in years times 50 milligrams, twice daily. (For instance, a 7-year-old would get a 350-milligram dose twice daily.) Reduce the dosage if diarrhea occurs. Consider using a buffered vitamin C powder (nonacidic) or liquid vitamin C. Both work well for infants and children and can be mixed in juice.

Herbal Remedy
Echinacea and goldenseal combination—Stimulates the immune system and prevents/treats infection of the skin.

Homeopathy
Pick the following remedy that best matches your child's symptoms. Unless otherwise indi-

cated, give your child 2 pellets of a 30C potency three times daily. (For infants, crush the pellets into powder and mix it with water.) Improvements should be seen within 48 hours. If there is no improvement within 48 hours, try another remedy. After you first notice improvement, stop giving the remedy unless symptoms begin to return.

Note: Lower potencies (6X, 12X, 6C) may need to be given more often (three or four times daily).

Belladonna—Use in the first stage of an abscess with fever, when the infected area is hot, bright red, and swollen with throbbing pain. Pus usually has not developed at this stage.

Hepar sulphuris—Use for a painful infection that is tender to the touch or made worse by cold air or cold applications. The discharge is thick and smells bad.

Lachesis—The abscess has a black or bluish-purple appearance. This is more common on the left side of the face.

Mercurius solubilis or vivus—Use when pus has formed and the child looks ill and is feverish, has increased salivation, and has bad breath. The discharge may also have a foul smell.

Silica 6X or 30C—Use when pus formation is slow to discharge or heal. Applications of warmth may help relieve pain.

Aromatherapy

Tea tree oil—Apply in a topical dilution, morning and night. Prevents infection and helps to draw the pus out.

Hydrotherapy

Alternate a hot and cold cloth over the affected area to help reduce pain and expel pus if the abscess is on the skin. Do 30 seconds hot followed by 30 seconds cold, and so on.

■ ADVANCED PLAN

Nutritional Supplements

Vitamin A—Supports the immune system. Available in liquid drops. Daily dosage: infants under 1 year, 1,875 international units (IU); children 1 to 3, 2,000 IU; kids 4 to 6, 2,500 IU; kids 7 to 10, 3,500 IU; males 11 and older, 5,000 IU; females 11 and older, 4,000 IU.

Note: These dosages are for short-term use (up to 10 days). Do not give higher dosages without a doctor's supervision.

Zinc—Supports the immune system and enhances skin healing. Dosage: children 2 and younger, 5 milligrams; ages 2 and older, 10 to 15 milligrams. Give once a day. Use for up to 2 weeks and then stop.

Colloidal silver—For abscess of the mouth. Silver particles in suspension are available at any health food store. Mix 5 drops in an 8-ounce glass of water. Swish in the mouth, and spit out. Repeat twice a day for 5 days.

Herbal Remedies

Burdock root—An excellent skin detoxifier and immune system supporter. Give your child a dose twice daily until the abscess is gone.

Calendula—Dilute ½ teaspoon in 2 teaspoons of water. Apply to the lesion once it has drained to promote healing and prevent infection.

Aromatherapy

Sweet thyme—Add 1 drop to a hot compress and apply twice daily to the skin abscess. You can do this even when the abscess is sensitive to heat, but if it is too painful, use the other options presented here. This helps to draw the pus out.

Acupressure

Large Intestine 4—Located in the webbing between the thumb and the index finger. This point is used for infections and for detoxification. The child can use the thumb of his other hand to apply mild pressure to the acupressure point, holding for 10 to 15 seconds. Repeat three times and then do the same on the other hand. Do this daily.

■ WHAT TO EXPECT

Natural treatments should bring a discharge of the pus. You'll notice improvements within 2 to 3 days, though it may take up to 7 days for total resolution.

Acne

The most common skin ailment in the world is not limited to adolescents. Some newborns develop red pimples during their first month as they undergo hormonal changes. They may appear on the chest, back, forehead, cheeks, or nose. Don't worry: The red rash and pimples disappear in infants within a few weeks and usually require no intervention. However, if the acne spreads throughout the body or worsens over time, it can be a sign of underlying food sensitivities or allergies.

Teenage acne is a very common condition affecting both sexes as they enter puberty. Among teens, especially males and those with naturally oily skin, the skin turns red and whiteheads and blackheads appear on the face, neck, shoulders, and back. Some pimples may be painful and can cause scarring.

Often, acne is caused by a surplus supply of sebum, an oily substance produced by the sebaceous glands of the skin. During puberty, increased hormone production can contribute to an increased production of sebum, as well as keratin, a protective protein that covers the skin. The combination can lead to a buildup of sebum, which blocks and infects pores and creates blackheads and pustules.

Nutritional deficiencies and poor digestion can make kids susceptible to acne. But acne is rarely the result of poor hygiene. For severe cases of acne, consult with a dermatologist.

Note: Don't pop pimples because they may scar. Also, don't let your child use greasy creams or cosmetics, which only further clog pores.

■ BASIC PLAN

Diet

For babies—Acne is normal for infants, but if it continues after the first month, it may be the result of foods that the breastfeeding mother is consuming. Try eliminating dairy and sugar products from the mother's diet for 2 weeks to see if the condition improves.

For older children and teenagers—Reduce intake of dairy, sugar, soft drinks, and fried foods. Avoid animal fats, hydrogenated fats such as margarine, and fried foods. Increase the intake of fresh fruits, vegetables, and whole grains. Grind 1 teaspoon of flaxseeds per 50 pounds of body weight (children weighing 30 to 50 pounds may also use 1 teaspoon). Give this amount daily for the essential fatty acids and fiber, along with 8 ounces of water.

Nutritional Supplements

The following dosages are for teenagers.

Zinc—Acts as a skin healer. Give 30 milligrams once a day. This should be balanced with 2 to 3 milligrams of copper. (Zinc/copper supplements are common; copper is also found in multivitamins.)

Flaxseed oil—Supplies essential fatty acids. If you don't add ground flaxseeds to your teenager's diet, this is the next best way to ensure that he gets this valuable oil. Give 1 tablespoon per day. Reduce the dosage if diarrhea occurs.

Herbal Remedies

A combination of the following herbs works well for teenage acne. It can take up to 2 months before improvement is seen.

Burdock root—20 drops extract or 1 capsule twice daily.

Oregon grape root—20 drops extract or 1 capsule twice daily.

Vitex—20 drops extract or 1 capsule twice daily.

Homeopathy

Pick the following remedy that best matches your child's symptoms. Unless otherwise indicated, give your child 2 pellets of a 30C potency twice daily. Improvements should be seen within 3 to 4 weeks. If there is no improvement within 4 weeks, try another remedy. After you first notice improvement, except where noted, stop giving the remedy unless symptoms begin to return.

Note: Lower potencies (6X, 12X, 6C) may need to be given more often (three times daily).

Calcarea sulphurica 6X—For chronic acne where there is a yellow discharge. Give 2 pellets three times daily for 1 month and continue if benefit is noted.

Hepar sulphuris 6X—For painful acne that is tender to the touch, with a yellow discharge. Give 2 pellets three times daily for 1 month and continue if benefit is noted.

Silica 6X—For pus formations and pimples that are slow to discharge or heal, with white pustular discharge. Give 2 pellets twice daily for 1 month and continue if benefit is noted.

Pulsatilla—For acne that begins during puberty for girls; acne breakout before or with the menstrual cycle. The girl tends to be shy and has low thirst.

Sulphur—For red blemishes and itchy pimples. The skin gets oily very easily.

Chronic acne and skin blemishes. The child is very warm and sweats easily, and has a high thirst for cold drinks.

■ ADVANCED PLAN

Nutritional Supplements

The following daily dosages are for teenagers.

Vitamin A—Males, 5,000 international units (IU); females, 4,000 IU. Higher dosages can be effective but should be under the supervision of a physician.

Vitamin E—100 IU per 50 pounds of body weight.

Chromium—200 to 400 micrograms. Also helps to decrease sweet cravings.

Vitamin C—Age in years times 50 milligrams.

Selenium—1 microgram per pound of body weight.

Probiotic—If antibiotics have been used for acne, then supplement with an acidophilus and bifidus formula for at least 2 months to help maintain the good bacteria in the digestive system that antibiotics might destroy. Give as directed on the container.

Aromatherapy

Tea tree oil acne formulas—Available as cream and facial washes. Use them for teenage acne; they act as a natural antiseptic to the skin. Follow the directions on the container.

Acupressure

Gently press the acupressure point with a thumb for 10 to 15 seconds. Do this for each of the points below. Perform on both sides of the body and repeat once each day.

Liver 3—Located on top of the foot, in the hollow between the big toe and second toe.

Large Intestine 4—Located in the webbing between the thumb and index finger.

■ WHAT TO EXPECT

Infant acne clears up on its own. Teenage acne requires long-term treatment. Many cases of teenage acne take up to 2 to 3 months before noticeable results are seen.

AIDS

Acquired immune deficiency syndrome (AIDS) results in the crippling of the immune system due to the human immunodeficiency virus (HIV). Once HIV infiltrates the body, it suppresses the action of white blood cells, known as T cells, which normally fight off infection. The HIV virus uses the genetic material of the T cells to reproduce itself, and as these cells die off, new HIV particles enter the bloodstream to infect more white blood cells.

For some individuals, the body's immune system weakens and can't stop opportunistic illnesses such as skin, blood, and fungal infections; some cancers; pneumonia; and various other infections from overpowering the body.

AIDS is not a disease but rather a syndrome, with varying signs and symptoms appearing within different people. The final stage of HIV infection occurs when the body's T cell count plunges to a level incapable of fighting off infections.

HIV is found in four body fluids: blood, breast milk, vaginal fluid, and semen. It can be transmitted to another person only if any or all of these infected fluids get into the body.

The modes of transmission of HIV are:

- Blood infusions (although blood products are now screened for HIV)
- From an infected mother to her infant during pregnancy or possibly breastfeeding
- From an infected hypodermic needle
- From unprotected sexual intercourse

Babies and small children will not get AIDS by sharing toys, drinking glasses, toothbrushes, or utensils with AIDS-infected siblings or day care center children. The virus is not transmitted through the air. The chances of a child contracting AIDS after being bitten by an AIDS-infected baby or child is very remote and highly unlikely.

However, the chances of a baby developing AIDS from her AIDS-infected pregnant mother ranges between 30 and 50 percent. Among babies born to HIV-infected mothers, between 10 and 15 percent contract HIV, according to the U.S. Centers for Disease Control and Prevention. Although there are more and more therapies developed to help treat HIV and AIDS, it remains incurable.

Conventional therapy is to use antiviral medications to help manage the HIV virus and to treat secondary infections aggressively. Natural approaches should be used as complementary treatment for children with HIV/AIDS. The immune system requires nutritional support to prevent secondary infections. It is the secondary infections (opportunistic infections) that are a serious threat to a person whose immune system is suppressed from the HIV virus.

■ BASIC PLAN

Diet

A whole-foods diet is recommended. (See "Diet" on page 4 for more information.) Avoid sugars due to their suppressive effect on the immune system. Fresh vegetable juice is excellent but should be taken with meals to avoid detrimental effects on blood sugar and immune cell activity. Extra protein (fish, soy, lean poultry, nuts, seeds) is recommended. Forty ounces of purified water a day is also recommended, along with organic foods. Ground flaxseeds are good for the immune system and help with elimination. Grind 1 teaspoon per 50 pounds of body weight (children weighing 30 to 50 pounds may also use 1 teaspoon) and give daily with 8 ounces of water.

Nutritional Supplements

Research is showing antioxidants to be very important with AIDS. In addition to a children's multivitamin, extra supplementation of the following vitamins and minerals with the help of a nutrition-oriented doctor are advised:

- Alpha lipoic acid
- Carotenoids
- Selenium
- Zinc
- Vitamin A
- Vitamin B$_{12}$
- Vitamin C
- Vitamin E

Whey protein powder—Increases the blood levels of the potent antioxidant glutathione and contains L-glutamine, which supports the health of the immune system. Children should take 5 to 20 grams daily or as directed by their health care professional.

Herbal Remedies

There have been no definitive studies on the efficacy of herbal medicines for persons with HIV. However, the following three herbs are worth using under the guidance of a doctor trained in herbal medicine.

Astragalus and reishi extract—Both of these herbs improve immune system resistance to secondary infections and have antiviral effects.

Licorice root—Supports immune function and has antiviral effects.

Homeopathy

See a practitioner for a constitutional remedy.

■ ADVANCED PLAN

Nutritional Supplements

Whole-food supplement—Contains super green foods and other nutrient-dense foods. Choose a formula designed for children. Give as directed on the container, indefinitely.

Microbial-derived enzymes—Taken with meals to help with digestion and absorption of food and nutrients. Give 1 to 2 capsules with each meal, indefinitely.

Essential fatty acid complex—Find a children's blend that is a balance of omega-3 and omega-6 fatty acids for immune support. Give as directed on the container, indefinitely.

Thymus glandular extract—Supports the immune system. Give one to two 250-milligram capsules or tablets daily, indefinitely.

Constitutional Hydrotherapy

Supports the immune system. Use it daily. (See Hydrotherapy for Children on page 115 for more information.)

■ WHAT TO EXPECT

Natural approaches as outlined in this chapter are highly recommended as a complementary treatment to support immune system function and lessen your child's susceptibility to secondary infections. Work to incorporate them with a natural health care practitioner or your child's doctor.

Allergies

An allergy, the most common disorder of the immune system, is a hypersensitive reaction to a normally harmless substance called an allergen. About one in every six children has one or more allergies.

Common allergens include pollens from

grasses and trees, plant oils, insect venom, molds, feathers, house dust, wool, and animal dander. The immune system reacts to these external environmental allergens and causes the release of inflammatory chemicals called histamines and other cell-derived chemicals. In their zealous pursuit to fight what they perceive as uninvited invaders, these chemicals set off a chain reaction inside the body. The tissues lining the nose or eyes swell, breathing becomes constrictive, mucus production increases and the skin becomes itchy.

The eyes, respiratory system, skin, and intestinal tract are among the body systems most vulnerable to allergic responses. Common symptoms of environmental allergies include watery and red eyes, stuffy or runny nose, itchy skin, fatigue, headaches, and sneezing. Allergic reactions may also include dry scaly rashes, blisters, hives, and itchy, swollen patches on the skin. A child may exhibit "allergic shiners"— dark, puffy circles under his eyes. Allergic shiners may also be the result of food allergies or kidney problems. See a naturopathic physician or health care practitioner for a proper diagnosis.

The condition can be chronic or seasonal, depending on the type of allergens causing the reaction. Two examples of chronic allergens are dust and animal dander. Seasonal allergies occur only during specific times of the year when pollen is released. During the spring, some children are vulnerable to hay fever due to pollens from grasses and trees. In the late summer and fall, they may be sensitive to ragweed pollen and molds.

Environmental allergens can lead to behavioral problems (such as bedwetting, irritability, depression, or attention deficit disorder) or chronic conditions (such as asthma, acne, ear infections, and sinusitis). The chance of a child developing allergies increases when there is a family history of allergies.

Sometimes, it can be difficult to pinpoint the cause of a child's allergy. A physician or natural health care practitioner can conduct tests to determine whether the child's allergy symptoms are the result of food allergies or environmental allergens. We rate electrodermal allergy testing or muscle testing over conventional blood or skin scratch allergy testing in identifying allergen sensitivities.

Conventional treatment involves identification and avoidance of the suspected allergens. Antihistamine medications are used to block the allergy response. Allergy desensitization shots are sometimes recommended for older children. We feel that in most cases, the following natural therapies are the best long-term approach for allergies.

■ BASIC PLAN

Diet

Identifying and eliminating a child's food sensitivities can take a burden off the immune system so that it can deal with environmental allergens more effectively. (See "Food Allergies and Food Sensitivities" on page 298 for more information.)

Increase the child's intake of fruits, vegetables, and fish such as salmon, halibut, mackerel, and trout for their omega-3 fatty acid content that has natural anti-inflammatory effects. Provide five to seven daily servings of fruits and vegetables, and three or four weekly servings of fish.

Also, make sure that your child is getting adequate water intake to prevent dehydration.

Nutritional Supplement

Vitamin C—Helps support the immune system and has mild anti-inflammatory effects. Choose a supplement that has bioflavonoids. Dosage: age in years times 50 milligrams, twice daily. Reduce the dosage if diarrhea occurs. Consider using a buffered vitamin C powder (nonacidic) or liquid vitamin C. Both work well for infants and children and can be mixed in juice.

Herbal Remedy

Nettle—Helpful for some children with environmental allergies by acting as natural antihistamine. Freeze-dried nettle capsules are useful, as is the tincture form. Dosage: children under age 10, 150 milligrams; 10 and older, 300 milligrams. Give as long as needed for relief of allergies.

Homeopathy

Pollen desensitization formula—Contains common pollens in a homeopathic mixture. Taking these formulas can desensitize the immune system to the offending pollens. Give as directed on the container. Start using at the beginning of the pollen season. Desensitiza-

tion formulas for dust, mold, cat hair, and more are also available.

Combination hay fever formula—If your child suffers from hay fever, a combination of the most common remedies for hay fever can be helpful. Give as directed on the container for 1 week; if improvement is noted, continue as needed for relief of symptoms.

Acupressure

Large Intestine 4—Relieves head congestion. Located in the webbing between the thumb and index finger. Press the acupressure point gently with a thumb for 10 to 15 seconds. Perform on both sides of the body and repeat two times each day.

Large Intestine 20—Reduces sneezing and nasal symptoms. Located on the lower, outer corner of each nostril. Press the acupressure point gently with a thumb for 10 to 15 seconds. Perform on both sides of the body and repeat two times each day.

■ ADVANCED PLAN

Nutritional Supplements

Quercitin—The daily dosage is 3 milligrams per pound of body weight.

Grape seed extract or pycnogenol—Give 1 milligram per pound of body weight daily.

Flaxseed oil—Daily dosages: children 2 and under, 1 teaspoon; kids 3 to 6, 2 teaspoons; kids 7 and older, 2 to 3 teaspoons. Cut back if loose stools occur.

Herbal Remedies

Astragalus—This Chinese herb helps to balance the immune system to react less against allergies.

Licorice root—Has anti-allergy effects; reduces inflammation of the sinus and respiratory tract.

Eyebright—For irritated eyes. Reduces inflammation, itching, and redness of the eyes. Also alleviates morning crust formation around the eyelids. Taken internally (capsule or tincture) or applied as drops to the eyes (put 5 drops in ½ ounce of saline solution, and put 2 drops of this solution in the eyes three times daily).

Homeopathy for Hay Fever

Pick the following remedy that best matches your child's hay fever symptoms. Unless otherwise indicated, give your child 2 pellets of a 30C potency twice daily. Improvements should be seen within 3 to 4 days. If there is no improvement within 4 days, try another remedy. After you first notice improvement, stop giving the remedy unless symptoms begin to return.

Note: Lower potencies (6X, 12X, 6C) may need to be given more often (three times daily).

Allium cepa—For watery eyes with burning nasal discharge. The child's nose runs "like a faucet." Sneezing is another symptom. Symptoms get better in the open air.

Ambrosia—For children who react to ragweed pollen. The child's head and nose are stuffed up. Works well taken preventatively for a month prior to and during hay fever season.

Arsenicum album—For burning eyes and runny nose that doesn't stop, causing the skin under the nose to get red and excoriated. The child is chilly and restless.

Euphrasia—For burning, tearing eyes that are bloodshot with a bland nasal discharge.

Sabadilla—For tremendous sneezing and runny nose. The child feels better in a warm room.

Wyethia—For intense itching on the roof of the mouth or behind the nose.

Constitutional remedy—See a homeopathic practitioner.

Aromatherapy

Melissa (lemon balm) and German chamomile—Add 1 drop of each to a vaporizer and have it in the room while your child sleeps. Both have an antihistamine effect. Do not use if your child is taking a homeopathic remedy, as the aromatherapy scents may neutralize the effects of the homeopathic agents.

■ WHAT TO EXPECT

Homeopathic treatment usually provides some relief within 3 to 5 days. Chronic allergies can take longer to clear up, but most children will notice improvement over the course of 2 to 4 weeks.

Anal Itching

This condition is characterized by persistent, annoying itchiness surrounding the anal area.

There may also be some redness and inflammation. Often, it is linked to other diseases of the gastrointestinal tract, local skin conditions, and food sensitivities.

This condition can be slow to heal and can require constant attention because of the wet, warm environment of the anal area. Repeated contact with waste further aggravates the situation.

Anal itching can be caused by many factors, among them:

- Pinworms, scabies, and other parasites
- Skin problems such as psoriasis or atopic dermatitis
- Allergic reaction to detergents and soaps, ointments, and medications
- Bacterial or fungal infection in the bowels
- Hemorrhoids
- Constipation
- Anal fissures
- Poor hygiene, resulting in leaving residual feces
- Wearing synthetic underwear or too-tight leggings or tights
- Failing to completely dry off after bathing
- Psychological response to anxiety

Conventional treatment depends on the cause of the itching. Generally, topical ointments are prescribed. Use a hypoallergenic soap when washing your child. Make sure to use a nonperfume, hypoallergenic detergent for sensitive skin. For babies, use unscented diapers. Your doctor can do lab tests for pinworms or other infections that may be causing your child's itching.

■ BASIC PLAN

Diet
Food sensitivities are often an underlying problem with anal itching. Acidic foods such as tomatoes and citrus fruits can be irritating to the rectal tissue. (See "Food Allergies and Food Sensitivities" on page 298 for more information.)

Nutritional Supplements
Zinc—Supports the immune system and enhances skin healing. Dosage: children 2 and younger, 5 milligrams daily; 2 and older, 10 to 15 milligrams daily. Use for 2 weeks and then stop.

Flaxseed oil—If dry skin is present, have the child take this daily, at the following dosages: children 2 and under, 1 teaspoon; kids 3 to 6, 2 teaspoons; kids 7 and older, 2 to 3 teaspoons. Reduce the dosage if diarrhea occurs.

Herbal Remedies
Calendula ointment—Soothing. Can be applied to the external area of the rectum. Apply twice daily.

Oatmeal bath—Add 1 cup of oatmeal powder such as Aveeno to your child's bath. It has a natural anti-itch effect on the skin. Pat the skin dry when your child gets out of the bath, to leave a film of oatmeal powder on the rectal area.

Homeopathy
Pick the following remedy that best matches your child's symptoms. Unless otherwise indi-

cated, give your child 2 pellets of a 30C potency twice daily. (For infants, crush the pellets into powder and mix it with water.) Improvements should be seen within 3 days. If there is no improvement within 3 days, try another remedy. After you first notice improvement, stop giving the remedy unless symptoms begin to return.

Note: Lower potencies (6X, 12X, 6C) may need to be given more often (three times daily).

Sulphur—For red, burning rectum, along with itchiness. The child often has diarrhea upon awakening in the morning.

Cina—For itchy rectum associated with pinworms. The child is irritable and constantly picking at her rectum and nose.

■ WHAT TO EXPECT

If the cause of the rectal itch is identified and treated, you'll notice improvement in a few days.

Anemia

This condition refers to a deficiency of red blood cells or hemoglobin, a pigment in red blood cells that carries oxygen throughout the body. Iron deficiency is one of the most common nutritional deficiencies worldwide and one of the most common causes of anemia. Other causes include nutritional deficiencies such as folate or vitamin B_{12} deficiency, hereditary defects in red blood cell production (for instance, thalassemia major and sickle cell disease), recent or current infection, lead poisoning, and chronic inflammation. A deficiency of hemoglobin leads to a decreased ability to transport oxygen to cells so that they can function and grow properly.

In infants up to 1 year and preschool children ages 1 to 5 years, iron deficiency anemia may result in developmental delays and behavioral disturbances such as decreased motor activity, social interaction, and attention to tasks. These developmental delays may persist past school age (that is, past 5 years of age) if the iron deficiency is not fully reversed.

Symptoms of anemia include paleness of the skin, lips, eyelid linings, and nail beds. Fatigue, sleep problems, chronic colds, inattentiveness, and irritability are also common. Children with anemia can exhibit signs of a condition known as pica, where they crave non-nutrient substances such as ice, clay, dirt, and cornstarch. Prolonged, untreated anemia can interfere with normal growth. A rapid rate of growth combined with inadequate intake of dietary iron places children under 2, particularly those 9 to 18 months old, at the highest risk of any age group for iron deficiency. The iron stores of full-term infants can meet an infant's iron requirements until 4 to 6 months of age, and iron deficiency anemia generally does not occur until approximately 9 months of age. However, compared with full-term infants of normal or high birth weight, preterm and low birth weight infants are born with lower iron stores and grow faster during infancy. Consequently, their iron stores are often depleted by ages 2 to 3 months and they are at greater risk for iron deficiency than are full-term infants of normal or high birth weight.

Anemia occurs when one or more of the following happens:

- Production of red blood cells is too low
- More red blood cells are destroyed than created
- There is low hemoglobin within red blood cells.

The two most common underlying causes of anemia in children are lack of iron in the diet (iron is needed for the production of hemoglobin) and ingesting cow's milk or products (such as formula) containing cow's milk too early. Cow's milk can cause irritation and bleeding of the intestinal wall, leading to blood loss. Immune system reactions to the milk protein casein can also lead to red blood cell destruction.

Introducing whole cow's milk before 1 year of age and consuming more than 24 ounces of whole cow's milk daily after the first year of life present risk factors for iron deficiency because this milk has little iron, may replace foods with higher iron content, and may cause occult gastrointestinal bleeding.

Because goat's milk and cow's milk have similar compositions, infants who are fed goat's milk are likely to have the same risk for developing iron deficiency as do infants who are fed cow's milk. Of all milks and formulas, breast milk has the highest percentage of bioavailable iron, and breast milk and iron-fortified formulas provide sufficient iron to meet an infant's needs. Iron-fortified formulas are readily available, do not cost much more than non-iron-fortified formulas, and have few proven side effects except for darker stools. Controlled trials and observational studies have indicated that iron-fortified formula causes no more gastrointestinal distress than does non-iron-fortified formula, and there is little medical indication for non-iron-fortified formula.

Note that even though breastfeeding provides the best form of food for an infant, it is still possible for anemia to occur.

Anemia is diagnosed through blood tests (also called a screening) by your child's doctor. We also recommend a ferritin measurement since it measures the storage levels of iron. This will tell whether the anemia has been occurring for a long time.

The U.S. Centers for Disease Control and Prevention make the following assessment and screening recommendations to fight anemia in children.

- In populations of infants and preschool children at high risk for iron deficiency anemia, the Centers suggest screening all children for anemia between ages 9 and 12 months; screening again 6 months later; and then screening annually from ages 2 to 5 years. High-risk groups include children from low-income families; children eligible

Food Sources of Iron

If you're trying to increase your child's intake of iron, consult this chart for ideas on how to get started. Unless otherwise noted, milligrams of iron listed are per 100-gram (3½ ounce) serving.

Food	Iron (mg)*
Kelp	100
Brewer's yeast	17.3†
Blackstrap molasses	16.1†
Wheat bran	14.9
Organic beef liver	8.8
Sunflower seeds	7.1
Millet	6.8
Parsley	6.2
Spirulina	5
Almonds	4.7
Beef	3.5
Lamb	3.5
Raisins	3.5
Light-meat turkey	1.6
Light-meat chicken	1
Egg, whole	0.72

*Serving size for spirulina is 1 tsp; for beef (non-liver), lamb, turkey, and chicken, 4 oz; for eggs, 1 whole egg.
†1 teaspoon twice daily is an average children's dosage.

- In populations of infants and preschool children not at high risk for iron deficiency anemia, screen only those children who have known risk factors for the condition. The next three bulleted items explain which children should be screened.
- Consider anemia screening before age 6 months for preterm infants and low birth weight infants who are not fed iron-fortified infant formula.
- At ages 9 to 12 months, and 6 months later (at ages 15 to 18 months), assess all non-high-risk infants and young children for risk factors for anemia. Screen the following children:

  Preterm or low birth weight infants

  Infants fed a diet of non-iron-fortified infant formula for more than 2 months

  Infants introduced to cow's milk before age 12 months

  Breastfed infants who do not consume a diet adequate in iron after age 6 months (that is, who receive insufficient iron from supplementary foods)

  Children who consume more than 24 ounces of cow's milk daily

  Children who have special health care needs (for instance, children who use medications that interfere with iron absorption, and children who have chronic infection, inflammatory disorders, restricted diets, or extensive blood loss from a wound, an accident, or surgery).

- Annually assess all non-high-risk children ages 2 to 5 years for risk factors for iron deficiency anemia. (Risk factors include a

for the Special Supplemental Nutrition Program for Women, Infants, and Children, or WIC; migrant children; and recently arrived refugee children.

low-iron diet, limited access to food because of poverty or neglect, and special health care needs.) Screen these children if they have any of these risk factors.

Conventional treatment of anemia focuses on iron-containing foods and iron supplementation.

■ BASIC PLAN

Diet

The Centers for Disease Control and Prevention have specific recommendations for the prevention of iron deficiency anemia. We agree with most of them:

- They encourage exclusive breastfeeding of infants (without supplementary liquid, formula, or food) for 4 to 6 months after birth.
- When exclusive breastfeeding is stopped, they encourage use of an additional source of iron (approximately 1 milligram per kilogram of body weight daily of iron), preferably from supplementary foods.
- For infants under 12 months who are not breastfed or who are partially breastfed, they recommend only iron-fortified infant formula as a substitute for breast milk. We do not entirely agree with this statement. If your child is partially breastfed, we recommend using a low-iron formula as a supplement. (See The Importance of Breastfeeding on page 123 for more information.)
- For breastfed infants who receive insufficient iron from supplementary foods by the age of 6 months (less than 1 milligram per kilogram daily), they suggest 1 milligram per kilogram of body weight daily of iron drops. We agree with using supplemental iron for infants only if the child has been tested for iron anemia and is deficient based on lab reports.
- For breastfed infants who were preterm or had a low birth weight, they recommend 2 to 4 milligrams per kilogram of body weight daily of iron drops (to a maximum of 15 milligrams per day) starting at 1 month after birth and continuing until 12 months after birth. We strongly recommend testing these infants for iron anemia periodically throughout their first year of life and only supplementing with iron if deficient based on lab results.
- They encourage the use of only breast milk or iron-fortified infant formula for any milk-based part of the diet (such as in infant cereal) and discourage the use of low-iron milks (such as cow's milk, goat's milk, and soy milk) until age 12 months.
- They suggest that children ages 1 to 5 years consume no more than 24 ounces of cow's milk, goat's milk, or soy milk each day.
- At ages 7 to 9 months, we recommend that infants be introduced to plain, iron-fortified infant cereal. Two or more servings per day of iron-fortified infant cereal can meet an infant's requirement for iron at this age.
- By about age 6 months, the Centers encourage one feeding per day of foods rich in vitamin C (such as fruits, vegetables, or

juice) to improve iron absorption, preferably with meals.

- They suggest introducing plain, pureed meats after age 6 months or when the infant is developmentally ready to consume such food.

For ideas on how to increase your child's iron intake from food, see "Food Sources of Iron" on page 155. It lists a number of animal and vegetable foods and their iron content. Eggs and beef are good animal sources of iron. They contain heme iron, which has a two to three times higher absorption rate than nonheme iron found in plant foods. Feed these three times weekly or more.

If your baby is on formula, switch to a nondairy formula that is iron-fortified.

For children, avoid giving cow's milk. Parents should provide alternatives such as rice, almond, and oat milk. Look for products that are calcium-enriched. Soy milk can be given to children over 1 year old, but for kids ages 1 to 5, give no more than 24 ounces of soy milk per day.

Nutritional Supplements

Iron supplements—Give as directed by your physician. A typical dosage is 3 to 6 milligrams per 2 pounds of the child's body weight daily for at least 1 month, following with half the dosage for 2 months. Never exceed a recommended dosage, since excess iron can be poisonous. Blood work should be rechecked 2 weeks after starting an iron supplement program.

Case History

Our own son, Mark, was about a year old when we noticed that he was paler than normal. He was being breastfed while gradually being introduced to solid foods. We had his blood tested and discovered that he was iron-deficient anemic. As naturopathic doctors specializing in nutrition, we thought that Angela's healthy diet and breastfeeding would keep Mark from being anemic. However, our son was born prematurely, which made him much more susceptible to anemia. We increased iron-rich foods in his diet and got him on a good liquid multivitamin and liquid iron (iron citrate with some B vitamins). We also gave him homeopathic Ferrum phosphoricum 6X and Calcarea phosphorica 6X so that his cells would incorporate the iron more efficiently. Incredibly, only 2 weeks later, a new blood test revealed that his red blood cell levels were back to normal. His pediatrician was impressed with his recovery.

Avoid iron sulfate (ferrous sulfate), which can be constipating and irritating to the digestive tract. Focus on iron bound to citrate, chelate, succinate, or glycinate. Iron drops can be put in juice containing vitamin C (such as orange juice) to enhance absorption. Avoid giving calcium, magnesium, and zinc at the same times as iron, since they can interfere with its absorption.

Vitamin C—Enhances the absorption of iron. Give 50 milligrams with each dose of iron.

Homeopathy

Ferrum phosphoricum 3X or 6X—Builds red blood cells and improves iron absorption. Give the child 2 pellets two or three times daily until your physician says that the anemia is gone. (For infants, crush the pellets into powder and mix it with water.) This usually takes a few months.

■ ADVANCED PLAN

Nutritional Supplements

Children's multivitamin—Give as directed on the container. Children's multivitamins are good preventatives for vegetarians, who are more susceptible to iron and B_{12} deficiencies.

Algae supplements—Natural sources of B_{12}. Examples include chlorella and spirulina. These are best used under the guidance of a nutrition-oriented doctor; 500 to 1,500 milligrams is a general dosage range for kids 3 and older.

Chlorophyll—Contains precursors for the formation of hemoglobin. Give 1 teaspoon daily or as directed on the container.

Herbal Remedies

Yellow dock—Contains iron and enhances absorption of iron. Use twice daily.

Nettle—Contains many minerals to help build the blood. Use twice daily.

Homeopathy

Calcarea phosphorica 3X or 6X—Give 2 pellets two or three times daily to support new red blood cell formation. (For infants, crush the pellets into powder and mix it with water.) You should see improvement within 2 to 3 weeks. Continue giving the remedy until your doctor says that anemia is no longer present.

Acupressure

Stomach 36—Located four finger-widths below the kneecap and one finger-width toward the outside of the leg (outside of the shinbone, on the muscle). Helps build red blood cells. Gently press the acupressure point with a thumb for 10 to 15 seconds. Repeat three times and then do the same on the other leg. Repeat daily.

Other Recommendations

Fresh air and sunlight help to build red blood cells.

■ WHAT TO EXPECT

The natural protocol given in this section should correct the iron deficiency anemia. Physical and lab test improvements should be seen within 2 weeks of treatment. Continue treatment until your doctor tells you otherwise. More severe and chronic anemias can take months to correct.

Anger

Anger is one of the natural emotions of children. Children should express their anger, as suppression is not healthy. Anger is often expressed in temper tantrums. Sometimes, biochemical imbalances can trigger feelings of anger in a child. Most children learn how to manage their anger as they mature, providing that they are surrounded with good role models. Therapy is indicated when chronic anger interferes with the emotional health of a child and/or interferes with his life. Conventional therapy commonly involves counseling. Relaxing music as well as regular exercise is recommended to help calm an angry child.

■ BASIC PLAN

Diet

Blood sugar imbalances can lead to fits of anger. Make sure that your child is eating regular meals (every 3 to 3½ hours) and avoiding sugar products (see "Hypoglycemia" on page 340). Food sensitivities can also change a child's mood and lead to feelings of anger (see "Food Allergies and Food Sensitivities" on page 298).

Nutritional Supplements

Calcium and magnesium—Have a relaxing effect on the nervous system. We recommend 500 milligrams of calcium and 250 milligrams of magnesium. Available in liquid preparations.

Homeopathy

Homeopathy should be considered a complementary treatment for anger, and should not take the place of counseling.

Pick the following remedy that best matches your child's symptoms. Unless otherwise indicated, give your child 2 pellets of a 30C potency twice daily. Improvements should be seen within 7 days. If there is no improvement within 7 days, try another remedy. After you first notice improvement, stop giving the remedy unless symptoms begin to return.

Note: Lower potencies (6X, 12X, 6C) may need to be given more often (three times daily).

Chamomilla—Use if the child is very impatient and sensitive to everything, or if the child is capricious: you give her what she wants and she throws it away. She may scream and cry when she does not get things on demand. Carrying of or rocking the child provides temporary relief.

Colocynthis—Use if the child is irritable and impatient. He may be offended very easily and constantly complain. Anger brings on bouts of digestive troubles such as abdominal cramps or diarrhea.

Ignatia—Use if mood is very changeable. The child seems calm and then breaks out into a fit of anger. Also use for anger from emotional trauma and suppressed emotions. The child may sigh a lot.

Nux vomica—Use for a competitive child who gets angry if she does not get her way. The child is very uptight and often suffers from constipation or digestive problem.

Stramonium—Use for anger that turns into fits of rage. The child curses and may have delusions.

Staphysagria—For suppressed anger. The child holds in anger that manifests itself in physical symptoms. Sensitive children who keep their anger and pain to themselves. Common remedy for children who have been abused.

Impatiens Bach Flower Remedy—Specific for anger issues. Give 2 drops twice a day for 2 weeks, then assess the child. Stop when improvement is noted, and use again if symptoms return.

■ ADVANCED PLAN

Homeopathy
See a homeopathic practitioner for a constitutional homeopathic remedy.

Aromatherapy
Rose is a remedy for anger. Lavender is relaxing as well. Add 2 or 3 drops of one of these oils to a vaporizer and allow the fragrance to fill the room, or add 2 drops to a bath. (See Aromatherapy for Children on page 109 for more information.) If the child is taking a homeopathic remedy, then use aromatherapy at a different time, as it may neutralize the effect of the homeopathic remedy.

Acupressure
Four Gates—Helps to release tension and pain. This is a combination of Liver 3, located on top of the foot in the hollow between the big toe and second toe, and Large Intestine 4, located in the webbing between the thumb and index finger. Two people push on all four points (both sides of the body) gently at the same time. Push on these points with mild pressure for 15 seconds. Repeat three times. Do this once daily.

■ WHAT TO EXPECT
Counseling should be the focus for chronic anger issues. Homeopathic remedies help to restore emotional balance for children with anger issues. Nutritional therapy should have a beneficial impact within 2 to 4 weeks.

Anxiety

Anxiety is that feeling of uneasiness, worry, or distress that we all get at one time or another, when faced with an unfamiliar, threatening, or challenging situation. Children can be particularly vulnerable to persistent or extreme feelings of anxiety and have difficulty identifying and communicating their distressed feelings. About 1 million children are diagnosed with obsessive-compulsive disorder, an anxiety condition characterized by repeated urges and repeated but purposeless behaviors.

Symptoms associated with anxiety in children include sweaty hands, nail biting, trembling muscles, heart palpitations, diarrhea, trouble sleeping, headaches, and shortness of breath. Some may regress when they feel anxious. They may exhibit clingy behavior, excessive tantrums, thumb sucking, and other actions beyond what would be expected at their developmental age. In some but not all cases, anxiety can be debilitating. Left untreated, it can develop into a full-blown panic attack.

On the plus side, anxiety can be used as an effective coping tool to help one work through problems or recognize a possible threat or conflict.

All of us experience anxiety occasionally, but when this emotion begins to interfere with day-to-day functioning in your child, it has evolved into a serious condition and requires medical intervention. Over time, anxiety taxes the nervous system.

Stress, constant change, and emotional events such as coping with death, a serious illness, or divorce can cause anxiety. In rarer instances, the cause may be physiological, such as an overactive thyroid gland. Natural medicines are helpful to relieve feelings of emotional and physical tension while underlying psychological issues are being addressed.

Conventional treatment focuses on psychotherapy and drug treatment (antidepressants and tranquilizing medications, although their use with children is not well-studied).

■ BASIC PLAN

Diet

Make sure that your child is not consuming too many stimulating foods. Consumption of caffeinated beverages such as soft drinks should be minimized. Limit sugar and refined carbohydrate intake. Regular meals (every 3 to 4 hours) to maintain balanced blood sugar levels helps to prevent anxiety.

Foods containing magnesium and calcium are good as they help to relax the nervous system. (See Vitamins and Minerals for Children on page 79 for lists of food sources for these minerals.)

Fish such as salmon, mackerel, and halibut are good for their omega-3 fatty acids, which studies show help anxiety and depression. Eat fresh, coldwater fish three or four times weekly.

Nutritional Supplement

Calcium and magnesium—Give 500 milligrams of calcium and 250 to 500 milligrams of magnesium daily. Available in liquid form. Usually taken together in a formula.

Herbal Remedies

Passionflower—An excellent herb that helps to relax the nervous system in children.

Chamomile—Helps to relax the nerves and calms an upset tummy as well.

Homeopathy

Pick the following remedy that best matches your child's symptoms. Unless otherwise indicated, give your child 2 pellets of a 30C potency twice daily. Improvements should be seen within 48 hours. If there is no improvement within 48 hours, try another remedy. After you first notice improvement, stop giving the remedy unless symptoms begin to return.

Note: Lower potencies (6X, 12X, 6C) may

need to be given more often (three times daily).

Kali phosphoricum 6X—Can be used as a nerve tonic. Have the child take 2 pellets two or three times daily.

Magnesia phosphorica 6X or 12X—Helps to relax the nerves. Can be used along with Kali phosphoricum. Give 2 pellets two or three times daily.

Aconitum napellus 30C—For acute attacks of anxiety. The child feels like he is going to die. This often starts after some type of shock, emotional or physical. The child has anxiety being in crowds. Not generally used on a long-term basis.

Argentum nitricum—For anxiety and fear of tests and speaking in public. The child is very nervous and hurried. The anxiety causes diarrhea or other physical problems.

Arsenicum album—The child is very nervous and restless and is a perfectionist. She may have anxiety about her health and the cleanliness of her environment.

Gelsemium—For anxiety that occurs from anticipating something such as speaking in front of the class, or before taking an exam. The child trembles and has diarrhea and headaches from anxiety.

Ignatia—The child holds emotions in. His feelings are hurt easily. He is worried and anxious about what people think about him.

Phosphorus—The child worries about others. She has many fears and anxiety about being alone in the dark, illness, thunder, and certain animals. She wants comfort and reassurance.

Bach Flower Rescue Remedy—Give the child a few drops every 5 minutes for acute anxiety, or twice daily as a preventative. Discontinue use when the problem is gone or if the remedy does not seem to help.

Aromatherapy

Roman chamomile and lavender—Mix with carrier oil and massage on the neck, or add 1 drop of each to a vaporizer or the child's bedsheets (See Aromatherapy for Children on page 109 for details.) If giving a homeopathic remedy, use aromatherapy at a different time to avoid neutralizing the effect of the homeopathic remedy.

Acupressure

Four Gates—Helps to release tension and pain. This is a combination of Liver 3, located on top of the foot in the hollow between the big toe and second toe, and Large Intestine 4, located between the webbing of the thumb and index finger. Two people push on all four points gently at the same time, for 15 seconds. Repeat three times. Do once daily.

■ ADVANCED PLAN

Nutritional Supplements

Children's multivitamin—Contains a base of vitamins and minerals.

Essential fatty acid complex—Choose a children's blend that contains omega-3 and omega-6 fatty acids. The child should get at least 100 milligrams of docosahexaenoic acid (DHA) daily. Flaxseed oil is also good. Give as directed on the container. Common dosages are 1 teaspoon daily for children up to age 2, 2 teaspoons for kids 3 to 6, and 2 to 3 teaspoons for those 7 and older.

Herbal Remedies

Hops—Has a nerve-relaxing effect.

Valerian—A stronger choice for reducing anxiety. Works well in herbal nerve relaxing formulas.

Acupressure

Pericardium 6—Relieves anxiety and palpitations. Located 2½ finger-widths below the wrist crease, in the middle of the forearm (on the palm side). Gently press the acupressure point with a thumb for 10 to 15 seconds. Repeat three times and then do the same on the other hand. Repeat daily or during times of anxiety.

■ WHAT TO EXPECT

Anxiety levels should decrease within 1 to 2 weeks of treatment. A children's counselor should treat moderate to severe cases of anxiety simultaneously with the natural therapies.

Appetite Loss

Poor appetite alone is usually not cause for concern, since minor emotional or physical issues can temporarily influence appetite. But if your child also shows symptoms of bloating, upset stomach, nausea, pain, constipation, or rapid weight loss, consult with your physician to rule out serious diseases.

In addition to many physical ailments, your child's no-thanks to food may also be linked to emotional issues such as anxiety, depression, grief, or stress. Or the cause may be food itself. Your child may be snacking on sugar-filled treats and soft drinks or fruit juices between meals, or eating large quantities of deep-fried foods that are difficult to digest.

But if your child suddenly develops a voracious appetite, pay close attention to its duration. Accelerating appetites may be linked to overexertion, growth spurts, or serious medical conditions such as diabetes or malfunctioning thyroids.

In general, low appetite in children comes and goes. Changeable eating patterns are common, especially in toddlers.

■ BASIC PLAN

Diet

Have a snack or nibbling tray on hand with small, bite-size foods that your child can munch on. Make it nutritious, fun, and age-appropriate. (See "Diet" on page 4 for more information.) For toddlers and older children, try cut-up vegetables such as carrots and celery sticks, pieces of cheese on whole wheat crackers, whole grain cereals, and slices of fruit such as apples or pears. Serve snacks between meals and after playing. Do not give snacks right before meals, since even healthful snacks can spoil a child's appetite.

Give your child a glass of water with some

fresh lemon squeezed in it. It can help increase appetite before meals. Just keep it to one glass: Drinking large amounts before or during a meal will make your child feel full so he won't eat as much.

Nutritional Supplement

Zinc—A deficiency in this mineral can result in a lower appetite. The child should take zinc as part of a children's multivitamin; consider an extra 5 to 10 milligrams daily for a 2-month period. This should include 1 to 2 milligrams of copper, which may be part of a multivitamin.

Herbal Remedies

Gentian root combined with skullcap—Helps to stimulate appetite. Put 5 drops of each herb in a small cup of juice or water before each meal. Alternatively, 5 drops of ginger root tincture can be used the same way, or fresh ginger root can be sprinkled over food.

Other helpful herbs include fennel and peppermint, either separately or combined as a tea, tincture, or capsule. Give before mealtime.

Homeopathy

Bach Flower Rescue Remedy—For low appetite caused by stress. Give 2 drops twice daily. Stop if there are no improvements after 2 weeks or if the problem resolves.

Ignatia 30C—For loss of appetite from emotional stress. Give 2 pellets twice daily for 1 week, and if improvement is noted, then use as needed.

■ ADVANCED PLAN

Aromatherapy

Bergamot, chamomile (Roman or German), and ginger—Add 1 drop of each of these appetite-stimulating oils to a humidifier. Or boil water, add the oils to the water, and let the scents come out with the steam and fill the air. If giving a homeopathic remedy, then use aromatherapy at a different time.

Acupressure

Stomach 36—Four finger-widths below the kneecap and one finger-width toward the outside of the leg (outside of the shinbone, on the muscle). Gently press the acupressure point with a thumb for 10 to 15 seconds. Perform on both sides of the body and repeat three times each day.

■ WHAT TO EXPECT

If your child has had a recent decrease in appetite, natural therapies should be helpful within 5 days. If no improvement is seen within this time, then consult with a doctor.

Arthritis

Juvenile arthritis is a type of rheumatoid arthritis causing chronic inflammation in the joints. The onset is before 16 years of age. It is estimated that 1 in 1,000 children is affected with chronic joint inflammation. Feet, ankles, knees, hips, wrist and finger joints, elbows, and shoulders are prime targets. X-rays will indicate any signs of soft tissue swelling, cartilage deterioration, and joint-space narrowing. The potential for joint damage and the presence of blood markers such as rheumatoid factor distinguish this type of arthritis from others, including osteoarthritis, which is the degeneration of cartilage of the joints, leading to pain and stiffness.

Symptoms include stiffness of involved joints, pain that is worse after exercise, and painful and tender joints that may also be red, swollen, and hot. Leg pain in children can indicate rheumatoid arthritis in some cases, especially if the following symptoms accompany the pain: low-grade fever, limping, morning aches, reduced appetite, weight loss, constant tiredness, and swelling of joints or muscles. As the condition worsens, the skin over the affected joints becomes reddish purple. The joints themselves may become deformed or destroyed. Symptoms may develop slowly and involve only one joint or may come on suddenly and involve several joints.

Medical evidence identifies rheumatoid arthritis as an autoimmune reaction, in which antibodies develop against joint tissue components. Theories suggest that heredity plays some role, but the exact genetic link has not yet been identified. Food allergies, microorganisms, and abnormal bowel permeability (poor digestion and absorption) are linked to arthritis as well. In addition, a deficiency of certain minerals (including calcium, zinc, magnesium, and copper) and essential fatty acid imbalance can also contribute to this disease.

Conventional treatment focuses on the use of nonsteroidal anti-inflammatory drugs (NSAIDs) such as aspirin, and on sulfasalazine, methotrexate, and corticosteroids. Physiotherapy may be used as well.

■ BASIC PLAN

Diet

Focus the child's diet on whole grains, legumes, fruits, vegetables, and fresh fish—salmon, halibut, tuna, trout, and so on. (See "Diet" on page 4 for more information.) Red cherry juice has natural anti-inflammatory benefits; drink one to two 8-ounce glasses daily. Eliminate processed foods, artificial colorings, dyes, and preservatives.

Eliminate dairy products and reduce sugar intake, and red meat. Also, eliminate products containing gluten (wheat, barley, and rye) for 1 month or longer to see if there is improvement.

Avoid tomatoes, all peppers except black pepper, white potatoes, and eggplant. These foods belong to the nightshade family and have been linked to arthritis symptoms. It may take up to 6 months for benefits to be noticed.

Have your child tested for food allergies. Some researchers feel that up to one-third of all rheumatoid arthritis sufferers can control the disease through the elimination of allergenic foods.

Nutritional Supplements

Essential fatty acids—Give these in the form of ground flaxseed, flaxseed oil, or fish oil. Or give a children's essential fatty acid complex that contains omega-3 and omega-6 fatty acids. Essential fatty acids, especially omega-3's, help to reduce inflammation in the body.

Dosages: Grind 1 teaspoon of flaxseeds per 50 pounds of body weight daily (children weighing 30 to 50 pounds may also use 1 teaspoon); give along with 8 ounces of water. Or give flaxseed oil, at 1 teaspoon for children up to age 2, 2 teaspoons for kids 3 to 6, and 2 to 3 teaspoons for kids 7 and older. Cut back if diarrhea occurs. For fish oil, give 1 gram per 50 pounds of body weight. For a children's essential fatty acid formula, give as directed on the container.

Methylsulfonylmethane (MSM)—A natural substance found in foods and the body that reduces the pain and inflammation of arthritis. Give 5 milligrams per pound of body weight twice daily; cut back if diarrhea occurs. Or give as prescribed by a practitioner.

Herbal Remedies

Bromelain—Give 3 milligrams per pound of body weight two or three times daily, between meals.

White willow—Give 1 drop per 3 pounds of body weight, two or three times daily.

Note: Do not use white willow during a fever or viral infection.

You can consult with a holistic doctor for formulas that contain these and one or more other natural anti-inflammatory herbs, such as licorice, turmeric, boswellia, ginger root, and/or devil's claw.

Homeopathy

Pick the following remedy that best matches your child's symptoms. Unless otherwise indicated, give your child 2 pellets of a 30C potency twice daily. Improvements should be seen within 7 days. If there is no improvement within 7 days, try another remedy. After you first notice improvement, stop giving the remedy unless symptoms begin to return.

Note: Lower potencies (6X, 12X, 6C) may need to be given more often (three times daily).

Arsenicum album—For burning pain, but the pain moves around to different body parts. Symptoms are worse after midnight. The child is often restless and has lots of anxiety.

Belladonna—For joints that are all hot, red, and swollen. Or for a throbbing sensation in the joints.

Causticum—For very stiff joints made worse by cold, dry weather. Useful when there is a lot of joint deformity, or if the child has difficulty rising from a seat.

Kali carbonicum—For right-sided joint symptoms. The child is very stiff and sensitive to cold. A stitching pain gets worse around 3:00 A.M. The pain feels better with movement.

Pulsatilla—Symptoms worsen as the day goes on; stiffness and soreness increase in the evening after sitting. Pains move around to different areas of the body and are very changeable.

Rhododendron—For arthritis that gets worse before a storm.

Rhus toxicodendron—For burning or

achy joints that become worse with cold and dampness and get better with heat and warm applications. The stiffness gets better from the first motion and continual motion throughout the day.

Constitutional Hydrotherapy

Do this daily. (See Hydrotherapy for Children on page 115 for details.) Reduces joint inflammation by improving circulation, digestion, and elimination. Good digestion and circulation are important to alleviate rheumatoid arthritis.

■ ADVANCED PLAN

Nutritional Supplements

Children's multivitamin—Give as directed on the label.

Thymus glandular extract—Give one to two 250-milligram tablets or capsules daily to balance the immune system.

Microbial-derived enzymes—Give 1 to 2 with each meal to improve digestion and absorption of nutrients.

Vitamin C—Has mild anti-inflammatory effects. The kind with bioflavonoids is preferable. The dosage is the child's age in years times 50 milligrams, given twice daily. Reduce the dosage if diarrhea occurs. Consider using a buffered vitamin C powder (nonacidic) or liquid vitamin C. Both work well for infants and children, and can be mixed in juice.

Vitamin E—Give 100 international units per 50 pounds of body weight.

Probiotic—If your child has been on an-tibiotics or steroid medications, then replenishing of good bacteria is needed, and acidophilus can help. Give a children's acidophilus supplement that also contains bifidus. Follow the directions on the container.

Herbal Remedy

Topical capsaicin cream—This is a nontoxic extract from cayenne pepper. Apply ⅛ teaspoon to the affected joint(s) one or two times daily to help relieve pain. Too much can be irritating, so use caution when applying.

Aromatherapy

German chamomile—Add to a carrier oil and rub over the affected area one or two times daily. If taking a homeopathic remedy, use aromatherapy at a different time.

■ WHAT TO EXPECT

Natural therapy can be very effective in reducing arthritic symptoms. If your child is on pharmaceutical treatment, incorporate the natural approach listed in this chapter. As improvement occurs over 1 to 2 months, you can work with your child's doctor to reduce or eliminate medications.

Asthma

Asthma is a respiratory illness that results in difficult or restricted breathing. This condition is characterized by constriction of the airway, swelling of the lungs, and overproduction of mucus that clogs the small air passageways. The child may exhibit coughing, wheezing, feelings of tightness in the chest, an increased respiratory rate, anxiety, and, of course, difficult breathing.

Asthma is most common in children under the age of 10. It affects twice as many boys as girls. The incidence of asthma continues to rise among children, due in part to greater pollution exposure from chemicals in the water, air, and food.

There are two main causes of asthma. First is allergic reactions to such things as dust, molds, pollens, animal dander, and chemical pollutants from cigarette smoke and processed foods. The immune system perceives these items as foreign and reacts with inflammatory chemicals.

The second category does not seem to be related to an allergic response but to other factors such cold air, exercise, and infections such as the common cold. In many instances, we have found that asthma may also have an emotional trigger, caused by stress or psychological trauma.

Some physicians feel that vaccines may contribute to asthma by not allowing the immune system to mature by fighting off childhood infections. It is felt that this may cause imbalances in the immune system and make it more reactive to allergens. Also, some researchers feel that vaccines may damage the immune system when given at too early of an age, or if a child is sensitive to one or more of the vaccines. (See Vaccinations on page 483 for more information.)

Most children with chronic asthma are prescribed bronchodilators. These drugs expand the airways to make breathing easier. They are usually inhaled to prevent or treat asthma. More serious cases of asthma require prescribed steroids, which decrease inflammation of the airways and suppress the immune response. Steroids have a much higher risk of side effects when taken long-term. The goal of a natural approach is to treat the underlying reason for the hyperreactivity of the immune system and airways. We have children who are on asthma medication stay on their drug medications while we implement natural therapies as part of their overall treatment program. As health improves and the child becomes less susceptible to asthma attacks, medications can be slowly weaned under the guidance of a doctor. Do not take your child off any prescribed medications yourself.

If your child has asthma, avoid allergens to which he is sensitive, such as animal hair, or try homeopathic desensitization drops to the offending allergen. You can also use the following tips to decrease or eliminate allergens around the house.

- Use HEPA air filters to clean the air in your home.
- Have air vents professionally cleaned.
- Wash bedding twice weekly to reduce dust, and cover the child's mattress, box spring, and pillows with plastic covers.
- Consider removing carpets and rugs and replacing them with wooden floors.

- Use nontoxic chemicals for housecleaning.
- Smoke of any kind should be forbidden in the home. This includes smoke from tobacco, fireplaces, and wood-burning stoves.
- Keep your child away from high-traffic roads, to lessen exposure to gas fumes.

Stress reduction is also important to prevent asthma. Work to reduce stress with exercise that is tolerable for the child; with play, prayer, and deep breathing; and also with counseling if emotional issues are a causative factor.

Caution: Acute asthma attacks are a potential life-threatening situation. Seek emergency medical help if your child is not responding to the usual treatment.

■ BASIC PLAN

Diet

Feed your child a whole-foods diet that focuses on vegetables, fruits, grains, fresh fish, and lean poultry sources. A vegan diet (a diet with no animal products) has been shown to provide significant improvement for people with asthma. The intake of food sources rich in omega-3 fatty acids may help reduce inflammatory reactions. Studies show that children who eat fish containing omega-3's more than once a week have one-third the risk of developing asthma compared with children who do not eat fish on a regular basis. Fish oil capsules have been shown to be helpful as well. Conversely, foods high in arachadonic acid (such as red meat) can increase inflammatory reactions.

Case History

Kelly was a 7-year-old girl who had had asthma since 2 years of age. She was prone to upper respiratory tract infections and sinus infections. She used an inhaler at least three times daily to prevent symptoms of asthma.

While giving us her health history, her mother revealed that Kelly's asthma had begun after her father left the family. She was still full of grief from this traumatic event. As part of her treatment, Kelly was prescribed the homeopathic remedy Pulsatilla. This remedy is helpful when conditions such as asthma have an emotional cause, such as abandonment. Kelly's mother was asked to keep her off of dairy products and sugar. Kelly had dramatic improvement over the next 6 months, and she now requires her bronchodilator only occasionally for acute flare-ups.

Eliminating food additives—artificial sweeteners, preservatives, and food colorings—can help, too. Tartrazine (yellow dye #5), red dye, sulfites (such as are found in dried fruits), benzoates, and monosodium glutamate (MSG) should be strictly avoided. Read labels and prepare meals with fresh food when possible.

Have your child tested for food allergies, or

eliminate common food allergens to see if there is improvement. Common allergens include dairy, wheat, eggs, chocolate, sugar, citrus fruit, shellfish, nuts, and peanuts.

Increase foods that are rich in flavonoids and carotenoids. Flavonoids and carotenoids are plant substances that have strong antioxidant and natural anti-inflammatory activities. Carotenoids are commonly found in dark green leafy vegetables and deep yellow and orange vegetables. Flavonoids are found in many plant-based foods, including garlic, onions, leeks, turnips, grapes, pineapple, apricots, almonds, walnuts, carrots, pumpkin, sunflower seeds, tangerines, molasses, sesame seeds, cauliflower, cherries, mangoes, elderberries, sprouted seeds and grains, and green leafy vegetables including mustard greens, collards, and endive.

Grind 1 teaspoon of flaxseeds per 50 pounds of body weight (children weighing 30 to 50 pounds may also use 1 teaspoon). Add this to cereal, sprinkle it on food, or mix it in a shake. Always give with 8 ounces of water. Flaxseeds contain omega-3 fatty acids, which help reduce inflammation.

Nutritional Supplements

Children's multivitamin—Give daily as directed on the container.

Vitamin C—Supports the immune system and has anti-allergy effects. The kind with bioflavonoids is preferable. Dosage: the child's age in years times 50 milligrams, twice daily. Reduce the dosage if diarrhea occurs. Consider using a buffered vitamin C powder (nonacidic) or liquid vitamin C. Both work well for infants and children, and can be mixed in juice.

Fish oil or flaxseed oil—For fish oil, give 1 gram per 50 pounds of body weight daily. Or give flaxseed oil at the following daily dosages: 1 teaspoon for children 2 and under, 2 teaspoons for kids 3 to 6, and 2 to 3 teaspoons for those 7 and older. Reduce the dosage if diarrhea occurs. Give this in addition to the dietary recommendations above, as kids with asthma need the extra essential fatty acids.

Herbal Remedies

The following herbs are best used when prescribed as formulas by a practitioner.

Licorice root—Soothing to respiratory passageways; has natural anti-inflammatory effects.

Mullein—Soothing to respiratory passageways and helps expel mucus if it is present.

Caution: You may have heard that the herb ma huang (ephedra) can help with asthma. While it does dilate air passageways and can be helpful, it is an extremely powerful and potentially dangerous herb. Do not use it without a doctor's advice.

Homeopathy

Homeopathic remedies are best used to prevent asthma symptoms. Do not replace your child's use of medications with natural remedies, although the two can be used together. Proper homeopathic treatment can work well in strengthening a child's system so that she is not as susceptible to asthmatic attacks.

Pick the following remedy that best matches your child's symptoms. Unless otherwise indicated, give your child 2 pellets of a 30C potency every 15 minutes for acute asthma, and twice daily for low-grade asthma. (For infants, crush the pellets into powder and mix it with water.) Acute improvement should be seen within an hour, or you should try a different remedy. After you first notice improvement, stop giving the remedy unless symptoms begin to return.

Note: Lower potencies (6X, 12X, 6C) may need to be given more often (three times daily).

Aconitum napellus—Most useful at the beginning of symptoms of an asthma attack. The child is anxious and restless.

Arsenicum album—An excellent remedy for acute asthma. If your child needs to go to the emergency room for a bad asthma attack, give the child a dose or two of this remedy in the 30C potency on the way. The child is anxious, fearful, restless, wants to sit up and lean forward, and asthma comes on or is worse between 12:00 and 2:00 A.M. The child feels better with warm drinks and when sitting upright. Cold air may bring on an attack.

Ipecacuanha—For acute asthma, where child has a lot of mucus formation that causes coughing, gagging, and vomiting.

Kali carbonicum—For asthma that is worse from 2:00 to 4:00 A.M. The child is very chilly, sits up and leans forward to relieve asthma. Not as restless as a child needing Arsenicum album.

Lachesis—The child wakes up choking

Vital Fact

Secondhand smoke is the third leading preventable cause of death, and among children it causes lower respiratory infections, middle ear infections, sudden infant death syndrome, and asthma. Half the world's children may be exposed to environmental tobacco smoke, exacerbating symptoms in 20 percent of children with asthma. Studies have confirmed that tobacco smoke causes an onset of childhood asthma and exacerbation of symptoms throughout life.

with asthma; her throat and chest feels constricted. Gets better with fresh air. The child cannot stand any pressure on the throat or chest, and tends to be warm.

Lobelia inflata—For asthma characterized by nausea and vomiting. Cold brings on asthma.

Medorrhinum—For chronic asthma where the child is very prone to respiratory tract infections. The child craves citrus fruit.

Natrum sulphuricum—Asthma is worse in cold, damp weather. Symptoms are worse from 4:00 A.M. to 5:00 A.M.

Pulsatilla—The child desires company, wants to be held. Feels better in fresh and cold air. Low thirst. Symptoms worse in the evening. Hay fever or acute bronchitis may bring on the asthma.

Tuberculinum—For chronic asthma. The child craves milk. The asthma may be triggered by an allergy to cat hair. The child is very susceptible to respiratory tract infections.

■ ADVANCED PLAN

Nutritional Supplements

Pycnogenol or grape seed extract—Has a natural antihistamine effect. Give 1 milligram per pound of body weight daily.

Quercitin—Has a natural antihistamine effect. Give 3 milligrams per pound of body weight, two or three times daily, between meals.

Magnesium—A natural relaxant of the airways. Give 250 to 500 milligrams daily. Reduce the dosage if diarrhea occurs.

Vitamin B$_6$—The asthma medication theophylline can deplete vitamin B$_6$. Supplementation of vitamin B$_6$ between 100 and 200 milligrams daily has shown benefit in asthmatic children. Use this dosage only under the supervision of a physician.

Vitamin B$_{12}$—Talk to your doctor about the use of B$_{12}$ injections that can be quite helpful to reduce the effects of asthma. Oral supplements may be helpful as well.

N-acetylcysteine—Helps liquefy mucus. Give 2 milligrams per pound of body weight twice daily if mucus is present.

Acupressure

Gently press both of the following acupressure points simultaneously with a thumb for 10 to 15 seconds. Repeat three times. Do this daily to prevent asthma.

Lung 1—Helps to relax the lungs and ease asthma symptoms. Located on the outer portion of the chest, right below the collarbone

Pericardium 6—Helps to relax the chest. Located 2½ finger-widths below the wrist crease, in the middle of the forearm (palm side).

■ WHAT TO EXPECT

Natural therapy is more effective for the long-term management of asthma. You should find over the course of 1 to 2 months that your child's susceptibility to asthma is reduced. Mild asthma attacks may be managed with natural therapy. More severe cases should always be treated with asthma drugs or a combination of drug and natural therapy (such as homeopathy). In any case, a doctor's supervision is required. Work with a naturopathic doctor to find the underlying cause of the asthma.

Athlete's Foot

Athlete's foot, also known as tinea pedis, is a persistent and annoying fungal infection of the foot. It commonly occurs between the toes and toenails, but it can also occur on other areas of the foot. The affected area can appear red, cracked, and scaly. Sores and blisters can form on the soles of the feet and between the toes. The infected areas all too often burn or itch.

Moisture and warmth provide an environment for this fungus to thrive. Public or private showers, locker rooms, gym floors, and hotel bathrooms are common places for a child to contract this fungus. Children with sweaty feet are more susceptible to athlete's foot, since moisture provides a breeding ground for fungus. Some children have a natural resistance to athlete's foot, while others must be more careful with hygiene. Exposing feet to open air by wearing sandals or porous slippers around the home or outside (if the climate permits) can help. Use cotton socks. If your child's feet perspire a lot, change his socks twice daily. Have him wear waterproof slippers or sandals in locker rooms and showers. Make sure that his feet are washed with soap daily.

Most cases of athlete's foot can be treated at home. However, complications can arise when a bacterial infection sets in along with the existing fungal infection. If your child's athlete's foot does not improve with natural treatment, or if it gets worse, see a doctor for treatment. Conventional treatment generally involves antifungal creams.

■ BASIC PLAN

Diet
Avoid giving your child sugar products; sugar feeds the fungus. This includes soft drinks, candy, and processed foods such as sugar-sweetened cereal. Fruit juices should be diluted and kept to a minimum. Garlic, oregano, and onions have antifungal effects and can be included in prepared meals. Children under the age of 3 may experience digestive upset if too-high amounts of these foods are consumed. Plain cultured yogurt contains good bacteria that fight fungus.

Nutritional Supplement
Probiotic—Builds up good bacteria (acidophilus and bifidus) that help to fight a fungal infection and keep it from overgrowing. This is especially important if there is any history of antibiotic use, which destroys beneficial bacteria in the body. Choose a formula made for children, and give as directed on the container.

Herbal Remedies
Tea tree oil—The herb of choice for fungal infections. Studies confirm the usefulness of this herbal treatment for athlete's foot. There are a couple of ways to apply it to the infected area of the foot:

- Add 10 drops of tea tree oil to 1 quart of warm water. Have your child soak his feet for 10 minutes. Then, dry the feet thoroughly with a towel and hair dryer. To increase compliance, have your child read a book or watch TV during this process.
- Wash your child's feet with soap and water, then dry thoroughly. Apply diluted tea tree oil or tea tree oil salve with a cotton swab to the affected area. Try to get under the nail as much as possible. Repeat daily.

Echinacea—Taken internally to support the immune system's response to the fungal infection.

Homeopathy

Pick the following remedy which best matches your child's symptoms. Unless otherwise indicated, give your child 2 pellets of a 30C potency twice daily. Improvements should be seen within 2 weeks. If there is no improvement within 2 weeks, try another remedy. After you first notice improvement, stop giving the remedy unless symptoms begin to return.

Note: Lower potencies (6X, 12X, 6C) may need to be given more often (three times daily).

Graphites—For cracked skin that oozes a thick, yellow fluid.

Silica—For red feet that sweat profusely and smell offensive.

Sulphur—For chronic athlete's foot, intense itching and burning of feet.

Thuja occidentalis—For long-standing fungal infections of the skin.

■ ADVANCED PLAN

Nutritional Supplements

Vitamin C—Supports the immune system and has mild anti-inflammatory effects. The type with bioflavonoids is preferable. Dosage: the child's age in years times 50 milligrams, twice daily. Reduce the dosage if diarrhea occurs. Consider using a buffered vitamin C powder (nonacidic) or liquid vitamin C. Both work well for infants and children, and can be mixed in juice.

Zinc—Supports the immune system and enhances skin healing. Dosage: children 2 and younger, 5 milligrams daily; 2 and older, 10 to 15 milligrams daily. For long-term use, take with 1 milligram of copper.

Herbal Remedy

Calendula—Soothing and healing to dry and cracked skin. Apply a cream or a tincture (1 teaspoon of tincture in 4 teaspoons of water) twice daily to the affected area.

■ WHAT TO EXPECT

Tea tree oil usually works quite well for athlete's foot. Your child should notice a decrease in the pain and inflammation within 2 weeks of treatment. You may notice the skin becoming drier for a period of time and then increasing in flaking as old, infected skin dies. Long-standing fungal infections may take a month or two of treatment. For fungal infection of the toenails, make sure to trim the nails twice weekly so that the tea tree oil can penetrate into the fungus.

Attention Deficit Hyperactivity Disorder (ADHD)

ADHD is the most common behavioral disorder in children. It is estimated that 5 to 10 percent of school-age children have this behavioral disorder, which can also affect teens and adults. It usually is not diagnosed until around first grade.

There is no laboratory or physical test that

diagnoses ADHD. Instead, it is diagnosed by a clinician based on a clinical history given by the parents, teachers, and child. There are specific criteria for the diagnosis of ADHD as outlined in the American Psychiatric Association's *Diagnostic and Statistical Manual of Mental Disorders, Fourth Edition.* They include the following:

- Abnormal and persistent inattention, from at least six symptoms continuing over a minimum of 6 months, OR abnormal and persistent hyperactivity-impulsivity, also from at least six symptoms over 6 months.
- Hyperactive-impulsive or inattentive symptoms that cause impairment must have been present before age 7 years.
- The symptoms are present in two settings (for instance, home and school).
- The symptoms interfere with developmentally appropriate social, academic, or occupational functioning.
- The symptoms are not the result of some other disorder.

There are three subtypes that can be diagnosed as well: ADHD Combined Type, where both inattention and hyperactivity-impulsivity exist for at least 6 months (this type is most common in children); ADHD Predominantly Inattentive Type, which mainly involves symptoms of inattention; ADHD Predominantly Hyperactive-Impulsive Type, which mainly involves symptoms of hyperactivity-impulsivity.

Symptoms range from mild to severe. Children with ADHD tend to be hyperactive, im-

Vital Fact

In the 5-year period from 1991 to 1995, the number of 15- to 19-year-olds being treated with Ritalin jumped 311 percent. Among children ages 2 to 5 and those 5 to 14 years old, the increase was approximately 170 percent.

pulsive, and inattentive. They are unable to focus for any extended length of time. They fidget in their chairs, blurt out answers in class, and don't wait their turns in games. This leads to problems within home, school, and social settings. A hyperactive child also feels isolated from his peers and can't figure out why he is so different.

Between 30 and 40 percent of children with ADHD have learning disabilities, although it is important to note that the ADHD child is not mentally retarded and in many cases is quite bright.

Boys are three times more likely to develop ADHD than girls. By the teen years, about 30 percent of children with ADHD outgrow this disorder.

The cause of ADHD remains unknown, but frequent ear infections and use of antibiotics, as well as premature birth and family history, are associated with a greater likelihood of developing this disorder. From a holistic viewpoint, causative factors may include food additives and food allergies, environmental allergens, and heavy metal toxicity such as lead, mercury, and aluminum poisoning. Some researchers suspect that vaccines may contribute to ADHD and learning disorders in susceptible children. There is also a connection between a poorly functioning digestive system and ADHD. Poor digestion and absorption leads to an increase in metabolic toxins and the subsequent release of inflammatory mediators which can disrupt neurotransmitter balance. Nutritional deficiencies are also suspect in the underlying cause of this condition—particularly deficiencies of essential fatty acids, B vitamins, and several minerals, including iron. Since iron deficiency anemia can cause attention problems, have your doctor test for it. Family problems or emotional disturbances may also be a factor.

Conventional treatment focuses on pharmaceutical treatment such as Ritalin, and/or behavioral therapy. Biofeedback and counseling can also be helpful for children with ADHD.

Note: Rule out heavy metal toxicity (lead, mercury, aluminum, and others). This can be done through hair, blood, or urine tests by your doctor. Learning and behavior disorders are linked to heavy metals.

■ BASIC PLAN

Diet

The effects of diet on behavior and attention vary with each child. Like many nutrition-oriented doctors, we have found that dietary improvements can make profound differences in many children with ADHD. Diet should be the base of a comprehensive approach to improving this condition. The whole-foods diet that focuses on vegetables, fruits, grains, fresh fish, and lean poultry sources is ideal. (See "Diet" on page 4 for help putting together a healthful diet for your child.)

There are six main areas to focus on with diet:

1. Avoid food additives. There are more than 5,000 additives in the food supply. Depending on the child's sensitivity, these additives can cause biochemical imbalances. Examples of additives include food preservatives such as nitrites and sulfites, colorings such as yellow dye #5 (tartrazine), and flavorings such as monosodium glutamate. It is almost impossible to completely eliminate all food additives, but you can limit them by preparing meals with whole foods and by reading labels. Benjamin Feingold, M.D., a longtime expert in hyperactivity, stated that up to 50 percent of hyperactive children are sensitive to artificial colorings and flavors, preservatives, and naturally occurring salicylates and phenolics.

2. Identify food allergies. Food allergies and sensitivities can cause behavior and attention problems. The most common food reactions we see are to cow's milk, cheese, sugar, wheat, corn, peanuts, chocolate, and citrus fruit. Children often crave foods to which they are sensitive. Start by eliminating one or two of the foods that your child eats frequently, such as sugar and milk, and take note of any changes in your child's behavior and moods. Continue this process every 2 to 3 weeks until you have identified the reactive foods. Other symptoms of food allergies include dark circles under the eyes, skin rashes, headaches, and digestive problems. These symptoms may improve as well, giving an indication that there was a reaction to the food that you eliminated. (For more information, see "Food Allergies and Food Sensitivities" on page 298.)

3. Consider testing. Many natural health care practitioners offer testing procedures such as electrodermal food testing (which measures reaction to different foods), NAET (Nambudripad's Allergy Elimination Techniques), blood tests (IgE and IgG4), and muscle testing. These offer a quicker way to identify food allergies. Conventional tests for food sensitivities (for instance, skin scratch tests) are generally not very helpful.

4. Keep blood sugar balanced. Many children feel better and have fewer fluctuations in behavior and attention span when their eating patterns support balanced blood sugar levels. This is done by avoiding simple sugars and refined carbohydrates such as candy, white bread and white rice, undiluted fruit juices, and soft drinks. Adequate protein intake is important too; good sources include nuts, fish, lean poultry, soy, and legumes. Fiber also helps to stabilize blood sugar levels. Vegetables are the main source of fiber that should be included with meals and snacks.

Have your child eat smaller, more frequent meals and snacks (every 2 to 3 hours) throughout the day instead of two or three larger meals. Make sure that your child does not miss any meals, especially breakfast, which can lead to concentration and memory problems.

5. Serve brain-healthy foods. Foods that contain essential fatty acids are very important for brain health—for both learning and mood. Brain cells contain high amounts of omega-3 fatty acids. Fish such as salmon, halibut, and trout are good sources. Fresh fish two or three times weekly is recommended. Flaxseeds can be ground up and sprinkled on salads or put in shakes; they are high in the essential fatty acids needed for proper brain function. Grind 1 teaspoon of flaxseeds per 50 pounds of body weight (children weighing 30 to 50 pounds may also use 1 teaspoon) and give this amount daily with 8 ounces of water.

6. Make sure that your child drinks purified water. Like other tissues, the brain needs a constant supply of water to function properly. Soft drinks and fruit juices do not supply the water that your child needs. Six to eight 8-ounce glasses of water daily are recommended.

Nutritional Supplements

Essential fatty acid complex—Choose a children's blend that contains the omega-3 fatty acids DHA (docosahexaenoic acid) and EPA (eicosapentaenoic acid), as well as omega-6 fatty acids. Give as directed on the container.

It should provide at least 100 milligrams of DHA per day.

Calcium and magnesium—Both minerals help to calm the nervous system. Give them together in a formula or separately throughout the day. Recommended dosage: 500 milligrams of calcium and 500 milligrams of magnesium.

Phosphatidylserine—A substance found in high concentrations in brain cells that helps the neurons (brain cells) to communicate with one another effectively. Recommended daily dosages: for children 25 to 75 pounds, 100 milligrams; for kids 75 to 100 pounds, 200 milligrams; for those 100 pounds or heavier, 300 milligrams.

Herbal Remedies

To improve concentration and memory, take these herbs individually or in formulas:

> **Ginkgo biloba**—10 to 20 drops
>
> **Gotu kola**—5 to 10 drops
>
> **Lemon balm**—3 to 5 drops

Calming herbs include passionflower, chamomile, and hops. Five to 10 drops can be added to the formula of one of these herbs.

Homeopathy

Pick the following remedy that best matches your child's symptoms. Unless otherwise indicated, give your child 2 pellets of a 30C potency twice daily. Signs of improvements should be seen within 10 days. If there is no improvement within 10 days, try another remedy. After you first notice improvement, stop giving the remedy unless symptoms begin to return. Consultation with a naturopathic doctor or homeopathic practitioner is advised. *Note:* Lower potencies (6X, 12X, 6C) may need to be given more often (three times daily).

Anacardium orientale—The child can be cruel to animals and people. He has low self-esteem, so he tries to prove things to people. Antisocial and absentminded; curses and swears.

Hyoscyamus niger—The child is very impulsive and can be very violent, especially toward a younger sibling from jealousy. He is very talkative and may be sexually precocious.

Medorrhinum—The child has major temper tantrums and is violent toward other kids. Has a hard time concentrating and is always looking for trouble. He gets warm very easily, and craves oranges, ice, and unripe fruit. He wants to stay up all night.

Stramonium—The child has many fears, such as the dark, animals, or being alone. There are fits of anger and rage where the child destroys things. He may have night terrors.

Tarentula hispanica—The child is very hurried and restless, constantly on the move. He is mischievous and destructive, very impulsive and out of control. He loves music and dancing.

Tuberculinum—The child is very demanding and impatient. He gets bored very easily. He can have a violent temper and be destructive, hitting and biting other kids and adults. He may be cruel to animals. He craves milk and smoked meats. He may have a ritual of banging his head on the floor or on hard surfaces.

■ ADVANCED PLAN

Nutritional Supplements

Vitamin B$_6$—Studies have shown that hyperactive children whose serotonin levels are low may respond to supplementation with this vitamin. Try 100 milligrams daily for children 5 and older, but no more. Higher dosages should be used only under the supervision of a doctor knowledgeable in nutrition. Otherwise, side effects such as neuropathy and other disorders of the nerves can occur.

B complex—Liquid forms are available. Give as directed on the container—25 milligrams daily for children under 7, 50 milligrams daily for ages 7 and up.

Children's multivitamin—This provides a base of vitamins and minerals for proper brain function. Give as directed on the container.

Zinc—A deficiency of this mineral can lead to ADHD symptoms. Daily dosage: for children 2 and younger, 5 milligrams; age 2 and older, 10 to 15 milligrams. For long-term zinc therapy, add 2 milligrams of copper daily.

Amino acids—Single amino acids or combinations of amino acids from a nutrition-oriented doctor can be helpful in balancing your child's brain chemistry. They are best taken between meals.

Probiotic—Increases the levels of good bacteria such as lactobacillus acidophilus and bifidus. Poor intestinal health, such as *Candida* overgrowth and poor absorption, is linked with ADHD. Choose a children's probiotic formula and give as directed on the container.

Homeopathy

Kali phosphoricum 6X and Magnesia phosphorica 6X—This combination is calming to the nervous system. Give 2 to 3 pellets of each three times daily for 1 month, to help concentration and to relax the nervous system. Continue indefinitely if improvement is noted.

Aromatherapy

Peppermint and frankincense—Peppermint helps to improve concentration, and frankincense is calming. These can be used singly or together. Put 1 drop of each in a vaporizer and put it in the child's room while he sleeps. If your child is taking a homeopathic remedy, then use aromatherapy at a different time.

■ WHAT TO EXPECT

If your child is not on medication, benefits of natural treatment should be observed within 4 to 8 weeks. Optimally, 3 months should be allowed to appropriately assess the benefit or the potential benefit of a natural protocol. Natural therapy is also recommended for children on drug therapy to address the underlying cause. However, do not stop any of your child's medications. Work with a nutrition-oriented doctor to wean your child off of the medications if possible.

Autism

First appearing in infancy or childhood, this behavioral mental disorder can last a lifetime.

Infantile autism shows signs within the first 30 months of a baby's life. The baby fails to cuddle, make eye contact, or want to be part of the family. Among young children with autism, the tendency is to refuse or limit speech and spend the majority of time alone and apart from other family members, peers, and members of the community. An autistic child engages in repetitive movements such as rocking or head banging. She also strongly resists any changes, even slight ones, to daily routines. For example, the child may wash her hands only at the bathroom sink and only if a certain towel is available to dry them.

Recent studies find a correlation between this condition and brain defects, fetal alcohol syndrome, and toxic metal poisoning from lead. Some evidence suggests that poor nutrition and food allergies may play roles. Various researchers and physicians are suspicious of a connection between the MMR (measles, mumps, and rubella) and pertussis vaccines and the onset of autism. It is imperative to improve digestive health in these children. Proper bowel function and nutrient absorption are often imbalanced in children with autism. We realize that getting an autistic child to follow the treatments suggested here may be a challenge, but do the best you can. Natural therapies are not a cure-all for this condition by any means, but they may help.

■ BASIC PLAN

Diet

Follow a whole-foods diet that focuses on vegetables, fruits, grains, fresh fish, nuts, seeds, and lean poultry sources.

Avoid food additives as much as possible, since they can cause biochemical imbalances. Food additives include nitrite and sulfite preservatives, colorings such as yellow dye #5 (tartrazine), and flavorings such as monosodium glutamate. It is nearly impossible to completely eliminate all food additives, but you can limit them by preparing meals with whole foods and by reading labels.

Eliminating food allergies and food sensitivities has been shown to improve symptoms of autism. Sugar, milk, and wheat appear to be the most common problem foods. Many natural health care practitioners offer testing procedures such as electrodermal food testing (which measures reaction to different foods), NAET (Nambudripad's Allergy Elimination Techniques), blood tests (IgE and IgG4), and muscle testing. These offer a quicker way to identify food allergies. (See "Food Allergies and Food Sensitivities" on page 298 for more information.)

Many children feel better and have fewer fluctuations in behavior and attention span when their eating patterns help to keep their blood sugar levels balanced. Avoid simple sugars and refined carbohydrates such as candy, white bread and white rice, undiluted fruit juices, and soft drinks. Adequate protein intake is important too; look to nuts, fish, lean poultry, soy, and legumes as good sources of protein. Fiber also helps to stabilize blood sugar levels. Vegetables are the main source of fiber that should be included with meals and snacks. Have your child eat smaller, more frequent meals and snacks (every 2 to 3 hours) throughout the day instead of two or three larger meals.

Foods with essential fatty acids are important for brain health. Fresh fish two or three times weekly is recommended. Flaxseed, which is high in essential fatty acid, can be ground up and sprinkled on salads or put in shakes. Grind 1 teaspoon of flaxseeds per 50 pounds of body weight (children weighing 30 to 50 pounds may also use 1 teaspoon), and give this amount daily along with 8 ounces of water.

Eggs, another brain-healthy food, contain docosahexaenoic acid (DHA), choline, and B vitamins for proper brain function.

Nutritional Supplements

Vitamin A—Supports the immune system. Daily dosage: infants under 1 year, 1,875 international units (IU); children 1 to 3, 2,000 IU; kids 4 to 6, 2,500 IU; kids 7 to 10, 3,500 IU; males 11 and older, 5,000 IU; females 11 and older, 4,000 IU.

Note: These dosages are for short-term use (up to 10 days). Higher dosages may be used

Vital Study

For a study published in *Magnesium Bulletin,* researchers looked at 52 autistic children and 11 nonautistic children who were treated with vitamin B_6 (30 milligrams per 2.2 pounds of body weight a day), magnesium (10 to 15 milligrams per 2.2 pounds of body weight), B_6 and magnesium, or a placebo. The combination of B_6 and magnesium was most effective, with a significant decrease in autistic behavior.

only under a doctor's supervision. Available in liquid drops.

Vitamin B_6—This is the most well-studied vitamin for autism. It is involved in the formation of many neurotransmitters such as serotonin and dopamine, which may benefit children with autism. Studies have shown that some children with autism benefit from high-dose B_6 supplementation. Extremely high dosages were used in studies: 30 milligrams per 2.2 pounds of body weight. Dosages such as these should be used only under the supervision of a doctor. If you are supplementing B_6, give a multivitamin as well, to maintain balance with the rest of the B vitamins.

Magnesium—Studies have also looked at combining vitamin B_6 and magnesium, with positive results. This makes sense, as vitamin B_6 increases the body's ability to use magnesium more effectively. Recommended dosage: 10 milligrams per 2.2 pounds of body weight daily. Reduce the dosage if diarrhea occurs.

Herbal Remedies

Formulas that contain one or more of the following are helpful for concentration. Use with the guidance of a holistic practitioner. Give such a formula two times daily.

Ginkgo (24 percent extract)—One drop of tincture per 3 pounds of body weight or 3 milligrams of capsule per pound, not exceeding 30 drops or 60 milligrams per dose.

Gotu kola—Ten to 20 drops or 30 to 60 milligrams per dose.

Lemon balm—A maximum of 5 drops per dose.

Homeopathy

Use constitutional homeopathy as prescribed by a practitioner.

■ ADVANCED PLAN

Nutritional Supplements

Essential fatty acid complex—Choose a children's complex containing the omega-3 fatty acids DHA (docosahexaenoic acid) and EPA (eicosapentaenoic acid), as well as omega-6 fatty acids. The formula should contain at least 100 milligrams of DHA. Give as directed on the container.

Phosphatidylserine—A substance found in high concentrations in brain cells that helps them to communicate with one another effectively. Recommended daily dosages: for children 25 to 75 pounds, 100 milligrams; 75 to 100 pounds, 200 milligrams; 100 pounds or more, 300 milligrams.

Aromatherapy

Peppermint and frankincense—Peppermint helps to improve concentration, and frankincense is calming. One or both can be used in a vaporizer. Use 1 drop of each during the day. If your child is taking a homeopathic remedy, use aromatherapy at a different time.

■ WHAT TO EXPECT

Many nutrition-oriented doctors find that the avoidance of food allergens such as wheat and cow's milk makes a dramatic difference in some autistic children. This can take 2 to 3 months to see if it is helpful. Constitutional homeopathy is a nontoxic therapy worth trying, and improvements can be seen within 4 to 6 weeks, although years of treatment may be required. Some practitioners also find bodywork, such as craniosacral therapy, to be helpful. (See "Craniosacral Therapy" on page 503 for more information.)

Backache

Children with backaches complain of aching, stiffness, or soreness in the area between the neck and the tailbone and anywhere along the spine. The cause may be muscular strain or sprain, overuse of back muscles, obesity, poor posture, out-of-shape stomach muscles, a fall, injury, or a medical condition such as arthritis. Internal conditions such as a kidney or bladder infection can also cause back pain. Correcting the underlying problem of chronic backaches in children can prevent more serious conditions in adulthood.

See a doctor if your child is unable to stand up or move freely, if he has radiating pain (spreading from a specific spot such as his neck or back to his arms or legs), if he has changes in urination or bowel movements, or if he has fever with the backache.

■ BASIC PLAN

Diet

To ensure proper nutrition for healing, a whole-foods diet is recommended. (See "Diet" on page 4 for more information.) Avoid sugar and caffeine products, as they can interfere with the healing process.

Nutritional Supplements

Calcium and magnesium—These minerals reduce muscle spasms. Give 500 milligrams of calcium and up to 500 milligrams of magnesium daily, available as a liquid calcium/magnesium blend.

Herbal Remedies

Bromelain—When taken between meals, bromelain has natural anti-inflammatory effects. Available in capsule form. Give 3 milligrams per pound of body weight two or three times daily, between meals.

Turmeric—This spice has anti-inflamma-tory effects. Give a maximum of 250 milligrams two or three times daily.

Homeopathy

Backache combination formulas are available for muscle spasm and pain. They are sold in ointment or tablet form. Give as directed on the container.

Or pick the one of the following remedies which best matches your child's symptoms. Unless otherwise indicated, give your child 2 pellets of a 30C potency three times daily. Improvements should be seen within 48 hours. If there is no improvement within 48 hours, try another remedy. After you first notice improvement, stop giving the remedy unless symptoms begin to return.

Note: Lower potencies (6X, 12X, 6C) may need to be given more often (four times daily).

Arnica montana—Use if the back pain occurred from a fall or trauma and bruising occurs.

Bryonia alba—For a backache that is aggravated from the slightest motion. There is stitching or aching pain in the back. Pain makes the child irritable. The back pain feels better with pressure.

Calcarea fluorica 6X—For children whose backs are always "going out" due to lax ligaments and tendons. Give 2 pellets twice daily.

Hypericum perforatum—For sharp shooting nerve pain due to a fall or blow to the back, especially when it is directly to the spine.

Magnesia phosphorica 6X—Specific for muscle spasms that accompany back pain.

Give one dose three times daily or as needed for relief of muscle spasms.

Nux vomica—For muscle cramps and spasms in the lower back. The pain wakes the child up at night; she must sit up to turn over. Pain is worse with motion and cold, and better with warmth and pressure. The child is very irritable from the back pain.

Rhus toxicodendron—The most common remedy for backache that results in stiffness. The child's back loosens up after movement and then tightens up again at the end of the day. She feels better lying on a hard surface and with warm applications; she feels worse from cold. The child is restless.

Ruta graveolens—For strained back ligaments. The back feels bruised and achy.

Silica 6X—For chronic lower back weakness. Give 2 pellets twice daily.

■ ADVANCED PLAN

Nutritional Supplements

Silica—This mineral strengthens the back's connective tissue. Give 4 milligrams per pound of body weight daily.

Flaxseed oil—Supplies essential fatty acid for tissue healing. Give at the following daily dosages: children 2 and under, 1 teaspoon; kids 3 to 6, 2 teaspoons; kids 7 and older, 2 to 3 teaspoons. Reduce the dosage if diarrhea occurs.

Vitamin E—Has a mild anti-inflammatory effect and helps with tissue healing. Give 100 international units per 50 pounds of body weight daily of natural vitamin E.

Vitamin C—Promotes healing of ligaments, tendons, and connective tissue. Dosage: the child's age in years times 50 milligrams, twice daily. Reduce the dosage if diarrhea occurs. Consider using a buffered vitamin C powder (nonacidic) or liquid vitamin C. Both work well for infants and children, and can be mixed in juice.

Herbal Remedies

St. John's wort and arnica _(Arnica montana)_—Apply these as oils or creams topically. Do not apply to broken skin.

Aromatherapy

Roman chamomile and lavender—Add these oils to a carrier oil, warm it up, and massage it into the back. If the child is taking a homeopathic remedy, use aromatherapy at a different time.

Acupressure

Small Intestine 3—Located on the outer side of the little finger, below the knuckle (toward the fingertip side). Press the acupressure point gently with a thumb for 10 to 15 seconds. Repeat three times and then do the same on the other hand. Do this daily.

■ WHAT TO EXPECT

Acute back pain should improve within 24 to 48 hours with use of the natural therapies. In some cases, relief is noticed within minutes. The remedies listed work best in conjunction with muscoskeletal treatment (such as massage, chiropractic, naturopathic, osteopathic, craniosacral, physiotherapy, or acupressure) from a qualified practitioner. Proper exercise should also be incorporated for a total treatment plan. See a doctor if the back pain does not improve within 5 days.

Bad Breath

Bad breath, also known as halitosis, is as embarrassing for children as it is for the rest of us. This condition can lead to ridicule by a child's peers and the development of low self-esteem. The offensive odor is usually the result of fermented bacteria accumulating in the mouth during the night.

Unlike with adults, it is unusual for a child to wake up in the morning with a case of chronic bad breath. Often, the odor is due to the fact that the child habitually breathes through his mouth, which can cause dry mouth tissues and bad breath.

It is critical to determine why a child is not breathing through his nostrils. The reasons include allergies, blocked sinuses, a stuffy nose, and swollen tonsils or other medical conditions. If the child has any foul-smelling, yellowish nasal discharge, or a fever, weight loss, or diarrhea, consult your physician immediately—these are signs of infection.

Most cases of bad breath in children are not the result of a serious disease. But if the bad breath persists for days, it may be a sign of illness. Common causes of offensive breath in children include:

- Poor dental hygiene, such as refusing to brush their teeth and not flossing
- Gum disease, tooth decay, mercury fillings, or infections in the mouth
- Undetected infection of the throat, such as tonsillitis or sinusitis
- Food or environmental allergies causing postnasal drip
- Poor digestion, including the effects of food allergies
- Flora imbalance (deficiency of good bacteria) from antibiotic use
- Systemic diseases such as diabetes or streptococcus infection

Conventional treatment focuses on ruling out infectious conditions of the mouth, throat, and sinus as well as systemic diseases. Make sure that you stress the importance of proper dental hygiene: Brush teeth and tongue, and floss after meals, and make sure that your child has regular dental exams.

■ BASIC PLAN

Diet
Reduce or eliminate sugar products in the diet, such as candy and soft drinks. Have your child eat yogurt with live cultures to improve the flora balance in his mouth. Do not give your child breath mints that contain sugar, as they provide an environment for bacteria to grow.

Nutritional Supplement
Probiotic—Look for a children's acidophilus supplement with bifidus. Give as di-

rected on the container for at least 2 months to improve flora balance of the mouth. This is especially important if antibiotics have been used in the past.

Herbal Remedies

Echinacea, myrrh, and calendula mouth rinse—The following herbal mouth rinse can be used in cases where bad breath is due to inflamed or infected gums or dental infections. It is to be used in addition to the recommendations of a dentist. Add 5 drops each of echinacea, myrrh, and calendula to 2 ounces of water. Have the child swish it in his mouth and swallow. Repeat twice daily for up to 2 weeks.

Chlorophyll—Nature's great breath freshener. Available in liquid form. Have your child take ½ teaspoon after each meal or as directed on the container.

Homeopathy

Pick the following remedy that best matches your child's symptoms. Unless otherwise indicated, give your child 2 pellets of a 30C potency twice daily. Improvements should be seen within 5 days. If there is no improvement within 5 days, try another remedy. After you first notice improvement, stop giving the remedy unless symptoms begin to return.

Note: Lower potencies (6X, 12X, 6C) may need to be given more often (three times daily).

Mercurius solubilis or vivus—For symptoms of bad breath, excessive salivation, and a thick-coated tongue.

Nux vomica—The child's breath has a sour odor. He has a bitter taste in his mouth and suffers from digestive problems.

Other Recommendations

Have your child stick out his tongue, and scrape its top with an upside-down spoon. This helps to manually remove bacteria that contribute to bad breath.

■ ADVANCED PLAN

Nutritional Supplements

Whole-food supplement—Look specifically for a supplement designed for children that contains fruits and vegetables. It helps to gently detoxify the body. Give as directed on the container.

Microbial-derived enzymes—When taken with meals, these help with the digestion and assimilation of foods. Use as directed if digestion is a problem.

Herbal Remedy

Peppermint and ginger herbal tea—Have the child drink these teas after meals. The ginger is soothing to the digestive system, while peppermint freshens the breath. Make ¼ to ½ cup of either one or a combination of these two readily available teas.

Aromatherapy

Myrrh and lemon rinse—Add 1 drop of myrrh and 2 drops of lemon to a glass of water. Have the child swish it in his mouth and spit it out.

Note: Use this only with children over 10 years of age. If your child is taking a homeopathic remedy, use aromatherapy at a different time.

■ WHAT TO EXPECT

Natural treatments should improve chronic bad breath. If there is no breath improvement within 2 weeks, consult with a dentist or doctor.

Bedwetting

This condition is characterized by a child wetting or soiling the bed at night or clothing during the day well past the age when he has gained control over his bladder and bowels. Medically, bedwetting at nighttime is termed nocturnal enuresis and during the day is called diurnal enuresis. This is an embarrassing situation for any child and a cause of frustration and concern for parents.

Nearly 7 million children beyond their toilet training years wet their beds. About 1 in every 3 children ages 4 or 5 wets the bed, and 1 in 10 boys still have a problem by age 12.

The reasons may be physical or behavioral. The child's bladder may be too small or underdeveloped, making it impossible to hold urine throughout the entire night. (A child's bladder must be strong and large enough to hold 12 ounces of urine at night to be able to withstand wetting the bed.) Or, the child may have a urinary tract infection that interferes with normal functioning of the bladder. Underlying conditions such as diabetes may also be involved.

Bedwetting may be triggered by a scary or stressful incident such as moving into a new neighborhood, parents going through a divorce, or conflicts with other children at day care or school. These incidents tend to be temporary. It is important not to ridicule or embarrass a child with this condition, as that approach generally makes things worse and heightens an already emotionally sensitive child.

Sometimes, food sensitivities can be at the root of bedwetting, too.

Children may slip up and wet their beds occasionally. A doctor should examine your child if he consistently displays any of these symptoms:

- Wakes up in the middle of the night with extreme thirst
- Complains of backache, stomachache, or fever
- After age 5, wets the bed during day naps as well as night
- Experiences pain during urination
- Begins wetting the bed again after staying dry for several months

Most cases left untreated will result in the child developing complete control over time.

Conventional treatment focuses on behavioral techniques, for example, putting a child on a regular bathroom schedule during the day. Alarms may be set at night to wake the child to void her bladder. Rewards are given to the child as a means of positive reinforcement. Another technique is to use a special device that senses urine in the underwear and sets off an alarm. The child is gradually conditioned to wait until morning to go to the bathroom. This technique is used in children ages 6 and older.

Children who are in a rush when they go to the bathroom must be taught to slow down and void completely. At the beginning, have the child return to the bathroom 5 minutes after voiding to "try again" to void the remaining urine.

Bodywork that improves spinal health and thus proper nerve flow can help treat the underlying cause of bedwetting in many children. Chiropractic and craniosacral therapies are excellent. (See pages 502 and 503 for more on these techniques.)

Counseling may be required for a kid who experiences bedwetting as a result of mental or emotional stress. It is important that the child is not reprimanded or ridiculed for a problem that is not her fault. This can make the situation worse due to the psychological stress put on the child. A patient, supportive, and understanding approach will help the child improve more effectively.

Drug therapy is also used in resistant conditions. The medication desmopressin acetate, a nasal spray, helps the kidneys reabsorb water so that there is not as much urine production. DDAVP is one brand. Special diapers are also available that hold urine and prevent soaking of the bed.

■ BASIC PLAN

Diet

Many children will benefit from identifying foods to which they are sensitive and from eliminating these foods or becoming desensitized to them. The most common food reactions we see in kids that have problems with bedwetting include milk, sugar, citrus fruits, and apple juice. Depending on the child, other foods can be a problem. (See "Food Allergies and Food Sensitivities" on page 298 for ways to identify them.) A natural health care practitioner can help you identify the reactive foods. Note that a bedwetting child should not drink fluids for 2 hours before bedtime.

Nutritional Supplements

Calcium and magnesium—Help to relax the nervous system. Magnesium works to relax the bladder wall and prevent bedwetting. Give 500 milligrams of calcium and 250 to 500 milligrams of magnesium daily with breakfast or lunch.

Herbal Remedies

Horsetail—A tonic for the urinary tract. Have the child take 5 drops two or three times daily for at least 3 weeks to see if there is improvement.

Oatstraw—Helpful for a child who is anxious and stressed. Give 5 to 10 drops three times daily.

Homeopathy

Pick the following remedy that best matches your child's symptoms. Unless otherwise indi-

cated, give your child 2 pellets of a 30C potency twice daily. Improvements should be seen within 7 days. If there is no improvement within 7 days, try another remedy. After you first notice improvement, stop giving the remedy unless symptoms begin to return.

Note: Lower potencies (6X, 12X, 6C) may need to be given more often (three times daily).

Causticum—The child has a history of holding the urine during the day and then urinating at night. She loses urine when sneezing. The child may be very sympathetic and have low confidence and many fears. Urinary muscles are weak.

Equisetum hyemale—When there is no apparent cause for bedwetting, this homeopathic can be helpful.

Ferrum phosphoricum—The child wets her pants during the day while standing.

Ignatia—For bedwetting since an emotional stress. The child is very uptight and moody. She cries easily and wants to be by herself.

Lycopodium—The child has low confidence and worries what others think about her. The embarrassment of bedwetting leads to increased problems with bladder control.

Phosphorus—The child has large thirst for cold drinks and may be drinking too much during the day. Very outgoing child.

Pulsatilla—For a child who is very sensitive emotionally. She may react to fruits and may also be prone to urinary tract infections. She feels the urge to urinate whenever she lies on her back in bed.

Sepia—The child wets the bed the first 1 to 2 hours after going to sleep. She may also lose urine from coughing or laughing.

Acupressure

Kidney 3—Helps to strengthen the kidneys. Located in the depression between the inside ankle bone and the Achilles tendon. Press the acupressure point gently with a thumb for 10 to 15 seconds. Perform on both sides of the body and repeat three times each day.

Aromatherapy

Cypress oil—Add it to a carrier oil and rub it over the lower back and abdomen. Repeat daily. German chamomile can also be used. If the child is taking a homeopathic remedy, use aromatherapy at a different time.

■ WHAT TO EXPECT

Improvement should be noticed within 2 weeks of treatment. If there are not signs of improvement, switch to a different therapy.

Bee Stings

When a bumblebee or honeybee attacks, it leaves its stinger and its attached venom sac in the child's skin. In most cases, the sting creates only slight pain, swelling, and irritation, and is more of a nuisance than a concern. But look for signs of an allergic reaction, such as swollen eyelids or hands, difficulty breathing, wheezing, dizziness, fainting, nausea, vomiting, and the appearance of a hivelike rash. For these symptoms, take your child immediately to the emergency room or your pediatrician's office. Bee stings can be fatal in children who are allergic to bee venom.

Other insects, including fire ants, paper wasps, hornets, and yellow jackets, are capable of stinging but do not leave stingers in their victims.

■ IMMEDIATE TREATMENT

1. Have someone stay with the child to make sure that he does not have an allergic reaction.

2. Wash the site with soap and water.

3. The stinger can be removed using a 4-inch gauze wiped over the area, or by scraping a fingernail or credit card over the area. Never squeeze the stinger or use tweezers. It will cause more venom to go into the skin and injure the muscle.

4. Apply ice to reduce the swelling.

5. Do not scratch the sting. Scratching causes the site to swell and itch more, and increases the chance of infection.

6. If your child is having a severe allergic reaction, seek emergency medical attention. Epinephrine is given by injection to stop allergic reactions.

■ BASIC PLAN

Nutritional Supplement

Vitamin C—Supports the immune system and has mild anti-inflammatory effects. The kind with bioflavonoids is preferable. Dosage: the child's age in years times 50 milligrams, twice daily until the sting has completely healed. Reduce the dosage if diarrhea occurs. Consider using a buffered vitamin C powder (nonacidic) or liquid vitamin C. Both work well for infants and children, and can be mixed in juice.

Homeopathy

Pick the following remedy that best matches your child's symptoms. Unless otherwise indicated, give your child 2 pellets of a 30C potency every 15 minutes for up to three doses. (For infants, crush the pellets into powder and mix it with water.) If there is no improvement within 2 hours, try another remedy. After you first notice improvement, stop giving the remedy unless symptoms begin to return.

Note: Lower potencies (6X, 12X, 6C), if used, should be given every 10 minutes.

Apis mellifica—The first remedy to use for bee stings. The affected area has stinging pain, redness, and swelling.

Carbolic acid—For severe reaction to a bee sting, where the child goes into a severe allergic reaction or coma. This homeopathic can be used in addition to but not in place of emergency medicine.

Bach Flower Rescue Remedy—For emotional upset and anxiety from a bee sting. Give 2 drops every 30 minutes, for up to three doses.

Bites

At any time, a baby or child may be bitten by another child, the family dog or cat, a wild animal, a spider, a snake, or any of a host of insects. The first step is to properly identify the source of the bite to determine the level and immediacy of the treatment required.

Of the 3 million dog bites reported each year, 60 percent of the victims are children, according to the Humane Society of the United States. Dogs and cats may attack when they are disturbed or provoked or when they feel threatened. If possible, you need to verify whether the animal has been vaccinated against rabies. The child may have to undergo a series of injections to keep from developing rabies or tetanus.

Depending on the source of the bite, the skin may be red, swollen, itchy, burning, cut, or bleeding. Animal and human bites carry the risk of infection since the mouth harbors countless bacteria and, sometimes, viruses. Insect and spider bites and stings can be mild or life-threatening, depending on the insect and the victim's sensitivity to an allergic reaction.

Although there are hundreds of different types of snakes found in the United States, only four are poisonous. They are copperheads, coral snakes, rattlesnakes, and water moccasins (also called cottonmouths). The poisonous venom can cause tissue damage, breathing difficulties, dizziness, headaches, nausea, and shock. The amount of venom injected into the victim depends on how recently the snake has eaten.

Medical evaluation and treatment is necessary for all types of bites. Natural therapies can help treatment.

■ BASIC PLAN

Diet

Have your child avoid sugar products while being treated for the bite. Sugar can impair the immune system.

Nutritional Supplements

Vitamin C—Promotes healing of ligaments, tendons, and tissue, and has an anti-inflammatory effect. Dosage: the child's age in years times 50 milligrams, twice daily. Reduce the dosage if diarrhea occurs. Consider using a buffered vitamin C powder (nonacidic) or liquid vitamin C. Both work well for infants and children, and can be mixed in juice.

Zinc—Supports the immune system and enhances skin healing. Daily dosage: children 2 and younger, 5 milligrams; 2 and older, 10 to 15 milligrams. Use for 2 weeks and then stop.

Herbal Remedies

Immune-supportive herbs such as echinacea are a good complementary approach to prevent infection. Goldenseal, lomatium, and other immune-supportive herbs are also indicated. (Follow the herbal dosage information for acute conditions on page 139.)

Homeopathy

Pick the following remedy that best matches your child's symptoms. Unless otherwise indicated, give your child 2 pellets of a 30C potency every 15 minutes for up to three doses. (For infants, crush the pellets into powder and mix it with water.) If there is no improvement within 2 hours, try another remedy. After you first notice improvement, stop giving the remedy unless symptoms begin to return.

Note: Lower potencies (6X, 12X, 6C), if used, should be given every 15 minutes.

Ledum—For puncture wounds from any source. The first remedy to use.

Hypericum perforatum—For puncture wounds where the nerve has been damaged. Sharp, shooting, radiating pain.

Crotalus horridus—A remedy for rattlesnake bites. Use in addition to antivenom from the hospital.

■ WHAT TO EXPECT

Most bites heal well with proper conventional and natural therapies.

Bladder Infection

Also know as irritable bladder, this bacterial infection can affect the entire urinary tract, which consists of the urethra, ureters, kidneys, and bladder.

The bladder is the body's reservoir for urine. Its muscular walls are designed to contract and force the urine from the body through the urethra. Under normal conditions, as the bladder fills with urine, nerve fibers inside its walls detect stretching and alert the brain to the need to empty the bladder.

Children with bladder infections need to urinate frequently. They may complain of burning, stinging pain during and immediately after urination, or foul-smelling urine. Other symptoms include stomachaches, fevers, and wetting the bed at night. Girls are more susceptible to bladder infections than boys because of the structure of the female urinary tract. In girls, the urethra is located close to the rectum, and bacteria from the rectum or lower intestines can easily reach the urethra.

The infection can develop slowly or suddenly. In some cases, the child also experiences cramping pains that intensify over time. Seek immediate medical attention if your child also has blood in the urine, fever, chills, vomiting, or severe lower back pain. These are signs that the infection may have spread to the kidneys. Conventional treatment involves antibiotic therapy.

■ BASIC PLAN

Diet

Fluid intake should be increased to help flush out the bacterial infection. Unsweetened cranberry juice is excellent, as studies show that it prevents bacteria from adhering to the bladder wall. Have your child drink 8 to 16 ounces of cranberry juice throughout the day and for 5 days after the infection has cleared. The taste may be too strong for younger kids and should be diluted in water. Cranberry juice extract tablets are also available. Purified water should also be increased to six 6-ounce glasses of water daily. Avoid sugar products of any kind, as they can lower immunity. Fruit juices (especially citrus fruits if the problem is chronic) other than cranberry should be limited, and if used should be highly diluted: 4 parts water to 1 part juice.

Chronic bladder or urinary tract infections can be the result of food sensitivities. Common sensitivities for this condition include citrus fruit, milk, and sugar. (See "Food Allergies and Food Sensitivities" on page 298 for more information.)

Nutritional Supplement

Vitamin C—Supports the immune system. Dosage: the child's age in years times 50 milligrams, twice daily. Reduce the dosage if diarrhea occurs. Consider using a buffered vitamin C powder (nonacidic) or liquid vitamin C. Both work well for infants and children, and can be mixed in juice.

Herbal Remedy

Combine the following:

Echinacea and goldenseal combination—Supports the immune system to get over an infection. Helpful for both bacterial and viral infections. 15 drops.

Uva-ursi or horsetail—Uva-ursi is one of the best herbs to fight infections of the urinary tract. Horsetail is an an antiseptic herb for the urinary tract. 10 drops.

Marshmallow root—Soothing to the bladder and urinary tract. 10 drops.

Add the mixture to water or diluted juice (preferably cranberry) and serve. Give this

Vital Fact

Approximately 3 percent of girls and 1 percent of boys have had a urinary tract infection by age 11.

remedy every 2 to 3 hours throughout the day. Continue giving the remedy until 1 week after the infection seems to have cleared.

Homeopathy

The following are remedies for acute bladder infections. Pick the one which best matches your child's symptoms. Unless otherwise indicated, give your child 2 pellets of a 30C potency every 2 hours. Improvements should be seen within 8 hours. If there is no improvement within 8 hours, try another remedy. After you first notice improvement, stop giving the remedy unless symptoms begin to return.

Note: Lower potencies (6X, 12X, 6C) may need to be given more often (every hour).

Aconitum napellus—Give at the very first symptoms of a urinary tract infection. The child may be spiking a fever and crying and/or screaming from the pain. Urination is hot and painful.

Apis mellifica—For stinging and burning pain with urination. Also helpful when the child is not able to urinate with the bladder infection. The pain gets worse with heat or warm applications (such as a warm bath) and better with cold.

Cantharis—The most common remedy for bladder infections. If it is hard to tell which homeopathic remedy to use, start with Cantharis and see if it helps. Symptoms include burning and cutting pains with urination, and a sense of urgency to urinate. Only small amounts of urine may come out at first when the child tries to empty her bladder. Blood may be present.

Mercurius corrosivus—The urine contains blood and pus and has an offensive odor. The child has great burning pains.

Pulsatilla—For the frequent urge to urinate. The child wants attention and to be held. She cries easily.

Sarsaparilla—For burning pain that occurs at the end of urination.

Constitutional Hydrotherapy

This stimulates the immune system and reduces inflammation of the urinary tract. (For directions, see Hydrotherapy for Children on page 115.)

■ ADVANCED PLAN

Nutritional Supplements

Zinc—Supports the immune system. Daily dosage: children 2 and younger, 5 milligrams; 2 and older, 10 to 15 milligrams. Use for 2 weeks and then stop.

Vitamin A—Helps support the immune system. Available in liquid drops. Daily dosage: infants under 1 year, 1,875 international units (IU); children 1 to 3, 2,000 IU; kids 4 to 6, 2,500 IU; kids 7 to 10, 3,500 IU; males

11 and older, 5,000 IU; females 11 and older, 4,000 IU.

Note: These dosages are for short-term use (up to 10 days). Higher dosages may be used only under a doctor's supervision.

Thymus glandular extract—Give one to two 250-milligram tablets or capsules daily.

Probiotic—In cases where antibiotics have been used, make sure to give a supplement of children's acidophilus with bifidus for a minimum of 2 months to replace good bacteria. Give as directed on the container.

Cranberry extract—Inhibits bacteria from attaching to the bladder wall. Give 10 milligrams per pound of body weight daily, in tablet or capsule form. Helpful to prevent chronic bladder infections.

Aromatherapy

Eucalyptus and sandalwood—Add these essential oils to a carrier oil and rub it over the lower abdomen. If taking a homeopathic remedy, use aromatherapy at a different time.

Acupressure

Press the acupressure point gently with a thumb for 10 to 15 seconds. Do this for each of the following points. Perform on both sides of the body and repeat three times each day.

Kidney 3—Located in the depression between the inside ankle bone and the Achilles tendon.

Large Intestine 4—Located in the webbing between the thumb and the index finger.

■ WHAT TO EXPECT

Your child will most likely be prescribed antibiotics. Natural therapies should be used as a complementary treatment to quicken recovery. Improvements should be noticed within 24 to 48 hours.

Blisters

Blisters are fluid-filled sacs just under the top layer of skin. Most are harmless and more of a source of nuisance or curiosity for children. As a blister forms, clear fluid fills in a pocket formed between the separated layers of skin; this is known as a friction blister. If a small blood vessel is broken as the blister forms, the fluid will contain blood instead of clear fluid and is known as a blood blister.

Left alone, the fluid in a friction blister will be gradually reabsorbed by the body. The blistered skin will fall off and be replaced by healthy new skin forming below it.

In newborns, blisters can occur on the upper lips. Known as sucking pads, these blisters form from breast- or bottlefeeding or from sucking on a pacifier. They are normal and often last until 1 year of age. They do not bother the baby and should be left alone.

In children, blisters can result from an injury to the skin caused by continual friction, allergic reactions, or chemical burns. Blisters on feet are often due to improperly fitting shoes or to not wearing socks with shoes. Blisters on hands are the result of too much friction between your child's hand and an object such as a baseball bat. Exposure to poison ivy, poison oak, or poison sumac can result in seeping blisters.

See a physician about any blister that shows these signs of infection:

- Prolonged pain
- Redness beyond the blister area
- Oozing pus
- Red lines streaking away from the blister site
- Fever
- Yellow crusting around the blister

■ BASIC PLAN

To prevent infection, do not open up small blisters. If it appears that a blister is going to burst, puncture it with a sterilized needle (sterilize the needle by holding it over a flame) and cover it with a bandage. Remove the bandage at nighttime to allow the blister to dry out.

If blisters are recurring on your child's feet, check the fit of shoes to make sure that they aren't too wide or too narrow. New shoes should be broken in for short periods of time over the first week of use. If your child is involved in a lot of activities and his feet sweat a lot, have him change socks more often.

Diet

We recommend a diet that increases the nutrients involved in skin healing. Essential fatty acids are found in flaxseeds; in coldwater fish such as salmon, halibut, and trout; and in fresh nuts and seeds. Fresh vegetables and fruits provide vitamins C and A, flavonoids, and minerals involved in skin healing. Sugar products should be limited to optimize skin regeneration.

Nutritional Supplement

Vitamin C—Promotes healing of skin. Dosage: the child's age in years times 50 milligrams, daily. Reduce the dosage if diarrhea occurs. Consider using a buffered vitamin C powder (nonacidic) or liquid vitamin C. Both work well for infants and children, and can be mixed in juice.

Herbal Remedies

Calendula—Apply topically twice daily as a tincture or ointment to speed skin healing and prevent infection.

Tea tree oil—Apply topically to blisters that appear infected (they are red and may have yellowish fluid). Also see a physician if an infection is present.

Homeopathy

Pick the following remedy that best matches your child's symptoms. Unless otherwise indicated, give your child 2 pellets of a 30C potency twice daily. Improvements should be seen within 5 days. If there is no improvement within 5 days, try another remedy. After you first notice improvement, stop giving the remedy unless symptoms begin to return.

Note: Lower potencies (6X, 12X, 6C) may need to be given more often (three times daily).

Apis mellifica—For a fluid-filled blister that burns and/or stings. The blister feels better with warm applications.

Cantharis—For blisters that occur from heat burns.

Causticum—For blisters that occur from chemical burns.

Silica—For blisters that appear to be filled with white fluid and are about to discharge.

■ ADVANCED PLAN

Nutritional Supplement

Zinc—Supports the immune system and enhances skin healing. Daily dosage: children 2 and younger, 5 milligrams; 2 and older, 10 to 15 milligrams. Use for 2 weeks and then stop.

Herbal Remedy

Aloe vera gel—Apply this topically to aid skin healing. Choose a product that is as close to 100 percent aloe vera as possible.

■ WHAT TO EXPECT

Healing should take approximately 5 to 10 days, as long as the irritating cause has been removed (for instance, a poorly fitting shoe). If there are signs of infection, see a doctor.

Blocked Tear Duct

By 3 weeks of age, most newborns' eyes begin tearing. Normally, the tears drain through tiny tear ducts at the inside corners of the eyes into the nose. A newborn has a thin membrane that covers these ducts. It usually breaks open soon after birth and allows proper drainage of the tears. If this membrane does not open fully, dacryostenosis, a blockage of the tear ducts, occurs, and infection is common. Resulting symptoms include a yellow, sticky discharge around the eyes and a watery discharge that is worsened by wind, dust, and nasal congestion.

Conventional treatment is to recommend massage of the blockage and antibiotics as necessary for infection. Hot and cold cloths can be alternated over the affected area to improve circulation and reduce congestion. Cases that do not resolve are treated by using a probe to open the obstructed membrane(s).

■ BASIC PLAN

Gently massage the tear duct that drains the eye, located in the inner, lower corner of the eye (where you see a little red bump). Massage in an upward direction, toward the nose, five times. Repeat this process three or more times during the day. This helps to open up the membrane that is clogging the passageway for tears to drain.

Nutritional Supplements

Vitamin C—Supports the immune system to prevent infection. Dosage: the child's age in years times 50 milligrams, daily. Reduce the dosage if diarrhea occurs. Consider using a buffered vitamin C powder (nonacidic) or liquid vitamin C.

Vital Fact

Blocked tear duct affects as many as 15 percent of newborns. The blockage resolves on its own by age 6 in 50 to 90 percent of children. There is a 70 percent chance that a 6-month-old will experience complete resolution of this problem by age 1.

Colloidal silver—If an infection is present, use 1 drop in the affected area twice daily. Silver particles in suspension are available at any health food store.

Herbal Remedy

Echinacea—Stimulates the immune system to help prevent infection. Echinacea is taken internally.

Homeopathy

Silica 6X—The most common remedy for blocked tear ducts. Give 2 pellets of Silica 6X three times daily. (For infants, crush the pellets into powder and mix it with water.) Try it along with massage for up to 12 weeks; if there is no improvement, then surgery may be necessary.

Hydrotherapy

Apply a warm, soft washcloth to the infant's eye for 2 minutes. Follow with a cold application for 2 minutes. Do three times daily.

■ WHAT TO EXPECT

Most blocked tear ducts resolve on their own. Massage and homeopathic treatment can be very effective. Try this approach for up to 2 months. Consult with your child's doctor if infection is present.

Bloody Nose

Inside a child's nose are tiny, delicate blood vessels that can easily rupture and lead to a bloody nose. The amount of blood from a nosebleed can be just a trickle or a steady stream.

Some nosebleeds are the result of rough-and-tumble play in which the nose is accidentally smacked. They can occur because of too-vigorous blowing with a tissue or from aggressively picking inside the nostrils with a sharp fingernail.

Dry winter air, a cold, or an allergy can also cause the tiny capillaries inside the lining of the nose to swell and rupture. Medical conditions such as hemophilia, high blood pressure, or leukemia can also lead to nosebleeds.

Nosebleeds usually are not painful, but they can be very frightening to a child, especially if she wakes up in the middle of the night with a bloody nose. At night, a child may swallow some blood and later vomit it up or pass a dark stool after the bleeding has stopped.

Nosebleeds are rarely serious. However, seek emergency medical care for the following situations:

- You cannot stop your child's nosebleed.
- The bleeding occurs frequently and lasts longer than 15 minutes per episode.
- Your child is bleeding from other areas of the face, including the gums.
- A severe blow to the head triggered the nosebleed.
- Your child has difficulty breathing.

■ IMMEDIATE TREATMENT

Have the child sit up and lean forward so that she does not swallow blood. Hold a towel or bowl below the child's mouth so that blood can be spit out if necessary. Insert a wet cotton ball or tissue into the bleeding nostril. Tightly pinch the soft parts of the nose together for 10 minutes. Tell the child to breathe through her mouth. If the bleeding does not resolve in 30 minutes, or if the nosebleed falls into one of the emergency categories, see a doctor. Petroleum jelly applied to the inside center wall of each nostril can help relieve dryness that is causing repeated bleeding of the nose.

Homeopathy

Pick the following remedy that best matches your child's symptoms. Unless otherwise indicated, give your child 2 pellets of a 30C potency every 10 minutes for up to three doses. If there is no improvement within 30 minutes, see a doctor. After you first notice improvement, stop giving the remedy unless symptoms begin to return.

Note: Lower potencies (6X, 12X, 6C), if used, should be given every 5 minutes.

Arnica montana—For nosebleed from trauma.

Phosphorus—For nosebleed from dry air or for children prone to repeated nosebleeds for no apparent cause. Give twice daily for 2 to 3 weeks as a preventative. Can also be used to treat acute nosebleeds. Give a dose every 10 minutes until the nosebleed stops.

Acupressure
Governing Vessel 26—Located two-thirds of the way up from the upper lip to the nose. Press the acupressure point gently with a thumb for 10 to 15 seconds. Repeat three times each day.

■ WHAT TO EXPECT
Acute, gushing nosebleeds should clear within 5 to 15 minutes. See a doctor if chronic nosebleeds are a problem.

Brittle Nails

Nails are made of skin cells hardened by a protein called keratin. The different parts of a fingernail include:

- The nail plate (the visible covering)
- The nail bed (the skin underneath the nail plate)
- The cuticle (the fold of skin at the base of the nail plate)
- The matrix (located under the cuticle)
- The lunula (the white, half-moon-shaped portion of the nail matrix)

Nails, with their hard shells, protect the tissue underneath and assist in manual dexterity. Fingernails are constantly at risk of being nicked, torn, or bruised or exposed to chemicals and infections.

The health of fingernails mirrors the health of the body. Skin conditions such as psoriasis or fungal infections can cause nails to become flaky and brittle. Fingernails are influenced by nutritional habits and digestive health. Children who do not eat a healthy diet are prone to brittle or splitting nails. Brittle nails that break easily can be deficiency signs for protein, vitamin A, vitamin B_{12}, iron, sulfur, silica, calcium, and other minerals in a child's diet.

■ BASIC PLAN

Diet
Follow a whole-foods diet. (See "Diet" on page 4 for more information.) Quality protein sources are important, such as fish, legumes, nuts, and lean poultry. In addition, foods rich in B vitamins such as whole grains should be increased. Sulfur-rich foods such as broccoli, garlic, onions, and sea vegetables should also be included in the diet. Calcium-rich sources such as carrots, broccoli, and calcium-enriched rice or soy milks are recommended; give only limited amounts of dairy products. Decrease the consumption of sugars and soft drinks, which leach minerals out of the body.

Nutritional Supplement
Children's multivitamin—Provides many of the nutrients involved in nail formation. Give as directed on the container daily.

Herbal Remedies

Children with weak digestion can benefit from herbs such as fennel, ginger root, and gentian root. Give one or a combination of these herbs with meals to tonify the digestive system and improve absorption.

Homeopathy

Pick the following remedy that best matches your child's symptoms. Unless otherwise indicated, give your child 2 pellets of a 30C potency twice daily. Improvements should be seen within 14 days. If there is no improvement within 14 days, try another remedy. After you first notice improvement, stop giving the remedy unless symptoms begin to return.

Note: Lower potencies (6X, 12X, 6C) may need to be given more often (three times daily).

Silica 6X—A specific remedy for tissue and nail health. Have the child take 2 pellets two or three times daily for 2 months or longer.

Calcarea carbonica—A remedy for large, flabby children whose nails break and peel easily.

■ ADVANCED PLAN

Nutritional Supplements

Biotin—A deficiency of this B vitamin can cause brittle nails. Especially indicated if your child has cradle cap and brittle nails. Recommended dosages for brittle nails: children 3 and under, 100 micrograms; kids ages 4 to 9, 200 micrograms; kids 10 and older, 300 micrograms.

Probiotic—Choose a children's formula that contains acidophilus and bifidus. These good bacteria are required to synthesize biotin and other minerals. Give as directed on the container.

Methylsulfonylmethane (MSM)—A good source of the mineral sulfur. Give 5 milligrams per pound of body weight daily. Cut back if diarrhea occurs. Available in liquid form.

Silica—Available as colloidal silica or horsetail extract. Give 4 milligrams per pound of body weight daily.

Homeopathy

Cell salt combination—Choose a combination of the 12 cell salts in one formula such as Bioplasma 6. Have the child take 2 pellets twice daily for at least 2 months.

■ WHAT TO EXPECT

Natural treatment should improve the health of the nails visibly within 1 to 2 months.

Broken Bones

A bad fall, a hard blow, an automobile collision, a sports injury, or an underlying medical condition can cause broken bones, or fractures, in children. Parents need to realize that bones are living, growing tissues that contain an ample supply of blood vessels and nerves.

When a bone breaks, it not only triggers pain, swelling, bruising, and immobility but it also causes trauma and shock throughout the entire body. Fractures located near joints are sometimes misidentified as simply bad sprains.

There are varying degrees of fractures. Here are definitions and causes for some types of fractures.

Partial (incomplete)—A break across the bone is incomplete.

Complete—The bone is broken in two pieces.

Closed (simple)—The broken bone does not protrude through the skin.

Open (compound)—The broken bone protrudes through the skin.

Comminuted—The bone is splintered at the broken area and many smaller fragments of bone are found between the two main pieces.

Greenstick—Only occurs in children and is defined by having one side of the bone break and the other side just bend. Often seen on the radius (forearm bone).

Spiral—Breaking force twists the bone apart.

Transverse—Occurs at right angles to the bone.

Impacted—One fragment is forcibly driven into the other.

Colles'—Fracture of the distal end of the radius (a wrist fracture), and the fragment is displaced posteriorly (toward the back of the wrist).

Potts'—Fracture of the distal end of the fibula (the lower portion of the leg) with serious injury of the distal tibia articulation (where the leg bone connects with the ankle).

Non-displaced—Correct anatomical alignment of the bone is maintained.

Displaced—Correct anatomical alignment of the bone is not maintained.

Stress—Partial fracture resulting from the inability of the bone to withstand repeated stresses, such as doing aerobics on hard surfaces or running long distances for prolonged periods of time. Almost one-fourth of stress fractures occur in the fibula.

Pathologic—A fracture that is a result of normal stress on a weakened bone. It occurs in such diseases as osteoporosis, neoplasia, osteomyelitis, and osteomalacia.

Natural therapies can help increase bone healing and decrease pain and discomfort.

■ BASIC PLAN

Diet

A diet focused on whole grains and vegetables will provide many of the minerals needed for healing a broken bone. Consume foods rich in the following for bone healing:

Calcium—Found in low-fat dairy products (unless your child is sensitive to them), collard greens, almonds, carrots, tofu, broccoli, wheat bran, kale.

Magnesium—Found in whole grains, tofu, nuts and seeds, and green leafy vegetables.

Boron—Found in nuts and seeds.

Vitamin K—Found in green leafy vegetables.

Case History

It was midnight when Dr. Mark's sister called. Her 4-year-old son, Ryan, had broken his wrist after falling out of bed. He had been x-rayed and given a cast at the hospital. Ryan's mother had already given him the homeopathic remedy Arnica montana to help with the initial pain and swelling. Dr. Mark had her follow with Symphytum, the number one homeopathic remedy for broken bones. Symphytum works so well that homeopathic practitioners advise patients to make sure that the bone is properly set, because it stimulates bone healing quickly.

Ryan's mom also continued giving him his liquid calcium-magnesium supplement as well as a children's multivitamin. This ensured that all the nutrients required for bone healing were present. On a follow-up visit, Ryan's doctor commented that his fracture had healed in half the time it usually takes for a fracture of this type to heal.

Silica—Found in rolled oats, which can be eaten as porridge or in Swiss muesli cereal.

Green leafy vegetables and whole grains provide a variety of other minerals that are good for bone health.

Protein is important, too; fresh fish such as salmon, halibut, and mackerel are good. They also contain vitamin D necessary for bone healing. Soy products are also good sources of protein, as is lean poultry.

Vitamin D is helpful as well. Expose your child to direct sunlight for at least 15 minutes daily for vitamin D. This nutrient is also found in dairy products, green leafy vegetables, and eggs.

Avoid soft drinks, as phosphoric acid leads to calcium excretion. Limit sugar, as it can interfere with the healing process. Limit red meat, too; high amounts can lead to calcium loss.

Nutritional Supplements

Calcium and magnesium—Give 500 to 1,000 milligrams of calcium and 250 to 500 milligrams of magnesium daily. Available in liquid form. Almost always bought in a formula, but can be given separately.

Children's multivitamin—Ensures that all the vitamins and minerals for bone healing are present. Give as directed on the container.

Homeopathy

Pick the following remedy that best matches your child's symptoms. Unless otherwise indicated, give your child 2 pellets of a 30C potency three times daily. Improvements in pain should be seen within 48 hours. If there is no improvement within 48 hours, try another remedy. After you first notice improvement, stop giving the remedy unless symptoms begin to return.

Note: Lower potencies (6X, 12X, 6C) may

need to be given more often (four times daily).

Arnica montana—Give 2 pellets immediately after the trauma has occurred. This will help reduce pain, shock, and swelling. Give the highest potency available. If a lower potency such as 12X or 12C is what is available, then repeat it every 15 minutes while going for medical attention.

Bryonia alba—To be given when the child is very irritable with the fracture and the slightest movement aggravates his pain. Can be alternated with Symphytum (give 2 pellets of one remedy, then give 2 pellets of the other remedy 3 hours later). The first remedy to give for rib fractures.

Calcarea phosphorica 6X—Specific for fractures that are taking longer than normal to heal. Give 2 pellets two or three times daily until the fracture has healed.

Symphytum—The number one homeopathic remedy for fractures. To be given after a fracture has been diagnosed and set into place. Speeds up the healing of fractures. Give 2 pellets of a 30C potency twice daily for 5 days.

Hydrotherapy

Alternate hot and cold towels over the opposite of the body part affected. For example, if the left arm is broken, alternate a hot towel (2 minutes) with a cold towel (2 minutes) over the right arm, repeat three times, and perform twice daily. There is a reflex action whereby circulation will be increased in the opposite body part, which increases nutrition to the healing bone.

■ ADVANCED PLAN

Nutritional Supplement

Vitamin C—Required for bone and soft tissue. The type with bioflavonoids is preferable. Dosage: the child's age in years times 50 milligrams, twice daily. Reduce the dosage if diarrhea occurs. Consider using a buffered vitamin C powder (nonacidic) or liquid vitamin C. Both work well for infants and children, and can be mixed in juice.

Herbal Remedies

Nettle—Contains silica and other minerals involved in bone healing. Give a dose twice daily until bone has healed.

Horsetail extract—An excellent source of silica. Give a dose twice daily until the bone has healed.

■ WHAT TO EXPECT

Homeopathic treatment can often reduce the discomfort associated with a fracture, but painkillers are generally still required. Children following the listed natural protocol recover significantly faster than children who are not given natural therapy.

Bronchiolitis

Bronchiolitis is an acute viral infection of the lower respiratory tract that primarily affects babies between 2 and 8 months old. Babies less than 6 months old or those with a family history of allergies are at even greater risk of developing this condition. About 11 in 100 children under age 1 develop bronchiolitis each year. Premature babies are at a higher risk of developing complications from this virus.

Early symptoms mimic a cold but then progress into a hacking cough, wheezing, and rapid, shallow breathing. The inflammation can become widespread and cause the airways to swell, spasm, and contract. Some babies develop fevers, lose their appetites, become irritable, and feel lethargic.

In severe cases of bronchiolitis, a baby's breathing is rapid, his face is slightly bluish, and his lungs are unable to expand fully with each inhalation. This condition can lead to pneumonia and respiratory failure.

The primary cause of bronchiolitis is respiratory syncytial virus (RSV), which tends to occur between the late fall and early spring. It typically develops after a baby has a few days of a cold and the symptoms start to worsen. Allergies can also contribute to this condition.

Conventional treatment focuses on the use of bronchodilators. More serious cases require hospitalization and the administration of oxygen and fluids. The antiviral drug ribavirin and/or immunoglobulin may be given to infants who have a preexisting lung disease. RSV vaccine is recommended by conventional doctors for high-risk infants.

■ BASIC PLAN

Infants should be kept from close contact with children or adults who are in the early or later stages of respiratory infections.

Diet

Mucus-forming foods should be avoided, including dairy products such as cows' milk and cows' milk–based formulas, cheese, and bananas. Eliminate refined sugar products, as they can lower immune function. Liquid foods such as soup are helpful.

Make sure that the infant drinks lots of fluids. If he is breastfed, continue normal feedings and nurse as often as possible.

Nutritional Supplements

Vitamin A—Supports the immune system. Daily dosage: infants under 1 year, 1,875 international units (IU); children 1 to 3, 2,000 IU; kids 4 to 6, 2,500 IU; kids 7 to 10, 3,500 IU; males 11 and older, 5,000 IU; females 11 and older, 4,000 IU.

Note: These dosages are for short-term use (up to 10 days). Higher dosages may be used only under a doctor's supervision. Available in liquid drops.

Vitamin C—Provides support to the immune system. Dosage: the child's age in years times 50 milligrams, twice daily. Reduce the dosage if diarrhea occurs. Consider using a buffered vitamin C powder (nonacidic) or liquid vitamin C. Both work well for infants and children, and can be mixed in juice.

Herbal Remedy

Echinacea or larix (L. occidentalis)— Echinacea has antiviral properties and supports the immune system. Larix, also known as Western larch, is immune-supportive as well.

Homeopathy

Any one of the following homeopathic remedies can be crushed, mixed in ¼ cup of water, and given orally. In cases where the child is in the hospital and intubated, a few drops can be rubbed on the chest. You can use a combination bronchitis formula, which contains a mixture of common homeopathics for bronchial symptoms. Or pick one of the following remedies that best matches your child's symptoms. For the remedies below, unless otherwise indicated, give your child 2 pellets of a 30C potency three times daily. Improvements should be seen within 48 hours. If there is no improvement within 48 hours, try another remedy. After you first notice improvement, stop giving the remedy unless symptoms begin to return.

Note: Lower potencies (6X, 12X, 6C) may need to be given more often (four times daily).

Arsenicum album—For symptoms of wheezing, chilliness, and restlessness.

Antimonium tartaricum—The chest rattles with mucus, but the child is unable to expectorate it. The child is weak and has difficulty breathing.

Phosphorus—For a cough that is worse on exposure to cold air and better after drinking cold drinks.

■ WHAT TO EXPECT

Natural treatment can help reduce the severity of the bronchiolitis as a complementary treatment and does not interfere with any conventional therapy.

Bronchitis

There are two types of bronchitis: acute and chronic. Acute bronchitis is an inflammation of the main airways of the lungs, bronchi, and trachea (the windpipe) that lasts less than 2 weeks. Symptoms begin with a dry, shallow cough that worsens into a deep cough that brings up yellow or gray phlegm or mucus from the lungs. There is shallow breathing, wheezing, upper chest pain, coughing, a runny nose, and a mild fever.

It is usually caused by a viral infection, sometimes in combination with a bacterial infection. The main viral culprits include influenza, respiratory syncytial virus (RSV), and the common cold.

Children are most susceptible to acute bronchitis in the winter or if they have developed a common cold or sore throat. Exposure to air pollutants and chilly weather as well as poor nutrition can increase their risk. Other factors include exposure to tobacco smoke or pungent fumes (ammonia, chlorine, sulfur dioxide, and bromine) and allergies to molds, pollens, dander, and dust.

Chronic bronchitis is a persistent inflammation of the airways that worsens with time. Its telltale sign is a mild but constant mucus-producing cough that can last 3 months or longer during the winter season. Coughing is worse in the morning. Wheezing and breathlessness are also common symptoms.

Over time, this condition can thicken and distort the linings of the bronchioles and bronchi, possibly narrowing or blocking the airways. The constant coughing causes pain in the lungs and respiratory system. Ignored, chronic bronchitis can lead to pneumonia, pulmonary hypertension, and heart failure.

Exposure to heavy concentrations of dust, irritating fumes, air pollution, and other nonspecific bronchial irritants can worsen symptoms.

Seek medical attention if your child has any of the following symptoms:

- A cough that has not improved in 3 days
- The child is an infant who is coughing often
- A high fever (above 103°F)
- Trouble breathing, or wheezing is present, or the chest is moving up and down unusually
- Lethargy
- Change of skin color, such as a blue tinge on the lips or tongue

Conventional treatment focuses on rest, increased fluids, antibiotic treatment for secondary bacterial infections, and bronchodilators. Prop the child's head up with pillows at night to help her breathe easier. Encourage productive coughing. Coughing is a reflex that enables mucus and infections to be expelled from the respiratory passageway. Gentle patting on the back can be helpful for infants. Suppression of a cough can lead to a more serious illness, such as pneumonia.

■ BASIC PLAN

Diet
Have your child go on a low-mucus diet by avoiding foods such as dairy products and ba-

nanas. Eliminate refined sugar products, as they can lower immune function. Soups, stews, and steamed vegetables are preferred foods. Garlic, fresh ginger, and onions are also good to help relieve congestion.

If the bronchitis is chronic, food sensitivities are often a problem. (See "Food Allergies and Food Sensitivities" on page 298 for more information.)

Increase the child's fluid intake. Have her drink fluids every 2 to 3 hours. The temperature of the child's environment should be based on her preference.

Nutritional Supplements
Vitamin A—Supports the immune system. Daily dosage: infants under 1 year, 1,875 international units (IU); children 1 to 3, 2,000 IU; kids 4 to 6, 2,500 IU; kids 7 to 10, 3,500 IU; males 11 and older, 5,000 IU; females 11 and older, 4,000 IU.

Note: These dosages are for short-term use (up to 10 days). Higher dosages may be used only under a doctor's supervision. Available in liquid drops.

Vitamin C—Supports the immune system. Dosage: the child's age in years times 50 milligrams, twice daily. Reduce the dosage if diarrhea occurs. Consider using a buffered vitamin C powder (nonacidic) or liquid vitamin C. Both work well for infants and children, and can be mixed in juice.

Herbal Remedies
Children's herbal cough formula—Cough formulas often include one or more of

the following herbs: echinacea, goldenseal, mullein, wild cherry bark, horehound, and licorice. They may also contain essential oils such as peppermint leaf extract or menthol oil to help open up the respiratory passageways. Follow the instructions on the container.

Echinacea and goldenseal—If a children's herbal cough formula is not available, then use this combination. (Follow the herbal dosage information for acute conditions on page 139.)

Homeopathy

There are many remedies that can be used for bronchitis. It is easiest to use a combination cough formula, or you can choose the single remedy that matches your child's symptoms. If you opt for the latter, pick the following remedy that best matches your child's symptoms. Unless otherwise indicated, give your child 2 pellets of a 30C potency three times daily. Improvements should be seen within 24 hours. If there is no improvement within 24 hours, try another remedy. After you first notice improvement, stop giving the remedy unless symptoms begin to return.

Note: Lower potencies (6X, 12X, 6C) may need to be given more often (four times daily).

Aconitum napellus—For a short, dry cough from exposure to dry, cold air. The child has great restlessness and anxiety, hot skin, and feels better lying on her back. The child is thirsty. Useful in the initial stage of a cough—the first 4 hours of symptoms.

Antimonium tartaricum—For a deep, rattling cough. The child has trouble expectorating mucus and may find it hard to breathe at times. She feels better in a cool room with the window open. Used in the more advanced stages of bronchitis.

Arsenicum album—For a cough with burning pain. The cough is worse at night (midnight to 2:00 A.M.) and gets better with warm applications and warm drinks. The child is restless and anxious.

Bryonia alba—For a dry cough that is very painful. Worse with any movement or when taking a deep breath. The child feels better in the open air, has a high thirst for cold drinks, and is irritable.

Coccus cacti—For a cough that produces stringy mucus. The child constantly clears her throat. The cough leads to vomiting.

Drosera—For a dry, barking cough that may end in gagging. The cough is worse lying down and tends to come on after midnight.

Hepar sulphuris—For a rattling, barking cough that comes on after exposure to dry, cold air. The child coughs when she is uncovered or gets undressed. Yellow mucus discharge. The child is irritable.

Ipecacuanha—For a cough with a lot of mucus that makes the child nauseated, gag, or vomit. The mucus may have tinges of blood in it.

Kali bichromicum—Thick, stringy, ropy, yellow or yellowish-green mucus is coughed up. The child gets worse from eating and drinking.

Phosphorus—For a cold that turns into bronchitis. A dry, tickling cough. The child may have burning in her chest and feels better with cold drinks. The cough is worse lying on the left side. The child is hoarse and desires company when sick.

Pulsatilla—For a cough with green or yellow-green mucus. The child is warm and clingy; she feels better in fresh air and when held. The cough is often worse at night and while lying down. The child is thirstless.

Rumex crispus—For a dry cough that begins when lying down. A tickling sensation in the throat leads to a cough. The cough is worse in cold or open air.

Spongia tosta—For a dry, barking cough that is better with warm foods or liquids. The child is hoarse.

Hydrotherapy

Constitutional hydrotherapy is excellent, as it reduces congestion in the bronchial tubes and brings good immune cells into the infected area. The second option is foot hydrotherapy. (See Hydrotherapy for Children on page 115 for directions on these treatments.) Perform either treatment one or two times daily.

You can also go into the bathroom, turn the shower on, and allow steam to fill up the room. Then sit in the bathroom with the child for 5 minutes. This will help her breathe easier.

■ ADVANCED PLAN

Nutritional Supplement

Zinc—Supports the immune system. Dosage: children 2 and younger, 5 milligrams; 2 and older, 10 to 15 milligrams. Use for 2 weeks and then stop.

Herbal Remedies

Peppermint tea—Can help reduce irritating coughs. Use it if a child is feverish or has digestive upset.

Ginger tea—Good for bronchitis where the child is chilly and has mucus production.

Aromatherapy

Eucalyptus, tea tree oil, and frankincense—Add these to a carrier oil and apply to the child's chest, or add 2 or 3 drops to a vaporizer and allow the fragrance to fill the room. Or add 2 drops of each oil to a bath. (See Aromatherapy for Children on page 109 for more information.) If your child is taking a homeopathic remedy, use aromatherapy at a different time.

Acupressure

Pericardium 6—Relaxes the bronchial passageway. Located 2½ finger-widths below the wrist crease, in the middle of the forearm (palm side). Gently press the acupressure point with a thumb for 10 to 15 seconds. Perform on both sides of the body and repeat three times each day.

Lung 1—Reduces cough. Located in the front of the shoulder area, in the space below where the collarbone and shoulder meet. Gently press the acupressure point with a thumb for 10 to 15 seconds. Perform on both sides of the body and repeat three times each day.

■ WHAT TO EXPECT

Improvement should be noticed within 2 days of treatment. Except where noted, do not discontinue therapy once the child has shown initial signs of improvement; continue until the condition has completely resolved.

Bruises

A bruise is an injury caused by a blow or bump that does not cut the skin but breaks blood vessels underneath the skin. Blood seeps out of these vessels, producing the telltale black-and-blue discoloration as well as swelling and soreness. Black eyes are also nothing more than bruises.

The deeper the bruise, or contusion, the longer it will take to heal. Leg bruises, for instance, can linger for up to 4 weeks because leg vessels have greater blood pressure than arm vessels.

Bruises also change in color, first starting off red, then turning blackish blue and finally yellowish green. The final color is a sign that the body has worked to remove the dead cells and tissues and replace them with healthy, new cells which will restore the color to the skin.

Falls, sprains, pinches, and suction can cause bruises. These are occupational hazards for active children who love to run, jump, bike, climb, or skate. Children who are anemic or obese tend to bruise easily. Sometimes, unexplained bruising can be a clue to parents that the child's blood vessel walls are brittle or that the child has insufficient blood clotting factors. Bruising can also signal the onset of serious illnesses such as leukemia or hemophilia.

Parents should have their child's bruise examined by a doctor under the following circumstances:

- The bruise is located on the head or in the eye area.
- Bruising seems to show up without any apparent cause.
- A minor bump or blow creates a large bruise.
- Bruises are located in unusual places such as the back, the calves, or the backs of the arms.
- Your child has difficulty talking, walking, or seeing or appears drowsy and dizzy.
- A fever accompanies the bruising.

Easy bruising or bruises that do not heal may be the result of anemia. See a doctor for a blood test. (For more information, see "Anemia" on page 153.)

Conventional approaches to bruises include elevation of the affected area, pain medications, and rest. Ice applications also work well. For the first 24 hours, apply an ice bag to the bruised area for 5 to 10 minutes at a time. Do not apply ice directly to skin; wrap the ice in a cloth.

■ BASIC PLAN

Diet

Increase food sources of vitamin C and flavonoids. These can take the form of whole foods or fresh juices. Good fruit examples are apples, oranges, grapefruit, pears, blueberries, tomatoes, cherries, grapes, and strawberries.

Kale, broccoli, cauliflower, and carrots are good vegetable examples.

Papaya contains enzymes that help to heal bruises. Eat papaya or drink fresh papaya juice on an empty stomach.

Nutritional Supplements

Vitamin C—Speeds up tissue healing and has mild anti-inflammatory effects. The kind with bioflavonoids is preferable. Dosage: the child's age in years times 50 milligrams, twice daily. Reduce the dosage if diarrhea occurs. Consider using a buffered vitamin C powder (nonacidic) or liquid vitamin C. Both work well for infants and children, and can be mixed in juice.

Methylsulfonylmethane (MSM)—Helps tissue healing and reduces pain and inflammation. Give 5 milligrams per pound of body weight internally each day (mix with juice), or apply as a cream topically.

Herbal Remedy

Arnica oil or gel—This can be applied topically to the bruise to reduce pain and speed up healing. Do not apply if the skin is broken.

Homeopathy

Arnica montana—Arnica is the best remedy for bruises as the result of trauma. Give 2 pellets of Arnica montana 30C two or three times within 24 hours after the initial injury. (For infants, crush homeopathic pellets into powder and mix it with water.)

Bellis perennis—For bruising of the in-ternal organs. Give 2 pellets of a 30C potency two or three times within 24 hours after the initial injury.

■ ADVANCED PLAN

Nutritional Supplements

Pycnogenol or grape seed extract—Supplies a concentrated source of flavonoids that help with tissue healing. Give 1 milligram per pound of body weight daily.

Children's multivitamin—Provides all the nutrients involved in tissue healing. Give as directed daily.

Herbal Remedies

Bromelain—Works as a natural anti-in-flammatory. Give 3 milligrams per pound of body weight two or three times daily, be-tween meals.

St. John's wort oil—When applied to un-broken skin, it helps to speed up the healing of bruises.

Aromatherapy

Lavender oil—Add to a carrier oil and rub over the bruise. If the child is taking a homeo-pathic remedy, then use aromatherapy at a dif-ferent time.

Acupressure

Gently press each of these acupressure points with a thumb for 10 to 15 seconds. Perform on both sides of the body and repeat three times each day.

Large Intestine 4—Located in the webbing between the thumb and index finger.

Stomach 36—Located four finger-widths below the kneecap and one finger-width toward the outside of the leg (outside of the shinbone, on the muscle).

Hydrotherapy

After 24 hours, alternate hot and cold cloths for 1 minute each over the affected area. Repeat four times. Improves circulation to the injury site and speeds up healing.

■ WHAT TO EXPECT

You should notice reduced pain and swelling within 2 days of treatment. Discoloration and tenderness may not resolve for a week or longer depending on the severity of the bruise.

Burns

A child's skin may be burned by heat, steam, scalding liquids, the sun, chemicals, or electricity. Treatment is based on the type of burn and its severity, location, and source. Severe burns can destroy all skin layers and damage the underlying muscle and fat.

Heat burns can be caused by wet heat, such as scalding hot water, or by dry heat, caused by a flame. These burns are classified by degree. A first-degree burn affects only the skin surface and is considered the most minor of all burns. The skin is usually red and moist and slightly swollen. A second-degree burn affects the skin surface and the layer just beneath it. Blisters and swelling may occur. A third-degree burn, the most serious, results in white, blackened, or bright red skin layers.

Chemical burns are caused by caustic substances that can be either acidic or alkaline. Symptoms of chemical burns include redness, blistering, swelling, and peeling.

Electrical burns are caused by electric shock. It is important to realize that the body is electrically charged and that the heart functions on tiny pulses of electricity. Electrical burns have the potential to disrupt the heartbeat and cause cardiac and respiratory arrest. Be aware that severe electrical burns quite often do not display much damage on the surface layer of skin. The real damage is deeper, in the layers underneath.

Consult your doctor about your child's burn for the following circumstances:

- All electrical burns
- Any burn located on the face, mouth, hands, or genitals
- Any burn that covers more than 10 percent of the body or that completely encircles an arm or leg
- Any burn that blisters or turns the skin white
- Any burn that remains red or oozes beyond 24 hours and intensifies in pain

■ IMMEDIATE TREATMENT

Heat burn—Remove the child from cause of the burn. Put the burned area under running cold water for 10 minutes. If you are outside, use a garden hose. This helps lessen the depth of the burn and reduce pain. Seek medical attention for more serious burns.

Chemical burn—Remove the contaminated clothing and rinse the exposed part of your child's body with water to wash away and dilute the chemicals. Do not rub the skin. Seek medical attention if necessary.

Electrical burn—If the child is still in contact with a live wire, then you must first turn off the electricity (switch or breaker) or remove the wire with a nonconducting item such as a wooden broom handle. Provide CPR if necessary. Have someone call for emergency help.

■ BASIC PLAN

Diet

Encourage your child to drink lots of fluids (water and electrolyte drinks). To speed healing, increase her intake of vegetables, fruits, and quality protein sources. Limit sugar products, as they may slow healing.

Make a shake that combines a whole-foods green drink with whey protein powder that contains glutamine. (For more about green drinks, see "Green Drinks: A Supplemental Source" on page 102.) This combination mixes well with rice, soy, or cow's milk.

Nutritional Supplements

Vitamin C—Supports the immune system and speeds tissue healing. Dosage: the child's age in years times 50 milligrams, twice daily. Reduce the dosage if diarrhea occurs. Consider using a buffered vitamin C powder (nonacidic) or liquid vitamin C. Both work well for infants and children, and can be mixed in juice.

Vitamin A—Supports the immune system and tissue healing. Daily dosage: infants under 1 year, 1,875 international units (IU); children 1 to 3, 2,000 IU; kids 4 to 6, 2,500 IU; kids 7 to 10, 3,500 IU; males 11 and older, 5,000 IU; females 11 and older, 4,000 IU.

Note: These dosages are for short-term use (up to 10 days). Higher dosages may be used only under a doctor's supervision. Available in liquid drops.

Zinc—Supports the immune system and enhances skin healing. Dosage: children 2 and younger, 5 milligrams; 2 and older, 10 to 15 milligrams. Use for 2 weeks and then stop.

L-glutamine—Studies show that it is beneficial to prevent secondary infections from burns, and it is required for tissue healing. Give 3 milligrams per pound of body weight daily.

Herbal Remedies

Aloe vera gel and/or comfrey root salve—Help to speed healing of a superficial burn. This is a topical application.

Propolis—Speeds healing of a burn and prevents secondary infections. Available as a spray, salve, or tincture. Follow directions.

Manuka honey—This is commonly used in countries such as New Zealand to help heal burns. It is applied topically. Use it under the supervision of your doctor.

Homeopathy

Pick the following remedy that best matches your child's symptoms. Unless otherwise indi-

cated, give your child 2 pellets of a 30C potency every 30 minutes for up to three doses. (For infants, crush the pellets into powder and mix it with water.) If there is no improvement within 2 hours, try another remedy. After you first notice improvement, stop giving the remedy unless symptoms begin to return.

Note: Lower potencies (6X, 12X, 6C), if used, should be given every 15 minutes.

Arsenicum album—For severe burning pain. The child is restless, anxious, and fearful. The burn feels better with warm applications.

Cantharis—By far the most common remedy used with burns, especially when blistering occurs.

Causticum—Specific for chemical burns.

Phosphorus—For electrical burns. Give this treatment on the way to the hospital.

Urtica urens—For scalding burns with stinging and burning pain. Good for fluid-filled blisters from first-degree burns. Use if Cantharis is not helpful.

Aromatherapy

Lavender or myrrh compress—If the skin is not open, apply a compress with lavender essential oil. If the skin is open, apply a compress with myrrh essential oil. To make a compress, add 3 drops of the essential oil to 5 cups of warm or cool water. Dip in a facecloth or cotton cloth, wring it out so that it is not dripping, and lay it on the affected area for 5 to 10 minutes. Check the child's skin after the first 2 minutes to ensure that it is not irritated. If the child is taking a homeopathic remedy, use aromatherapy at a different time.

■ ADVANCED PLAN

Nutritional Supplements

Children's multivitamin—Provides all the nutrients involved with tissue healing. Give as directed daily.

Vitamin E—In addition to the multivitamin, give an extra 100 international units of vitamin E per 50 pounds of body weight daily for tissue healing. Give for 2 weeks or until the skin has healed. Can also be applied topically once blistering has cleared.

■ WHAT TO EXPECT

Natural therapies can relieve the pain of minor burns within minutes. Severe burns should be treated with natural therapies to speed healing and to help prevent secondary infection. Talk to your doctor about your wish to incorporate them into your child's treatment protocol.

Calluses and Corns

Calluses and corns comprise the thickened skin that appears on feet or hands due to excessive pressure or friction. They provide an extra cushion to parts of the feet that bear the brunt of body weight. On hands, calluses appear as the result of continued pressure (such as guitar strumming) or repeated injury to a small area.

Corns form the same way that calluses do. They thicken the outermost layer of skin in response to constant rubbing or external pressure over a bony prominence. The culprit is usually ill-fitting shoes—either too-small shoes or ones with pointed toes.

So, what's the difference between calluses and corns? Location. Calluses develop on the soles and heels of feet as well as the hands. Corns are smaller, usually pea-size, and occur on top of or in between toes. They can ache spontaneously or be tender to the touch due to the pressure they place on nerves.

■ BASIC PLAN

Make sure that your child's shoes fit properly. Tight-fitting shoes cause friction on the skin.

Nutritional Supplement

Vitamin E gel—Apply this topically once a day directly on the corn or callus, to soften it.

Herbal Remedy

Tea tree oil—Add 3 drops to a bucket of warm water and soak the affected area for 5 minutes once a day.

Homeopathy

Antimonium crudum 30C—Give 2 pellets twice daily for 1 week to see if there is improvement. Continue for another 2 weeks if improvement is evident.

Aromatherapy

Lemon oil—Apply one dab of undiluted oil with a cotton swab to the callus or corn once daily. Over time, the tissue will slough off.

Cancer

Cancer is a broad category encompassing a number of diseases that develop as a result of uncontrolled growth of certain cells within the body. Cancers are opportunistic invaders within defective, damaged, or genetically changed cells. Unable to function and divide normally, these cells begin to grow wildly. These cancer cells aggressively multiply and aggressively attack surrounding tissue. They are capable of spreading throughout the circulatory and lymphatic systems and the entire body.

Cancer can strike anyone at any age, including infants and children. It can take years or decades to develop, or it can form quickly.

Cancers fall into these broad categories:

Carcinoma—This category includes cancers of glands, internal organs, mucous membranes, and the skin.

Leukemia—This grouping includes cancers of the tissues that manufacture red blood cells, and is often commonly known as blood cancer. This is the most common cancer in children.

Lymphoma—Cancers of the lymphatic tissues and lymph nodes represent this type. This is among the most common types of childhood cancers.

Sarcoma—This group includes cancers of the bones, connective tissues, and muscles.

Certainly, symptoms will depend on the type, location, and severity of the cancer.

Generally, anemia, appetite loss, unexplained weight loss, and constant fatigue are all subtle signs of developing cancer. So are the emergence of lumps, persistent coughs, constant headaches, and numbness.

Yet, specific cancers also display their own telltale signs. Children with leukemia, for instance, may bruise easily, be prone to infections, be feverish, feel tired, and have pale skin and, possibly, bleeding gums. Children with lymphoma often have fevers, night sweats, loss of appetite, and lymph nodes that are swollen and tender to the touch.

Pinpointing the exact cause of a specific cancer can be difficult or impossible. However, scientific research indicates strong possibilities that cancer is linked to these environmental, hereditary, and nutritional suspects:

- Exposure to food additives, pesticides and herbicides, air pollution, tobacco smoke, heavy metals, radiation, and some medications (such as cyclosporine, used for organ transplants)
- A family history of cancer, which increases the risk of a child developing cancer due to an inherited predisposition
- Poor diets that are high in saturated fats and processed foods and low in fresh fruits and vegetables. Cured, pickled, and smoked foods and barbecued meats carry increased risks of containing carcinogens.

Conventional medicine focuses on one or a combination of therapies including chemotherapy, radiation, surgery, gene therapy, and bone marrow transplant. The success rate varies depending on the type of cancer, the stage of the cancer, and the type of treatment.

Many parents look for alternative or complementary approaches to treat their children's cancer, or at least to ease the symptoms associated with the disease and the side effects of its often harsh conventional treatment. Natural medicine should be included as a form of treatment from a knowledgeable doctor. Natural medicine can also help reduce the side effects associated with conventional therapy, and it can support immune function. Choose a pediatric cancer specialist who is willing to work with a natural health care provider such as a naturopathic doctor.

There are a multitude of ways to approach cancer. Counseling for both child and family is encouraged to reduce stress and improve mental outlook. Constitutional hydrotherapy can improve immune function and promote detoxification; use it daily. (See Hydrotherapy for Children on page 115 for more information.) Mental imagery has also been shown to improve immune function; see a professional trained in mental imagery.

Fortunately, integrative medicine is progressing so that children with cancer can be offered the best of conventional and natural medicine. Here, we'll provide an overview of the kinds of natural treatments available through qualified practitioners, as well as a few things you can do yourself to help your child.

■ BASIC PLAN

Diet

Feed your child a whole-foods diet rich in vegetables, fruits, whole grains, fresh fish, and legumes. Organic foods are important. Mushrooms that boost immune function include shiitake and reishi.

Reduce or eliminate meat products.

Fresh juicing helps to supply valuable enzymes and nutrients that help detoxify and support immune function.

Purified water must be used instead of regular tap water.

Nutritional Supplements

Inositol hexaphosphate (IP$_6$)—This supplement boosts the immune system to fight cancer cells. Give as directed by a doctor. Best taken between meals.

Vitamin C—Supports the immune system. The kind with bioflavonoids is preferable. Dosage: the child's age in years times 50 milligrams, twice daily. Reduce the dosage if diarrhea occurs. Consider using a buffered vitamin C powder (nonacidic) or liquid vitamin C. Both work well for infants and children, and can be mixed in juice.

Note: Much higher dosages of vitamin C are often used by natural health care practitioners; talk to your practitioner.

Herbal Therapy

Herbs that support immune function are helpful. They can be taken individually, or better yet, as part of immune formulas. Good examples include echinacea, astragalus, reishi, larix, cat's claw, maitake, and licorice root.

The herbal formulas Essiac and Hoxsey are used by many practitioners of natural medicine as part of a comprehensive treatment program for cancer.

Homeopathy

There is no one remedy to be used for the treatment of cancer. Consult a practitioner for individualized recommendations.

The following remedies are useful to help reduce the side effects of chemotherapy and radiation. They are best used immediately following a treatment. Pick the following remedy that best matches your child's symptoms. Unless otherwise indicated, give your child 2 pellets of a 30C potency twice daily. (For infants, crush the pellets into powder and mix it with water.) Improvements should be seen within 48 hours. If there is no improvement within 48 hours, try another remedy. After you first notice improvement, stop giving the remedy unless symptoms begin to return.

Note: Lower potencies (6X, 12X, 6C) may need to be given more often (three times daily).

Cadmium sulphuratum—The best remedy to use to prevent fatigue, vomiting, and loss of hair. Give 2 pellets prior to a chemotherapy treatment and immediately after.

Ipecacuanha—For constant nausea. Vomiting does not relieve symptoms.

Nux vomica—For symptoms of vomiting, nausea, heartburn, and constipation. The child looks and feels tired and irritable.

■ ADVANCED PLAN

Nutritional Supplements

Bovine or shark cartilage—Data are unclear as to the effectiveness of these supplements. Check with your natural health care practitioner in regard to their use.

Thymic extract—Give 250 milligrams daily of a thymus glandular or thymic protein A. Use under the care of a health practitioner.

Children's multivitamin—Provides a full range of nutrients for the immune system.

Antioxidant complex—Opinions vary on the use of antioxidants during chemotherapy treatment. Consult with your child's oncologist about using antioxidants during chemotherapy treatment. We recommend their use at least between treatments.

■ WHAT TO EXPECT

Natural therapy helps to reduce the side effects associated with conventional treatments and supports the immune system. Work with a doctor who is open to complementary natural treatments.

Candida

Candida, known medically as *Candida albicans,* is a yeast fungus that is harbored inside the intestinal tract. In small amounts, it is harmless. But in unhealthy children, it can grow and intensify. Candida can infiltrate all organs and tissues and has been linked to nearly all medical conditions, headlined by AIDS, arthritis, asthma, cancer, diabetes, the flu, heart disease, middle ear infections, and chronic sinusitis.

Symptoms vary by the location of fungal growth. Here are the five major areas of the body especially vulnerable to candida:

1. The skin. Candida manifests itself in the body's largest organ through such symptoms as excessive sweating, acne, psoriasis, eczema, and hives.

2. The nervous system. The fungus is associated with hyperactivity, autism, and learning disabilities as well as anxiety, moodiness, depression, extreme fatigue, forgetfulness, sleeplessness, and, in extreme cases, hallucinations and violent behavior.

3. The digestive system. Candida symptoms here include bloating, cramps, food allergies, gas, and a tendency to swing between bouts of constipation and diarrhea.

4. The endocrine system. The condition can cause children to develop both hypothyroidism and hyperthyroidism since it can harm the adrenal glands and the thyroid.

5. The genitourinary tract. Symptoms here vary by sex. Boys are prone to chronic anal or rectal itching, genital rashes, and jock itch. Girls may develop bloating, cramps, bladder or vaginal infections, and mood swings—particularly in those who have reached puberty.

The biggest cause of uncontrolled *Candida albicans* growth is the use of antibiotics. Antibiotics, especially the broad-spectrum variety, kill not only harmful but also healthy, friendly bacteria throughout the digestive, urinary, and respiratory tracts and mouth. This leads to an imbalance that enhances the growth of yeast organisms. Candida can also be caused by internal cortisone, chemotherapy drugs, or ionizing radiation. In addition, weak immune systems and hormonal imbalances can create an environment that is unable to stop the fungus. Poor digestive function can also feed the fungus and contribute to its proliferation.

Oral thrush is an overgrowth of yeast in a baby's mouth. It is characterized by white, cheesy patches on the inside of the cheeks, the roof of the mouth, and the tongue. It is not usually a sign of a dangerous condition, although conditions such as diabetes may be involved. It typically occurs after antibiotic use. It can be differentiated from milk deposits in that thrush does not wipe off as milk will. Children's acidophilus should be given to the baby. Apply it to a pacifier, the nipple of a bottle, or to the breastfeeding mother's nipple, or have your child suck it off the tip of your finger. Make sure to boil rubber nipples or pacifiers for 15 minutes once daily to prevent reinfection. A breastfeeding mother should avoid sugar products if her child has thrush. Most cases will resolve with natural treatment. If not, a doctor can prescribe an antifungal cream. (For more information, see "Thrush" on page 448.)

■ BASIC PLAN

Diet

A diet that limits the intake of sugar products is best, since sugar feeds yeast. This includes fruits and fruit juices for a period of time, until balance among the bacteria has been restored.

Food sensitivities may be depleting the immune system. (See "Food Allergies and Food Sensitivities" on page 298 for more information.)

Yogurt with live cultures supplies good bacteria, which keep yeast growth under control. Give your child a yogurt product that has no sugar added.

Nutritional Supplement

Probiotic—Supplies the good bacteria acidophilus and bifidus, which keep yeast overgrowth under control. Choose a children's formula, and give as directed on the container. The breastfeeding mother should take an adult formula in addition to giving the child's formula to her infant.

Herbal Remedy

Oregano—Has anti-yeast effects and is available in drops. Give as directed on the container. Best used under the guidance of a natural health care practitioner.

Homeopathy

Pick the following remedy that best matches your child's symptoms. Unless otherwise indicated, give your child 2 pellets of a 30C potency twice daily. (For infants, crush the pellets into powder and mix it with water.) Improvements should be seen within 7 days. If there is no improvement within 7 days, try another remedy. After you first notice improvement, stop giving the remedy unless symptoms begin to return.

Note: Lower potencies (6X, 12X, 6C) may

need to be given more often (three times daily).

Borax—For raised white patches on the tongue, roof of mouth, and gums.

Homeopathic Candida—Can be used to help the immune system mount a response against overgrowth of *Candida albicans* in the body. Give as directed on the bottle or under the guidance of a homeopathic practitioner.

You can also procure a constitutional homeopathic remedy from a homeopath.

■ ADVANCED PLAN

Herbal Remedies

Echinacea—Has been shown to have anti-yeast properties; supports the immune system.

Digestive tonic herbs such as gentian root and ginger root are helpful to improve digestion and alleviate yeast problems.

■ WHAT TO EXPECT

If a child has had candida for a long period of time, it can take a few months of treatment for complete recovery to occur.

Canker Sores

Canker sores, also known as aphthous ulcers, are painful mouth ulcers that are commonly misidentified as cold sores. Cold sores are caused by the herpes virus and are extremely contagious. Unlike cold sores, a canker sore first appears as a tiny red dot inside the cheeks or on the lips. It then develops into a vesicle with a milky white head and red outer rim that eventually ruptures. This ulcer can create secondary yeast or bacterial infections. Canker sores appear singly or in groups of two or three, and they can be very tiny or as large as 1 inch in diameter.

The condition can be aggravated by eating acidic or spicy foods, which make canker sores sting and burn. It can also make talking painful and difficult. Children with canker sores may be reluctant to eat.

Determining the cause behind a canker sore can be tricky. Medical evidence suggests that people with weakened immune systems, those who are deficient in iron or vitamin B_{12}, and those who have anemia are more prone to developing them. Stress, small cuts, food allergies, highly acidic foods, and chocolate can also trigger canker sores. Unfortunately, once a person gets a canker sore, his chances of recurring episodes are heightened.

Conventional treatment focuses on pain relievers.

■ BASIC PLAN

Diet

Food sensitivities are almost always at the root of canker sores. The most common food culprits include citrus fruits (such as oranges, lemons, and limes) and other acidic foods (such as tomatoes, pineapple, and apples) or juices made from them. Spicy foods such as garlic may be a trigger, too, as can wheat, chocolate, and sugar. If your child has recurring canker sores, do some elimination and reintroduction of these foods, and chances are, you will identify the problem. (See "Food Allergies and Food Sensitivities" on page 298 for more information.)

Have your child eat yogurt with live cultures, which is soothing to the mouth, while the canker sores are healing.

Soups and steamed foods are also good choices for your child to eat while his mouth is sensitive.

Nutritional Supplement

Vitamin C—Aids tissue healing. It's best to use nonacidic vitamin C for canker sores, such as calcium ascorbate or Ester C. Dosage: the child's age in years times 50 milligrams, once daily.

Herbal Remedy

Mix 2 drops of myrrh and 3 drops of goldenseal or calendula in ¼ cup of water. Have the child swish it in his mouth and spit it out. Repeat three times daily until the canker sores are gone.

Homeopathy

Pick the following remedy that best matches your child's symptoms. Unless otherwise indicated, give your child 2 pellets of a 30C potency twice daily. (For infants, crush the pellets into powder and mix it with water.) Improvements should be seen within 48 hours. If there is no improvement within 48 hours, try another remedy. After you first notice improvement, stop giving the remedy unless symptoms begin to return.

Note: Lower potencies (6X, 12X, 6C) may need to be given more often (three times daily).

Arsenicum album—For canker sores that cause burning pain. The child is thirsty and desires sips of warm water; he is restless and anxious.

Borax—For canker sores that occur along with thrush. The sores bleed easily.

Mercurius solubilis or vivus—For canker sores or ulcers in the mouth. The child has bad breath, a coated tongue, excess salivation, and a metallic taste in his mouth.

Natrum muriaticum—The child has cold sores on the lips and canker sores inside the mouth. The lips are dry. The child craves salty foods. Symptoms get worse from being in sunlight.

Natrum phosphoricum 6X—An acid-base balancer that aids recovery from canker sores. Have the child take it two or three times daily until canker sores are gone. Can also be used preventatively for chronic cases. Use this remedy if you are unsure of which one to use.

Sulphur—For canker sores that cause burning pain. The child is very warm and has a red face and a high thirst for cold drinks.

■ ADVANCED PLAN

Nutritional Supplements

Children's multivitamin—Supplies nutrients for tissue healing. B vitamins such as B_{12} contained in a multivitamin help to prevent and treat canker sores. Give as directed on the container.

Zinc—Supports the immune system and enhances skin healing. Dosage: children 2 and younger, 5 milligrams; 2 and older, 10 to 15 milligrams. Use for 2 weeks and then stop.

Probiotic—A children's acidophilus and bifidus supplement supplies friendly bacteria in the mouth to support tissue healing. Give as directed on the container.

Herbal Remedies

Propolis—Stimulates tissue healing. Use as a spray or tincture.

DGL—Also known as deglycyrrhizinated licorice root extract, this is a special form of licorice root. Dissolve in a glass of water, and have the child swish it in his mouth and spit or swallow. Repeat three times daily.

Acupressure

Large Intestine 4—Located in the webbing between the thumb and index finger. Gently press the acupressure point with a thumb for 10 to 15 seconds. Repeat three times, and then do the same on the other hand. Repeat daily.

Aromatherapy

Myrrh—With a cotton swab, dab undiluted myrrh onto the canker sore. Repeat three times daily.

■ WHAT TO EXPECT

You should see significant healing within 1 to 3 days.

Cat Scratch Disease

This bacterial infection occurs as a result of being scratched or clawed by a cat, although dogs can also be responsible for this disease in people. It doesn't matter whether the scratch or claw mark is barely visible or deep. Children under age 10 are the top reported group to develop cat scratch disease.

Within 3 to 10 days, the infected site looks like a small boil at first. Only about half of infected people show any symptoms other than swollen glands. Others exhibit symptoms including nausea, chills, loss of appetite, headache, low-grade fever, swollen lymph nodes, and, possibly, measles-looking rashes. Some children develop a crusting sore or blisterlike protrusion at the site of the scratch or clawing. Symptoms tend to persist for months, and in rare instances, cat scratch disease can lead to encephalitis (inflammation of the brain). If your child is exhibiting any symptoms of cat scratch disease, you should see a doctor early for an evaluation.

The conventional treatment is antibiotics and pain-relieving medicines.

■ BASIC PLAN

Diet
Avoid sugar products, as they can suppress the immune system. Make sure that your child drinks plenty of fluids.

Nutritional Supplement
Vitamin C—Supports the immune system. Dosage: the child's age in years times 50

milligrams, twice daily. Reduce the dosage if diarrhea occurs. Consider using a buffered vitamin C powder (nonacidic) or liquid vitamin C. Both work well for infants and children, and can be mixed in juice.

Herbal Remedies

Echinacea—Supports the immune system against infection.

Consider an herbal blend with a combination of immune-enhancing herbs, possibly including lomatium, reishi, astragalus, and licorice.

Propolis is also excellent to apply topically to the scratch to help fight infection.

Homeopathy

Pick the following remedy that best matches your child's symptoms. Unless otherwise indicated, give your child 2 pellets of a 30C potency every 15 minutes for up to four doses. (For infants, crush the pellets into powder and mix it with water.) If there is no improvement within 2 hours, try another remedy.

Belladonna—The area where the scratch occurred is red and inflamed. The child is developing a high fever. Useful in the first 24 hours.

Calendula—For an infected wound that is red and inflamed with stinging pain.

Pyrogen or pyrogenium—For a more serious infection where the wound is red and may have pus formation. The child looks very sick and has a high fever. This is not a common remedy in stores, so you may need to see a homeopathic practitioner.

■ ADVANCED PLAN

Nutritional Supplements

Vitamin A—Supports the immune system. Daily dosage: infants under 1 year, 1,875 international units (IU); children 1 to 3, 2,000 IU; kids 4 to 6, 2,500 IU; kids 7 to 10, 3,500 IU; males 11 and older, 5,000 IU; females 11 and older, 4,000 IU.

Note: These dosages are for short-term use (up to 10 days). Higher dosages may be used only under a doctor's supervision. Available in liquid drops.

Zinc—Supports the immune system and enhances skin healing. Dosage: children 2 and younger, 5 milligrams; 2 and older, 10 to 15 milligrams. Use for 2 weeks and then stop.

■ WHAT TO EXPECT

Your doctor will likely prescribe antibiotics. Natural therapy helps to fight the infection more effectively. Improvements should be noticed within 24 to 48 hours.

Cavities

Cavities are the consequences of tooth decay. The process known as dental caries occurs when the tooth enamel (the outer, compact layer of the tooth) and the dentin (the main body of the tooth, inside the enamel) slowly break down and decay.

Up to age 6, children have 20 primary teeth. Between the ages of 6 and 18, these primary teeth are gradually replaced by a permanent set of 32 teeth. This set is divided into 8 incisors in front (used for biting and cutting food), 4 canines (used to stabilize large bites of food), 8 premolars (used for grinding and crushing food), and 12 molars (also used for grinding and crushing food).

Signs of decay include discoloration or erosion around the crown or the root.

For a cavity to develop requires the concentrated and persistent presence of certain bacteria in the mouth that eat away at the surface of the teeth. Genetics, diet, and dental hygiene habits all contribute to the health of the teeth. Children born to parents who have poor teeth are more vulnerable to cavities. So are children whose diets are dominated by foods and drinks that are high in refined sugars and starches, sweetened carbonated beverages, and acidic foods. These substances provide a food source for the bacteria, which produce the tooth-damaging acid. Finally, children who do not brush their teeth or floss run the risk of developing cavities.

In infants, there is a form of tooth decay known as baby bottle syndrome. This results when a baby falls asleep with a sugar-filled juice bottle in his mouth. The sugars combine with plaque (the sticky film on teeth) to promote bacterial growth and tooth decay.

Children with cavities experience sensitivities to hot, cold, or sweet foods.

Conventional treatment focuses on prevention with proper oral hygiene. For existing cavities, dental cleanings and fillings are recommended. If fillings are needed, make sure to get composites and not mercury fillings, which are toxic to the nervous and immune systems.

■ BASIC PLAN

Start brushing your baby's teeth when the first teeth appear, around 6 to 7 months of age. Use a baby toothbrush, a piece of gauze, or a washcloth to clean the gums and teeth. A dab of a natural children's toothpaste can be used but is not necessary. When your child gets teeth, begin a habit of flossing once daily and brushing at least twice daily.

Diet

A child's diet should focus on vegetables, legumes, and whole grains. Avoid foods and drinks that are high in refined sugars and starches. Also avoid sweetened carbonated beverages and acidic foods.

Do not let your baby sleep with a bottle of juice or milk. Bacteria build up more quickly with these fluids in the mouth.

Nutritional Supplements

Calcium and magnesium—These encourage proper dental development. Give the child 500 milligrams of calcium and 250 to 500 milligrams of magnesium in a liquid complex daily.

Fluoride—We do not generally recommend that fluoride supplements be taken internally, as they can be toxic. There is a debate about whether internal consumption of fluoride may be harmful to the immune system. Fluoride toothpaste can be used by age 2, but children should not swallow the toothpaste.

We recommend external fluoride treatments by a dentist.

Homeopathy

Calcarea fluorica 6X—Used for brittle teeth that are loose and unhealthy. Give 2 pellets two or three times daily for at least 3 months.

Kreosotum 30C—For teeth that crumble and decay easily. Give 2 pellets twice daily for 1 month.

Acupressure

Large Intestine 4—Helps to relieve tooth pain. Located in the webbing between the thumb and index finger. Gently press the acupressure point with a thumb for 10 to 15 seconds. Repeat three times and then do the same on the other hand. Repeat daily.

■ WHAT TO EXPECT

Natural therapy should be able to prevent susceptibility to future cavities.

Celiac Disease

This chronic intestinal disorder is triggered by a hypersensitivity or intolerance to gluten, a cereal protein found in wheat, triticale, kamut, spelt, rye, barley, and possibly oats. The chances of developing this disease are 1 in 5,000 in the United States. It is usually diagnosed before a child reaches his second birthday. Blood tests by your doctor can help to diagnose this condition.

Inside the intestines, the body's immune system cells, known as T lymphocyctes, mistakenly regard gluten as an unwanted invader and attack it. During this battle, the lining of the small intestine is damaged, complicating the body's ability to absorb nutrients. This results in malnutrition. However, improvements begin within days of starting a gluten-free diet, and a child's small intestine is usually completely healed in 3 to 6 months.

Celiac disease may be asymptomatic, or it may be accompanied by such symptoms as anemia, pale stools, painful abdominal bloating, diarrhea, vomiting, loss of muscle tone, weight loss, and leg/foot swelling. Failure to grow and thrive, mouth ulcers, eczema, mood swings, and trouble concentrating can also be symptoms of this disease in children.

Heredity plays a major factor in this disease, especially in children of Irish descent. In Ireland, the chances of getting celiac disease are 1 in 300.

Some children do not have celiac disease but have a sensitivity to wheat products. In such cases, the child can tolerate only certain amounts of wheat or grain products before symptoms occur.

■ BASIC PLAN

Diet

A child with celiac disease should avoid gluten-containing foods such as wheat, triticale, kamut, spelt, rye, barley, and possibly oats. Foods such as rice, corn, nuts, vegetables, fruits, legumes, fish, and poultry can be eaten.

Make sure that your child is not also sensitive to dairy products. A wheat-free recipe book should be purchased for meal and recipe ideas. Utilize resources such as the Web site www.celiac.com to find a detailed list of foods that are safe or that should be avoided. Your doctor may also be able to put you in touch with a local nutritionist or dietitian who can provide you with a list.

Nutritional Supplements

Microbial-derived enzymes—Give 1 to 2 enzymes with meals to support digestion and absorption.

Note: These do not *allow* your child to eat gluten products, but if gluten products are unknowingly ingested, the enzymes may help to prevent an immune reaction.

Children's multivitamin—Provides a base of nutrients for children. Those with celiac disease are prone to vitamin deficiencies if gluten-containing products are eaten. Give as directed daily.

Herbal Remedies

Consider using herbs or combinations of herbs that support digestion. Examples include gentian root, ginger, and fennel.

■ ADVANCED PLAN

Nutritional Supplement

Probiotic—A children's acidophilus and bifidus supplement optimizes good bacteria in the child's digestive tract. Give as directed on the container.

Vital Fact

In Italy, all children are screened by age 6 for celiac disease so that children who have the disease, but no early symptoms, are identified. In the United States, the time between the first symptoms and diagnosis averages about 10 years.

■ WHAT TO EXPECT

Natural therapies can help to improve overall digestion, as people with this condition often react to other foods as well. Do not expect a "cure" for celiac disease.

Chapped Lips

Chapping is caused by dehydration. It is aggravated by a child's automatic tendency to lick her lips to restore moisture: As soon as the moisture dries, the lips are more parched.

Lips serve to protect teeth, but they take a lot of wear and tear. Surprisingly, lips do not contain the natural oils that keep the rest of your skin supple and moisturized. They lack a pigment called melanin, necessary to fend off sun damage. Healthy lips need to be well-hydrated. Otherwise, they become red and dry, form blisters, and crack, causing mild pain and irritation.

Small blisters on the upper lip of a newborn may be detected during her first month. This is a consequence of aggressive sucking and will disappear by her first birthday.

For all ages, chapped lips are caused by exposure to hot sun, biting winds, air-conditioning, and indoor dry heat. It may also be a sign that your child needs to drink a little more water. Chapped lips and dry skin all over the body can be a sign of essential fatty acid deficiency.

■ BASIC PLAN

Wet your child's lips with water and then apply petroleum jelly to lock in moisture.

Avoid flavored lip balms, which cause the child to lick her lips, causing more chapping.

Diet

Chapped lips combined with dry skin all over the body requires an increase of foods that are high in essential fatty acids. Examples include fish such as salmon and halibut, nuts, canola oil, flaxseed oil, and green leafy vegetables. Flaxseeds are another good source: Grind 1 teaspoon of flaxseeds per 50 pounds of body weight (children weighing 30 to 50 pounds may also use 1 teaspoon), and give daily along with 8 ounces of water. Also, make sure that your child drinks plenty of water throughout the day.

Nutritional Supplements

Flaxseed and borage/evening primrose oil—Flaxseed oil is a source of omega-3 and omega-9 fatty acids. Daily dosages are: children up to age 2, 1 teaspoon; kids 3 to 6, 2 tea-spoons; kids 7 and up, 2 to 3 teaspoons. Reduce the dosage if diarrhea occurs.

Combine the flaxseed oil with ½ to 1 teaspoon of borage oil, for omega-6 fatty acids. Or instead of borage oil, use evening primrose oil, at the following daily dosages: kids to age 2, ½ teaspoon; kids 3 to 6, 1 teaspoon; those 7 and older, 1 to 2 teaspoons. Give once a day with meals.

You could also substitute a daily children's essential fatty acid complex for all of these oils. It should contain omega-3 and omega-6 fatty acids. Follow the directions on the container.

Herbal Remedies

Calendula gel—Apply topically.

Herbal lip balm products are available at your health food store or pharmacy.

Homeopathy

Natrum muriaticum 6X—Give 2 pellets twice daily for 3 to 5 days, and continue as needed. (For infants, crush homeopathic pellets into powder and mix it with water.)

■ ADVANCED PLAN

Homeopathy

Pick the following remedy that best matches your child's symptoms. Unless otherwise indicated, give your child 2 pellets of a 30C potency twice daily. Improvements should be seen within 48 hours. If there is no improvement within 48 hours, try another remedy. After you first notice improvement, stop giving the remedy unless symptoms begin to return.

Note: Lower potencies (6X, 12X, 6C) may need to be given more often (three times daily).

Graphites—For lips that have cracked because the skin is so dry. Yellow fluid oozes from the cracks.

Petroleum—For rough, cracked, and red skin. The problem is worse at the corners of the mouth. Most of the skin is usually dry and cracked.

Aromatherapy

Roman chamomile—For moisturizing. Add it to a carrier oil and apply to the lips at night. If the child is taking a homeopathic remedy, use aromatherapy at a different time.

■ WHAT TO EXPECT

Improvements with the correct homeopathic remedy are usually seen within 1 week. Essential fatty acid deficiency can take several weeks of treatment to improve.

Chicken Pox

Caused by the varicella-zoster virus of the herpes family, this extremely contagious childhood disease can affect anyone at any age. Infected children can spread the disease to others through respiratory droplets—usually by talking, coughing, and sneezing.

The virus is contagious for up to 5 days before the rash appears and is not usually contagious beyond 5 days after the rash develops. It can take up to 2 weeks for symptoms to surface. Epidemics usually occur in winter and early spring.

Usually more annoying than harmful, chicken pox first appears like a little bug bite on your baby or child's belly. Then, the child may experience headaches, loss of appetite, and a mild fever. Next, an army of bumps surface, all displaying tiny, clear water blisters. For a week or so, symptoms include a mild fever, some blisters, rashes all over the body, and tormenting itching. Crusty scabs comprise the final stage and can last for up to 2 weeks before flaking off and being replaced by healthy, healed skin.

Since chicken pox can develop into encephalitis or Reye's syndrome, both life-threatening brain inflammations, it is critical to consult your pediatrician about any unusual, persistent, or severe symptoms that your child displays. Giving aspirin during chicken pox can also cause Reye's syndrome. Here are some signs to alert your pediatrician:

- Appearance of a few sores that are very swollen, red, or painful. They could be infected.
- A fever develops after the sores start to scab over and heal.
- Your child complains of pain when the neck is stretched.
- Your child develops mouth, vaginal, or rectal sores.
- The combination of a high fever, vomiting, confusion, convulsions, and severe headache is present.

Vital Fact

The fatality rate in U.S. schoolchildren who become infected with chicken pox is approximately 2 per 100,000 cases.

The one consolation about chicken pox is that once a child has had it, the chances of a second recurrence are extremely remote. Natural therapies help to make the child more comfortable, to prevent scratching so that scarring does not occur. It also helps prevent complications such as secondary bacterial infections of the skin.

Conventional treatment focuses on pain-relieving medications (not aspirin) and antihistamines to help reduce itching. Pediatricians commonly recommend the chicken pox vaccine as a preventive measure.

■ BASIC PLAN

Diet

A whole-foods diet is recommended. Avoid sugar products and undiluted fruit juices, which can hinder immune function. Steamed vegetables and homemade soups are excellent.

Make sure that your child is drinking plenty of fluids.

Nutritional Supplements

Vitamin C—Provides support to the immune system. Dosage: the child's age in years times 50 milligrams, twice daily. Reduce the dosage if diarrhea occurs. Consider using a buffered vitamin C powder (nonacidic) or liquid vitamin C. Both work well for infants and children, and can be mixed in juice.

Vitamin A—Supports the immune system. Daily dosage: infants under 1 year, 1,875 international units (IU); children 1 to 3, 2,000 IU; kids 4 to 6, 2,500 IU; kids 7 to 10, 3,500 IU; males 11 and older, 5,000 IU; females 11 and older, 4,000 IU.

Note: These dosages are for short-term use (up to 10 days). Higher dosages may be used only under a doctor's supervision. Available in liquid drops.

Herbal Remedies

Echinacea and goldenseal combination—Supports the immune system and prevents bacterial infection of the skin lesions.

Oatmeal bath—Add 1 cup of oatmeal powder such as Aveeno to a warm bath. The other alternative is to put regular oatmeal (such as Quaker Oats) into a cheesecloth bag, tie it with a string, and hang it under the faucet or float it in the tub. Have the child soak in the warm bath for 5 to 15 minutes. Then, pat the child dry so that a film of oatmeal is left on the skin. This film contains the anti-itch properties of the oatmeal. Aveeno itch ointment is also available over the counter.

Homeopathy

Pick the following remedy that best matches your child's symptoms. Unless otherwise indicated, give your child 2 pellets of a 30C potency twice daily. (For infants, crush the pellets into powder and mix it with water.) Improvements should be seen within 48 hours. If there is no improvement within 48 hours, try another remedy. After you first notice improvement, stop giving the remedy unless symptoms begin to return.

Note: Lower potencies (6X, 12X, 6C) may need to be given more often (three times daily).

Antimonium crudum—The scabs and discharge look like honey. The tongue has a white coating. Lesions burn and itch. Symptoms get worse in a warm room and better with fresh air.

Croton tiglium—Blisters are intensely itchy and painful when scratched. There are lesions on the face and genitals.

Pulsatilla—Blisters itch and crust over. The child is tearful and clingy. Even though there is fever, the child has little to no thirst. He feels worse when becoming too warm and better in the fresh air.

Rhus toxicodendron—Give to a child who has extreme itching and restlessness with weeping vesicle eruptions. The child craves milk.

Sulphur—For itching, redness, and burning. Useful if Rhus toxicodendron stops working or if Rhus toxicodendron does not help. The child scratches his skin until it bleeds.

Varicella—Give when you first find out that the child has chicken pox. Prevents serious bouts of chicken pox and speeds healing.

Caution: Do not use the herb white willow to help your child with pain relief. It contains active ingredients similar to aspirin. It could theoretically pose the same Reye's syndrome danger as aspirin, and should be avoided during viral infections.

■ ADVANCED PLAN

Nutritional Supplements

Zinc—Supports the immune system and enhances skin healing. Dosage: children 2 and younger, 5 milligrams; 2 and older, 10 to 15 milligrams. Use for 2 weeks and then stop.

Thymus glandular—For immune support. Give two 250-milligram tablets or capsules daily.

Vitamin E gel—Can be applied to any scars that form.

Herbal Remedies

Antiviral herbs can be given by themselves or in a formula. Examples include echinacea, lomatium, reishi, astragalus, licorice, and larix. Echinacea is a great herb to use by itself.

Gumweed (*Grindelia camporum*)—The tincture applied to the chicken pox lesions helps to reduce itching.

Calendula—Diluted (1 teaspoon of tincture in 4 teaspoons of water) and applied to the skin, this helps to prevent infection from developing.

Aromatherapy

German chamomile and lavender—Add these to the child's bath to help relax him before bed and reduce itching. Swish the bathwater and essential oils around before placing the child in the bathtub. If the child is taking a homeopathic remedy, use aromatherapy at a different time.

■ WHAT TO EXPECT

Natural treatment should help reduce the itching and severity of the illness. General improvement is usually noticed within 2 days of treatment. Immune-supportive treatments help to prevent serious respiratory tract and skin infections.

Cholesterol Problems

Cholesterol is a waxy, fatlike substance called a sterol that is found in animal foods, including meat, eggs, fish, and dairy products. Although it is often given a bad rap, cholesterol is essential for life. Every cell needs cholesterol.

The majority of cholesterol, about 80 percent, is made in your liver. Only about 20 percent is derived from food sources. Cholesterol is needed to manufacture hormones, it provides structural support in cell membranes, and it helps regulate blood pressure. It is also the main building block for vitamin D. Problems occur when there are too-high levels of cholesterol in the body, when there is an imbalance between the different types of cholesterol, or when cholesterol becomes oxidized.

Good cholesterol (known as high-density lipoprotein, or HDL) transports cholesterol from the arterial wall to the liver where it is recycled for future use or discarded from the body. Bad cholesterol (known as low-density lipoprotein, or LDL) also transports cholesterol throughout the body, but it litters blood vessel walls with tiny bits of cholesterol. Over time, the arteries can become blocked, leading to a heart attack or other heart condition.

A desirable total cholesterol measurement is less than 200 milligrams per deciliter for adults. In school-age children, the acceptable target is to be below 170 milligrams per deciliter. The risk of heart disease is related to the ratio of LDL to HDL, which should be less than 3.5. (There are many other markers besides cholesterol that are also now used to assess cardiac risk, such as lipoproteins and homocysteine.) Also, your doctor should rule out low thyroid, which can elevate cholesterol levels.

Although cholesterol-related problems such as heart disease and stroke commonly occur among adults, your child may be in the very early stages of cholesterol concern. His genetic makeup and the amount of saturated animal fat and cholesterol he eats chiefly determine the balance of the HDL and LDL cholesterol in his body. So does his activity level. Studies show that hardening of the arteries begins in childhood.

The American Academy of Pediatrics and the National Cholesterol Education Program Expert Panel advise getting your child's cholesterol checked if any of these risk factors exist:

- Either parent registers a cholesterol level over 240
- Your child is obese, has high blood pressure, or is exposed to secondhand cigarette smoke at home
- A parent, aunt, uncle or grandparent suffered a heart attack, stroke, angina, or other cardiovascular disease before age 55
- A parent, aunt, uncle, or grandparent underwent a balloon angioplasty or coronary artery bypass surgery before age 55

■ BASIC PLAN

Diet

Reduce the amount of saturated fat in your child's diet by reducing the intake of meat products such as beef, pork, chicken, lamb, and shellfish.

Focus on eating "good fats." These include the omega-3 fatty acids as found in coldwater fish such as salmon and in plant foods such as flaxseeds. Avoid "bad fats," which are found in fried foods and in processed foods that contain hydrogenated or partially hydrogenated oils or fats. Limit your oil use in cooking to oils such as olive and canola. Use butter instead of margarine. (See "Fats" on page 7 for more information on good and bad fats.)

Increase your child's intake of fiber-rich foods such as vegetables, fruits, whole grains, and legumes.

Note: If your child has high cholesterol and/or triglyceride levels, fruits should be eaten in moderation and with meals. Spiking of insulin levels from simple sugars, especially on an empty stomach, can lead to elevation of cholesterol and triglyceride levels (known as syndrome X, a common condition that affects approximately 25 percent of the population).

Candies, soft drinks, and simple sugar products should be eliminated or reduced.

Foods such as garlic, onions, and yogurt with live cultures help to protect the cardiovascular system.

Nutritional Supplements

High cholesterol levels in children should be treated by a doctor knowledgeable in natural medicine. The following are some of the more effective supplements.

Inositol hexaniacinate—This flush-free form of niacin lowers total cholesterol and improves HDL, LDL, and lipoprotein (a) markers. Consult with your holistic doctor about using this supplement.

Children's multivitamin—Contains vitamins and minerals such as vitamins C and E and selenium that prevent oxidation of cholesterol.

Herbal Remedy

Garlic extract—Helps reduce cholesterol levels. Give 200 milligrams daily for children 10 and under, and 400 milligrams daily for children 11 and older.

■ ADVANCED PLAN

Nutritional Supplement

Children's whole-food supplement—Contains vegetables and fruits, which have phytochemicals that help control cholesterol. Give as directed on the container.

■ WHAT TO EXPECT

By working with a nutrition-oriented doctor and following a program as outlined in this chapter, you should be able to control your child's high cholesterol levels. Don't forget that exercise and weight management are very important to control cholesterol.

Circumcision

At birth, boys have skin called the foreskin that covers the end of the penis. Circumcision is a surgical procedure in which the foreskin is removed, thus exposing the tip of the penis. This procedure is usually performed in the first few days of life. Some parents choose to have their sons circumcised so that they "look the same" as other boys, while others feel that circumcision is unnecessary. Circumcision is also done for religious, social, and cultural reasons. For example, followers of the Jewish and Islamic faiths practice circumcision.

From a medical viewpoint, there are some minor health benefits from circumcision. Following are the medical benefits as stated by the American Academy of Pediatrics (AAP):

- A slightly lower risk of urinary tract infections (UTIs). A circumcised infant boy has about a 1 in 1,000 chance of developing a UTI in the first year of life. An uncircumcised infant boy has about a 1 in 100 chance of developing a UTI in the first year of life.
- A lower risk of cancer of the penis. However, this type of cancer is very rare in both circumcised and uncircumcised males.
- A slightly lower risk of getting sexually transmitted diseases, including HIV, the AIDS virus
- Prevention of foreskin infections
- Prevention of phimosis, a condition in uncircumcised males that makes foreskin retraction impossible
- Easier genital hygiene

It should be noted, however, that the AAP states, "these benefits are not sufficient for the American Academy of Pediatrics to recommend that all infant boys be circumcised."

According to the AAP, the following are reasons why parents may choose to not circumcise their child:

- Possible risks. As with any surgery, circumcision has some risks. Complications from circumcision are rare and usually minor. They may include bleeding, infection, cutting the foreskin too short or too long, and improper healing.
- The belief that the foreskin is necessary to protect the tip of the penis. When the foreskin is removed, the tip of the penis may become irritated and cause the opening of the penis to become too small. This can cause urination problems that may need to be surgically corrected.

- The belief that circumcision makes the tip of the penis less sensitive, causing a decrease in sexual pleasure later in life.
- Almost all uncircumcised boys can be taught proper hygiene that can lower their chances of getting infections, cancer of the penis, and sexually transmitted diseases.

It is recommended that circumcision be performed only on healthy infants. It is also recommended that pain medications be used if circumcision is performed.

Finally, it should be noted, we chose to avoid circumcision with our son, based on our religious, philosophical, and medical beliefs. We do not recommend circumcision, especially if based on medical benefits only.

■ BASIC PLAN

Herbal Remedy

Calendula—Talk with your doctor about applying calendula cream or tincture (1 teaspoon diluted in 4 teaspoons of water) to the penis. This herb is safe, promotes healing, and acts as a natural disinfectant.

Homeopathy

Give your infant 2 pellets of Arnica montana 30C as soon as possible after the surgery. (For infants, pellets should always be crushed and mixed in water.) This helps to reduce pain and swelling. Four hours later, follow with 2 pellets of Staphysagria 30C, and repeat the dose in 4 more hours. This remedy also promotes healing and reduces pain that occurs from cutting.

Vital Fact

Sixty-three percent of newborn boys are circumcised in America.

Note: These homeopathic remedies do not interfere with any pain medications or anesthesia.

Colds

Medically called viral rhinitis, the common cold actually is a catchphrase for a variety of upper respiratory symptoms caused by one or more of hundreds of different viruses. The sheer number of these viruses is why there is not yet a cure for the common cold: The body's immune system isn't able to lodge a specific attack plan because it either misidentifies the viral invader or is fighting one when another appears. Natural therapies are quite effective in optimizing immune system function and preventing and alleviating the common cold. When taken at the first signs of a cold, natural therapies may prevent it from developing.

Symptoms include watery eyes, nasal discharge, sore throat, stuffiness, sneezing, achy muscles, headaches, low-grade fevers, and tiredness. The symptoms can last 7 to 10 days, peaking at day 3 or 4.

Infants and toddlers are highly susceptible

to colds because their immune systems are still developing and they have not yet built up immunity against some of the cold viruses. In infants, the nasal discharge will first appear watery, then thicken and turn yellowish.

In young children, repeated cold episodes can lead to ear infections. Parents are advised to check for any drainage from the ears or signs of irritability and sleeplessness in their children.

The real culprit is a susceptible immune system. Children who are always coming down with colds or who have a hard time shaking colds usually have nutritional deficiencies and are depleting their immune systems by eating foods to which they are sensitive.

The conventional approach is rest, fluids, decongestants, and pain relievers.

■ BASIC PLAN

Diet

Make sure that your child gets plenty of fluids to prevent dehydration. Stay consistent with breastfeeding or bottlefeeding for infants. Older children should drink at least six glasses of water throughout the day. Fruit juices, if used, should be diluted with water by at least 50 percent, as simple sugars can weaken the immune system. Homemade warm broths and soups are best, as they are easy to digest and moisten the respiratory tract. Good old chicken soup is effective during a cold. Fresh garlic added to the soup is helpful as long as your child is not sensitive to it. Do not give fried foods, as they are hard to digest. Avoid giving your child dairy products; they can contribute to mucus formation.

Nutritional Supplement

Vitamin C—Supports the immune system. Dosage: the child's age in years times 50 milligrams, twice daily. Reduce the dosage if diarrhea occurs. Consider using a buffered vitamin C powder (nonacidic) or liquid vitamin C. Both work well for infants and children, and can be mixed in juice.

Herbal Remedies

Echinacea—This herb has received the most study with regard to the common cold and upper respiratory tract infections. Look for a children's glycerin-based formula.

Larix—A good immune system enhancer. It is available in a powder form that blends into water and juice, sometimes with a mild, sweet taste.

Homeopathy

Use a combination cold formula, or pick the one of the following remedies which best matches your child's symptoms. For the remedies on the next page, unless otherwise indicated, give your child 2 pellets of a 30C potency three times daily. (For infants, crush the pellets into powder and mix it with water.) Improvements should be seen within 48 hours. If there is no improvement within 48 hours, try another remedy. After you first notice improvement, stop giving the remedy unless symptoms begin to return.

Note: Lower potencies (6X, 12X, 6C) may need to be given more often (four times daily).

Aconitum napellus—For a cold that comes on very quickly after the child is exposed to dry, cold weather. Useful in the first day of a cold. The child is restless and anxious, and she often has a dry cough and a high thirst for cold drinks. A high fever comes on quickly. One cheek may be red and the other pale.

Allium cepa—For clear, burning nasal discharge that irritates the nostrils and upper lip. The child's eyes water. Symptoms are worse in a warm room.

Arsenicum album—For profuse, clear watery discharge from the nose that makes the upper lip red. The child's nose may be stuffed up but still runs. Symptoms are worse between 12:00 and 3:00 A.M., when the child wakes up. The child is anxious, restless, and fearful with the cold. She feels very chilly and is thirsty for sips of water.

Ferrum phosphoricum—The child is feverish but does not act sick in the first stages of a cold. Her throat and face are red.

Gelsemium—The child feels droopy and drowsy and perhaps dizzy. She has chills up and down her back; her body feels very tired and her muscles ache. She has a headache at base of the neck.

Mercurius solubilis or vivus—The child is sensitive to both hot and cold temperatures. Her tongue is coated, and she has bad breath. She has a foul body odor and thick nasal discharge.

Nux vomica—The child is chilly and more irritable than normal. She has a hard time get-ting warm. There can be sneezing and a cough waking up in the morning.

Pulsatilla—The child is feverish. She becomes more clingy than normal and does not want an adult to leave her side. She is weepy and has low thirst and may develop yellow or green mucus from the sinuses. She feels better in the fresh air and worse in a warm room.

Constitutional or Foot Hydrotherapy

These therapies stimulate the immune system and relieve congestion of the upper respiratory passageways and sinus. (See Hydrotherapy for Children on page 115 for directions.)

Vital Fact

We have had many parents ask us what they can do for their children because they catch cold after cold in the wintertime. One of the simplest but most effective prescriptions has been to give extra vitamin C. This makes sense, as many children receive less fruit during the winter season and thus their vitamin C intakes decrease. A high percentage of the parents report that this simple vitamin makes a dramatic reduction in their children's frequency and duration of colds as compared with the previous winter. Taking vitamin C in addition to a children's multivitamin is even better, as so many vitamins and minerals are needed for proper function of the immune system.

Vital Study

For a study published in *Forum Immunologie*, researchers followed 108 people who had a high susceptibility to colds to see whether echinacea extract use made a difference. People selected had had at least three cold-related infections the previous winter. One group received 4 milliliters (120 drops) of echinacea twice daily, while the other group received a placebo. Blood tests to measure immune function were taken at the beginning of the study and at two other intervals. The groups were examined after 4 weeks and 8 weeks to see whether a cold infection had occurred. Clinical results showed that people treated with echinacea had a decreased frequency of infections. These people also developed milder infections and had a longer time interval before their first infection (40 days) compared with 25 days for the placebo group. In addition, the echinacea group had fewer infections that spread to the lower respiratory tract.

Acupressure

Gently press the acupressure point with a thumb for 10 to 15 seconds. Repeat three times and then do the same on the other side of the body. Repeat daily.

Large Intestine 4—Relieves head congestion and sinus discomfort. Located in the web-bing between the thumb and index finger.

Large Intestine 20—Reduces sneezing and nasal symptoms. Located on the lower, outer corner of each nostril.

■ ADVANCED PLAN

Nutritional Supplements

Zinc—For treatment of the common cold, zinc is best used in the form of a zinc gluconate lozenge. Studies have shown zinc gluconate to be effective for cold sufferers. Zinc lozenges should be used only with children who are old enough to suck on them without choking. They should not exceed 30 milligrams daily of elemental zinc for more than 5 days.

Thymus glandular extract—Give one to two 250-milligram tablets or capsules daily. Also available in a homeopathic liquid preparation (give 5 drops twice daily).

Herbal Remedies

There are several herbs that can be used to treat viral infections such as the common cold. We frequently recommend a formula called the virus cocktail that includes echinacea, astragalus, lomatium, reishi, and licorice root. It is safe to use with children. Echinacea is a good herb to start with.

Astragalus—One of the best Chinese herbs for the common cold. Supports the immune system and tonifies the lungs. Do not use when a fever is present.

Lomatium—A potent antiviral herb that inhibits the replication of viruses. Used by herbalists and naturopathic doctors for the common cold and flu.

Fresh ginger tea—This can help a cold and sore throat. It is also helpful to relieve chills that accompany a cold. Have your child sip a cup of warm ginger tea during the day. If using fresh ginger root, make a decoction. If using a tea bag, make an infusion. (See "Herbal Preparations" on page 30 for more on tea decoctions and infusions.)

Yarrow—This herb can be used if a high fever accompanies the cold.

Note: If your child is prone to colds during the winter, immune-supportive herbs can be used throughout the winter season. We typically recommend that echinacea, larix, or a combination of the herbs listed here be taken for 4 weeks on and then 1 week off. Repeat this cycle throughout the winter. This can be helpful for kids in a day care setting who are exposed to a higher concentration of cold viruses. It is of course important that diet and nutritional deficiencies be addressed as well.

Aromatherapy

Peppermint or tea tree oil—Add 1 drop of one of these oils to a vaporizer and use it in your child's room. If the child is taking a homeopathic remedy, use aromatherapy at a different time.

■ WHAT TO EXPECT

If natural therapies are started at the first signs of symptoms, the cold may be averted or the length and severity greatly reduced. Improvements should be seen within 48 hours of beginning natural therapy. The chance of a more serious illness developing is greatly reduced with the natural approaches outlined in this chapter.

Cold Sores

Cold sores, also known as fever blisters, are painful skin eruptions that form on or at the edge of the lips. In rarer instances, they can also appear on the nose, chin, cheeks, and other parts of the body.

These small, red, fluid-filled blisters are painful and itchy and yield tingling sensations. After a week or so, the blisters turn from red to a crusty yellow, a sign that healing has begun.

Cold sores are caused by the herpes simplex virus, which is highly contagious. Some estimates suggest that all of us come into contact with at least one strain of the virus before age 5. The virus can remain dormant in a nerve for a lifetime or become activated and replicate.

This condition is capable of recurring. That's because even though the sores disappear within 2 weeks, the virus is still alive and thriving inside the nerve root cells of the body.

Stress, tiredness, sunlight exposure, food sensitivities, or a secondary infection such as a common cold can reactivate the dormant herpes simplex virus and create a cold sore outbreak.

Generally, cold sores are unsightly and an-

Case History

Terry was brought to our clinic by his mother. Only 10 years old, he was constantly battling cold sores that kept reoccurring on his mouth. We tested him for food sensitivities and found that peanuts and citrus fruits came up highly reactive. His mother kept Terry away from these foods as much as possible over the next year, and he had only one outbreak after that—at a party when he ate some peanuts.

noying. But notify your pediatrician when your child:

- Develops cold sores before his first birthday
- Complains of vision problems when he has a cold sore. That could be a clue that the virus has spread to the eyes.
- Contracts his first outbreak of cold sores
- Has many cold sores on his lips and cheeks, and inside his mouth
- Has cold sores that last more than 2 weeks

Conventional treatment focuses on pain relievers (topical and internal). Applying ice during the initial outbreak of a cold sore can help to suppress its growth. Have the child rub ice on the affected area for a couple of minutes every hour. More aggressive conventional treatment involves use of the antiviral drug acyclovir.

■ BASIC PLAN

Diet

Foods containing the amino acid L-arginine may promote the growth of the herpes virus. Have your child minimize these foods if he has recurring outbreaks, or take them out of the diet when a cold sore has begun to form. Foods containing L-arginine include chocolate, nuts, cereal grains, carob, raisins, and corn.

Increase foods that contain the amino acid L-lysine, which suppresses the herpes virus. Foods with a high content of this amino acid include beans, potatoes, fish, eggs, and brewer's yeast.

Acidic foods such as oranges and tomatoes should be avoided during an outbreak. If your child suffers from chronic outbreaks, these foods should be avoided indefinitely.

Identify food sensitivities, which could be contributing to reoccurring outbreaks. (See "Food Allergies and Food Sensitivities" on page 298 for details.)

Soups are good to give a child to eat during a cold sore outbreak, especially since they don't require much chewing and thus avoid aggravating a tender cold sore.

Nutritional Supplements

L-lysine—This amino acid on an empty stomach helps to suppress the herpes virus. Children over 6 can take 250 milligrams twice daily on an empty stomach for 1 week.

Vitamin C—Supports the immune system and has mild anti-inflammatory effects. The type with bioflavonoids is preferable. Dosage:

the child's age in years times 50 milligrams, taken twice daily. Reduce the dosage if diarrhea occurs. Consider using a buffered vitamin C powder (nonacidic) or liquid vitamin C. Both work well for infants and children, and can be mixed in juice.

Herbal Remedies

Topical creams of either licorice root or melissa are very effective in alleviating pain that accompanies cold sores. They also suppress viral replication.

Echinacea and lomatium—Give your child one or both of these herbs for their antiviral and immune-enhancing effects.

Homeopathy

Pick the following remedy that best matches your child's symptoms. Unless otherwise indicated, give your child 2 pellets of a 30C potency twice daily. (For infants, crush the pellets into powder and mix it with water.) Improvements should be seen within 48 hours. If there is no improvement within 48 hours, try another remedy. After you first notice improvement, stop giving the remedy unless symptoms begin to return.

Note: Lower potencies (6X, 12X, 6C) may need to be given more often (three times daily).

Arsenicum album—For red lesions that burn intensely and feel better with warm applications. The child's cold sores are worse from eating citrus fruit.

Hepar sulphuris—For cold sore blisters that are very tender to the touch and feel worse with cold applications. Pus formation occurs rapidly. Fluid-filled blisters are infected.

Natrum muriaticum—For reoccurring cold sores, especially that occur on the upper lips. The lips are very dry and cracked, with a crack in the middle of the lower lip. The child has high thirst. Exposure to sun and cold brings on an outbreak. Also for herpes that occurs after emotional shock or grief, and for canker sores that occur along with cold sores.

Rhus toxicodendron—For red, itchy, fluid filled blisters that burn and crust over. The lips are swollen and inflamed.

■ ADVANCED PLAN

Nutritional Supplements

Zinc—Supports the immune system and enhances skin healing. Dosage: children 2 and younger, 5 milligrams; 2 and older, 10 to 15 milligrams. Use for 2 weeks and then stop.

Children's multivitamin—Provides a base of nutrients that optimize immune function. Should contain selenium, which prevents viruses from replicating.

Herbal Remedy

Calendula—Apply as a tincture (1 teaspoon mixed with 4 teaspoons of water) or cream to sores to speed up healing and prevent a secondary infection. Apply twice daily.

Homeopathy

Herpes simplex nosode—Useful when a child is prone to reoccurring cold sore outbreaks. Give the child a 30C potency twice daily for 3 days and stop. Helps to prevent future outbreaks.

Aromatherapy

Myrrh and lemon—Add these to a carrier oil, then apply to the cold sore with a cotton swab. Repeat two or three times daily.

■ WHAT TO EXPECT

You should see a reduction of symptoms within 2 days of treatment and healing of the lesions within 7 to 14 days. Natural therapy begun at the onset of an outbreak can greatly reduce the severity of the outbreak. Your child will be much less susceptible to future outbreaks if you follow the guidelines in this chapter.

Colic

Excessive crying, irritability, and apparent abdominal pain characterize the symptoms of colic. This condition is a cause of frustration and concern for many parents.

Pediatricians refer to this condition as "the rule of the threes." The Chinese describe this behavior as "the 100 days' crying." Colic tends to last at least 3 hours a day, 3 days a week, and 3 weeks in a month. These crying episodes usually occur between the first 3 weeks of life until the age of 3 months. They frequently begin in the late afternoon and last until the evening.

Colic is not hereditary or affected by birth order. The first baby may be colicky but her subsequent siblings may not be.

There are different theories as to what causes colic. Likely causes of colic are allergies to milk or formulas, foods that the breastfeeding mother is eating and passing through the breast milk, colon spasms, a hyperactive gastrointestinal tract, tension in the household, or parental anxiety. We find that colic is much less common in children who are breastfed. This is likely due to the components of breast milk that mature an infant's digestive tract.

Don't dismiss all crying as harmless colic. If your newborn exhibits these behaviors, you should contact a doctor:

- A dramatic change in her crying pattern that leads to more painful outbursts
- Crying that is long in duration and inconsolable during all times of the day
- Awakening in pain and crying

Note: Always follow your intuition if you suspect that your baby is experiencing pain somewhere on her body.

Our experience is that diet changes and natural remedies, especially homeopathy, are highly successful in alleviating or improving this condition.

Conventional treatment involves gas-relieving medications, sedatives, and antispasmodic medicines.

■ BASIC PLAN

Diet

Foods that a breastfeeding mother eats can cause digestive reactions in her infant.

Common offenders include dairy products such as cow's milk and cheese; caffeine-containing foods such as coffee and chocolate; spicy foods such as garlic, onions, and peppers; citrus fruits and juices; soft drinks; wheat and corn; and brewer's yeast. Gas-forming foods such as cauliflower, broccoli, cucumbers, and beans should be avoided as well to see if there is improvement. Cut out these foods if you are eating a lot of them, and see whether your baby improves over the period of a week. Steamed and cooked vegetables are preferable while you are breastfeeding, as they are broken down more efficiently.

Solely breastfeeding is recommended until at least 6 months of age, to prevent colic.

The formula that a bottlefed infant is using may cause colic. Switch to a non-cow's-milk formula. Hypoallergenic, predigested protein formulas are available in most pharmacies and grocery stores.

It is important for a mother to be relaxed while breastfeeding her infant, as tension can affect the taste and flow of breast milk. It's also important to use the proper position, whether feeding a baby from the breast or the bottle. Improper position can lead to the baby swallowing too much air.

Nutritional Supplements

Vitamin supplements that a breastfeeding mother takes can contribute to colic. They should be avoided for 2 weeks to see if there is improvement.

Probiotic—A children's probiotic supplement can be helpful to improve digestive function, especially if the baby was given antibiotics at birth. The formula should contain *Lactobacillus bifidus* and *L. acidophilus*. Add it to formula or put it on the breastfeeding mother's nipple before nursing. Or, have baby suck it off your finger. Follow the directions on the container.

Herbal Remedies

Four main herbs that are used for colic include fennel, chamomile, peppermint, and catnip. They can be used individually or in formulas.

Start with giving the baby fennel: 1 teaspoon of fresh tea three times daily or as needed for the relief of colic. If that doesn't seem to help after a day or so, switch to one of the other herbs (it's the same dose for all). Glycerin tinctures (nonalcoholic) can also be used at 3 drops per dose.

A breastfeeding mother can also drink 2 cups of ginger tea during the day to help her infant.

Homeopathy

Use a combination colic formula, or use whichever of the following remedies matches up best to the child's symptoms. For the remedies that follow, unless otherwise indicated, give your child 2 pellets of a 30C potency twice daily. (Crush the pellets into powder and mix it with water.) Improvements should be seen within 48 hours. If there is no improvement within 48 hours, try another remedy. After you first notice improvement, stop giving the remedy unless symptoms begin to return.

Note: Lower potencies (6X, 12X, 6C) may need to be given more often (three times daily).

Aethusa cynapium—The infant is unable to digest milk and vomits the milk up. This reaction to milk (breast milk and other kinds) leads to colic.

Calcarea carbonica—The infant fits the Calcarea carbonica constitutional type. (See "Constitutional Homeopathic Remedies for Children" on page 60). She is large and flabby, and sweats easily on her head. She spits up milk. There is a sour odor to her body.

Chamomilla—This is the most common remedy for colic. The infant is screaming, irritable, hard to console, and wants to be carried (less crying while carried but the relief is only temporary). She may also have greenish diarrhea. Symptoms are worse while teething.

Colocynthis—The child pulls her feet up to her abdomen. Better with warm applications, lying face downward, and with pressure. The child is irritable.

Dioscorea villosa—The infant arches backward during bouts of colic.

Ignatia—For continuous crying. Especially indicated when the mother is emotionally upset from mental or emotional stress (present or during the pregnancy). Can be used by both mother and infant.

Lycopodium—The infant has a lot of gas and bloating after 4:00 P.M. She does not like tight diapers or clothes around the abdomen.

Magnesia phosphorica—The child pulls her feet up to her abdomen and is better with warm applications.

Nux vomica—For colic that is related to constipation or a reaction to foods. The child is chilly and irritable, and may arch back. Better with warm applications.

Pulsatilla—The child fits the Pulsatilla constitutional type—clingy and wants to be cuddled by her mother constantly. (See "Constitutional Homeopathic Remedies for Children" on page 60.) She feels better being carried and talked to. She feels better in fresh air and worse in warm rooms.

Aromatherapy

German chamomile and ginger—Dilute this combination in a carrier oil such as grape seed, olive, or sweet almond oil, and rub it on the abdomen. If the child is taking a homeopathic remedy, use aromatherapy at a different time.

Other Recommendations

Every parent finds a technique that helps to relax a colicky child. It can be walking around your home and gently bouncing the baby in your arms. Some parents find that a quiet environment with dim lighting and soft music is helpful. Others find that baby bouncing seats help, or that holding a warm water bottle to the infant's belly helps to relieve colic.

■ ADVANCED PLAN

See a massage therapist for abdominal massage. (A therapist trained in infant massage is best.) You can also get a constitutional homeopathic remedy from a homeopathic practitioner.

■ WHAT TO EXPECT

We find that the correct natural treatment usually provides relief within 2 to 3 days. The correct homeopathic remedy often provides relief the same day it is first given. The diet recommendations in this chapter are important to follow to treat the underlying cause of many cases of colic.

Conjunctivitis

Better known as pinkeye, conjunctivitis results in the inflammation of the conjunctiva, the delicate tissue that protects the surface of the eyeball and the inner eyelid.

Conjunctivitis often starts in one eye and spreads to the other. The telltale signs include itchiness, redness of the eye, and swelling of the eyelid. Often, there is a sticky discharge or crusting from the eye. Sometimes, the lids will stick together, particularly when the child awakens. A child may complain of sensitivity to light, blurred vision, or a gritty feeling in his eye.

This is a highly contagious condition typically caused by a virus or, less often, by a bacterial infection. It readily spreads from child to child at schools and day care centers, much like a common cold. In the home, the condition can spread to family members who come into contact with contaminated bed linens.

Newborns whose tear ducts have not completely formed may develop a type of conjunctivitis.

Beyond viral and bacterial infections, common allergens such as cigarette smoke and pollen can cause allergic conjunctivitis.

This is usually not a serious disease. However, see your doctor if the symptoms do not disappear within a couple of days of treatment. Immediately notify your doctor if your child experiences blurred vision. That could be a symptom of a more serious health condition.

Conventional medicine focuses on antibacterial or anti-allergy eye drops.

■ BASIC PLAN

Diet

Have your child eat foods rich in vitamin A (carrots, sweet potatoes, parsley, kale, spinach, mangoes, broccoli, and squash) and vitamin C (citrus fruits, tomatoes, green peppers, dark green leafy vegetables, broccoli, cantaloupe, strawberries, Brussels sprouts, potatoes, and asparagus).

Avoid sugar products as they lower immune function.

Nutritional Supplements

Vitamin C—Helps support the immune system. Dosage: the child's age in years times 50 milligrams, twice daily. Reduce the dosage if diarrhea occurs. Consider using a buffered vitamin C powder (nonacidic) or liquid vitamin C. Both work well for infants and children, and can be mixed in juice.

Vitamin A—Helps support the immune system. Daily dosage: infants under 1 year, 1,875 international units (IU); children 1 to 3, 2,000 IU; kids 4 to 6, 2,500 IU; kids 7 to 10, 3,500 IU; males 11 and older, 5,000 IU; females 11 and older, 4,000 IU.

Note: These dosages are for short-term use (up to 10 days). Higher dosages may be used only under a doctor's supervision. Available in liquid drops.

Herbal Remedy

Euphrasia (eyebright) eye drops—Help relieve itching and fight infections of the eye. Add 5 drops of euphrasia to ½ ounce of saline solution. Place 1 or 2 drops in the infected eye(s) three times daily.

Homeopathy

Give Similisan or other combination homeopathic eye drops for irritation. Give as directed on the container.

Or pick the following remedy that best matches your child's symptoms. Unless otherwise indicated, give your child 2 pellets of a 30C potency three times daily. (For infants, crush the pellets into powder and mix it with water.) Improvements should be seen within 48 hours. If there is no improvement within 48 hours, try another remedy. After you first notice improvement, stop giving the remedy unless symptoms begin to return.

Note: Lower potencies (6X, 12X, 6C) may need to be given more often (four times daily).

Apis mellifica—For marked swelling of the inner eyelid with stinging, burning tears and itchy eyes. The eyes feel hot. The child feels worse in a warm room and better with cold applications to the eyes.

Argentum nitricum—For conjunctivitis in newborns. Discharge is thick.

Arsenicum album—For tremendous tearing of the eyes, which burn and throb. The child is restless.

Belladonna—For conjunctivitis that comes on very quickly, along with a red face and fever. The child feels throbbing pain and is sensitive to light. More common in the child's right eye.

Euphrasia—The child's eyes and eyelids are red. He has watery, burning tears and a runny nose. Good for allergy-related conjunctivitis.

Hepar sulphuris—For inflamed eyelids that are very sensitive to touch and cold. The eyes have a yellow, thick discharge.

Mercurius solubilis or vivus—For the middle to later stages of conjunctivitis, where there is lots of discharge. Burning pain is worse at night and worse with warmth. The eyes have foul-smelling discharge.

Pulsatilla—For yellow or greenish discharge from the eyes. Fresh air and cold water to the eyes provides relief. The eyes may be stuck when the child wakes up in the morning. The child is weepy and clingy. Eyes feel worse in a warm room.

Sulphur—For hot, red, dry eyes. The child feels burning pain. Symptoms are worse in a warm room and better in the fresh air.

■ ADVANCED PLAN

Nutritional Supplements

Zinc—Supports the immune system and enhances skin healing. Dosage: children 2 and younger, 5 milligrams; 2 and older, 10 to 15 milligrams. Use for 2 weeks and then stop.

Quercitin—Has anti-allergy affects that are helpful for conjunctivitis. Dosage: 3 milligrams per pound of body weight, twice daily.

Herbal Remedy

Echinacea and goldenseal combination—For immune support to fight a bacterial or viral infection.

Acupressure

Gently press the acupressure point with your thumb for 10 to 15 seconds. Perform on both sides of the child's body and repeat three times each day.

Yuyao—The indentation in the middle of the eyebrow (straight up from the pupil)

Gallbladder 20—Located below the base of the skull, in the space between the two vertical neck muscles.

■ WHAT TO EXPECT

Improvement should be seen within 48 hours of beginning natural therapy.

Constipation

If a child is having noticeably fewer bowel movements or difficulty and discomfort passing large, hard stools, it is likely that she is constipated.

Stools form in the large intestine, which removes moisture from wet, shapeless waste that has passed through the small intestine. Constipation commonly results from a diet lacking in fluids and/or fiber.

Insufficient fluids and fiber cause stools to become rigid and hard or to develop sharp, jagged surfaces that could painfully stretch or tear the rectal tissue during a bowel movement. Blood in the stool and a child's pain will more than likely be the result of a rectal fissure, or tear.

Some children are also reluctant to move their bowels away from home. A retained stool can become dehydrated and hard, making it difficult to pass.

After one month of life, most infants have three or four daily bowel movements, which usually follow feedings. Some breastfed babies, however, have one bowel movement a day, every other day or once a week, because they use the milk so efficiently that they don't have any waste. The most important thing is that the infant's stool is soft and discomfort does not seem to be a problem.

It is common for breastfed infants to have problems with constipation after being started on solid foods. This transition usually lasts only a week.

Bowel movement patterns differ from child to child. Some will move their bowels once every 2 to 3 days. Others will move their bowels once a day.

It's important for parents to familiarize themselves with their child's typical bowel habits and the consistency of stools. The most telling factor in determining whether your child is constipated is to gauge her comfort in passing a stool. Also, an aching or tender

Vital Study

Researchers at the University of Palermo Pediatric Hospital in Italy studied 27 infants (average age 20.7 months) who suffered from chronic constipation without a known cause, and looked at the role cow's milk played in their condition. The only change researchers made to the children's diet was the substitution of soy milk instead of cow's milk. During the diet that was free of cow's milk protein, there was a resolution of symptoms in 21 infants, and improvements were noticed within 3 days. When the cow's milk was reintroduced, the symptoms returned within 2 to 3 days.

stomach may signal constipation. Children should have at least one complete bowel movement daily.

Seek medical evaluation when:

- There is blood in the stool
- Your child is constipated and vomiting
- She has severe pain while passing a stool
- There is a loss of control over bowel movements
- There is anal or abdominal pain that lasts more than 2 hours
- There is no stool for 7 consecutive days
- Your child has chronic constipation

Conventional treatment focuses on increasing the child's intake of fluids and dietary fiber, on laxatives, and on behavior modification.

Note: Do not use enemas or suppositories without a physician's advice, as they can cause irritation or tearing in the rectum if done improperly.

Stress can be at the root of constipation. Holding in feelings can result in physical problems such as constipation. Help your child with underlying emotional and mental stress. Counseling may be necessary.

Abdominal massage also helps to improve bowel activity.

■ BASIC PLAN

Encouraging regularity is the best cure for constipation. Get your child in the habit of sitting on the toilet at the same time each morning to develop a pattern of bowel elimination. The child should sit on the toilet for a good 5 minutes without being in a hurry. Regular exercise helps to improve bowel elimination. If your child is not active physically, help her to choose some physical activities to do on a regular basis.

Diet

Start by increasing fluids in your child's diet. Water, diluted fruit juices, diluted herbal teas, and soups are ways to increase fluid intake. A glass of warm water and lemon in the morning helps to move the bowels.

Increase fiber intake as well. Vegetables and fruits are the best sources of fiber. Give pureed vegetables to infants, and give steamed and cooked vegetables such as broccoli, cauliflower, and carrots for children. Carrot sticks, celery, and cauliflower with dip as snacks between meals are helpful for older children. Whole grain foods such as oatmeal and whole wheat bread are also good sources of fiber for older children. Ground-up flaxseeds are an excellent source of fiber: Grind 1 teaspoon of flaxseeds per 50 pounds of body weight (children weighing 30 to 50 pounds may also use 1 teaspoon), and give this amount daily mixed with food, in a shake, or in juice. (Always accompany with 8 ounces of water.) Apples provide a good source of fiber. Cooked prunes, or prunes soaked overnight, and prune juice have a natural laxative effect. They should be used in moderation or for short-term relief of constipation. Bran muffins mixed with fruit such as raisins are popular with children, and they're a good way to increase fiber.

Avoid or reduce the intake of bananas and dairy products, which can be constipating.

A bottlefed infant suffering from constipation should be switched to a different formula to see if it makes a difference. Nondairy formulas usually work best.

Food sensitivities can be at the root of constipation. (See "Food Allergies and Food Sensitivities" on page 298 to learn how to identify them.)

Nutritional Supplement

Probiotic—Look for a children's probiotic supplement with acidophilus and bifidus, which can be helpful to improve elimination. It is especially important for infants who have been on antibiotics. Give as

directed on the container.

Caution: Parents should not give higher does of magnesium and vitamin C as "natural laxatives" for long-term treatment. These two nutrients do move the bowels, but in an artificial manner. Long-term use can result in dehydration and make the bowels "lazier."

Herbal Remedies

Laxative herbs such as cascara sagrada and senna should be used only on a short-term basis for the relief of acute bouts of constipation. They should not be used with infants.

Herbs such as fennel root, licorice, and yellow dock can be used on a long-term basis to tonify the digestive tract and make bowel elimination more efficient.

Homeopathy

Pick the following remedy that best matches your child's symptoms. Unless otherwise indicated, give your child 2 pellets of a 30C potency twice daily. (For infants, crush the pellets into powder and mix it with water.) Improvements should be seen within 2 to 3 days. If there is no improvement within 3 days, try another remedy. After you first notice improvement, stop giving the remedy unless symptoms begin to return.

Note: Lower potencies (6X, 12X, 6C) may need to be given more often (three times daily).

Alumina—The child goes many days without the desire to pass stool. She strains intensely to pass even a soft stool. Stools are usually hard and dry.

Bryonia alba—For dry, large stools. The

child is irritable and has high thirst for cold drinks. The colon feels better with pressure.

Calcarea carbonica—For constipation in children and infants who tend to be large, flabby, and sweat easily (especially on their feet and the backs of their heads). There are no urges for a bowel movement.

Natrum muriaticum—For children who tend to be more withdrawn and serious. They crave salt and drink lots of water but still have dry stools and constipation.

Nux moschata—For severe constipation; the child is very sleepy and drowsy. The child has low thirst.

Nux vomica—The child is irritable and suffers from constipation. Incomplete bowel movements. The child has a great urging to pass stool but passes only small quantities, which are painful.

Silica—The child has difficulty passing stool and often passes only small pieces of stool. The stool may partially come out and then recede back in. The child tends to be thin and delicate.

Acupressure

Gently press the acupressure point with a thumb for 10 to 15 seconds. Perform on both sides of the body and repeat three times each day.

Large Intestine 4—Relieves constipation. Located in the webbing between the thumb and index finger.

Stomach 36—Improves digestive function. Located four finger-widths below the kneecap and one finger-width toward the outside of the leg (outside of the shinbone on the muscle).

Aromatherapy

Roman chamomile and ginger—Add these to a carrier oil and rub it onto the abdomen once daily. If the child is taking a homeopathic remedy, use aromatherapy at a different time.

■ WHAT TO EXPECT

You should see the bowels becoming more regular within 1 week for children with chronic constipation. For acute cases, improvement should be seen within 24 to 48 hours.

Contact Dermatitis

This skin condition is inflammation resulting from contact with or exposure to a substance. Symptoms include blisters, intense itching, and a red, thick, flaky rash.

There are two types of contact dermatitis. The most common type is irritant contact dermatitis, which occurs when an external irritant touches the skin. The rash from hand eczema, for example, may be triggered by soaps, dishwashing detergents, and cleaning agents.

The second but more serious type is allergic contact dermatitis, which describes the reaction that follows exposure to a particular substance (an allergen). The first contact doesn't immediately spark the reaction. It sensitizes the child to the allergen, and subsequent exposures trigger the reaction.

An allergic reaction occurs when the body recognizes allergens and reacts by activating immune cells that release chemical mediators in the skin contact area. The combination of the allergen and the mediator produces the itching rash and oozing blisters within 8 to 72 hours after the exposure.

Common allergens are poison ivy, poison sumac, and poison oak; metals, such as nickel, in jewelry and watches; and some furry pets. Preservatives, fragrances, and other chemical additives found in lotions and makeup can also lead to an allergic reaction.

■ BASIC PLAN

Diet

Avoid known food sensitivities, which can further aggravate the skin rash. (See "Food Allergies and Food Sensitivities" on page 298 for more information.)

Nutritional Supplement

Vitamin C—Provides support to the immune system. Dosage: the child's age in years times 50 milligrams, twice daily. Reduce the dosage if diarrhea occurs. Consider using a buffered vitamin C powder (nonacidic) or liquid vitamin C. Both work well for infants and children, and can be mixed in juice.

Herbal Remedy

Calendula or aloe cream or gel—Apply topically to soothe and heal skin.

Homeopathy

Pick the following remedy that best matches your child's symptoms. Unless otherwise indicated, give your child 2 pellets of a 30C potency twice daily. (For infants, crush the pellets into powder and mix it with water.) Improvements should be seen within 48 hours. If there is no improvement within 48 hours, try another remedy. After you first notice improvement, stop giving the remedy unless symptoms begin to return.

Note: Lower potencies (6X, 12X, 6C) may need to be given more often (three times daily).

Arsenicum album—For a burning rash that is better with warm applications.

Sulphur—For skin irritation that is very red, burning, and itchy. Give a dose twice daily for 2 to 3 days.

■ WHAT TO EXPECT

Once the offending substance has been avoided, improvement should be seen within 3 to 7 days.

Cough

Coughs are part of the body's natural security system. These sudden bursts of air and sputum from the breathing tract are attempts to clear the windpipe and lungs of viruses, bacteria, dusts, chemical irritants, or foreign objects so that oxygen flows easily toward the lungs.

The sound of a cough often suggests its cause. A cough may be loud and barking, dry and scratchy, or moist and muted by mucus—as when it is a common symptom of a cold and related diseases of the ear, nose, and throat.

A cough can also be a symptom of a viral or bacterial respiratory tract infection, such as pneumonia, bronchitis, or croup. In some cases, a cough could suggest more serious conditions, such as a tumor, heart disease, cystic fibrosis, or asthma or epiglottitis.

A cough may come in fits—as when it signals choking or a reaction to environmental irritants, such as chemical fumes, dust, or cigarette smoke.

Since curiosity often drives young children to put small objects and toys in their mouths, watch them carefully to make sure that nothing gets swallowed or becomes an obstruction. See your doctor if you suspect that your child has swallowed an object.

A cool mist humidifier in your child's room may relieve dry coughs. Leave it on during the night. A hot shower can help with a stuffy nose and cough. This can help temporarily relieve his congestion and help him eat, drink, and get to sleep. Prop the child's head up with pillows at night to help him breathe easier. Encourage productive coughing: Coughing is a reflex that enables mucus and infections to be expelled from the respiratory passageways. Gentle patting on the back can be helpful for infants. Suppression of a cough can lead to a more serious illness, such as pneumonia.

■ BASIC PLAN

Diet

Have your child go on a low-mucus diet by avoiding foods such as dairy products and bananas. Eliminate refined sugar products, as they can lower immune function. Soups, stews, and steamed vegetables are good choices. Garlic, fresh ginger, and onions are also good; they help relieve congestion.

If your child often suffers from coughs, then food sensitivities could well be a problem. (See "Food Allergies and Food Sensitivities" on page 298 for more information.)

Increase your child's fluid intake. Have him drink fluids every 2 to 3 hours. Try to avoid concentrated fruit juices; use water or diluted fruit juice instead. The temperature of the fluid should be based on the child's preference.

Nutritional Supplements

Vitamin A—Supports the immune system. Daily dosage: infants under 1 year, 1,875 international units (IU); children 1 to 3, 2,000 IU; kids 4 to 6, 2,500 IU; kids 7 to 10, 3,500 IU; males 11 and older, 5,000 IU; females 11 and older, 4,000 IU.

Note: These dosages are for short-term use (up to 10 days). Higher dosages may be used only under a doctor's supervision. Available in liquid drops.

Vitamin C—Supports the immune system. Dosage: the child's age in years times 50 milligrams, twice daily. Reduce the dosage if diarrhea occurs. Consider using a buffered vitamin C powder (nonacidic) or liquid vitamin C. Both work well for infants and children, and can be mixed in juice.

Herbal Remedies

Children's herbal cough formula— Herbs in a formula often include one or more of the following: echinacea, goldenseal, mullein, wild cherry bark, horehound, and licorice. They may also contain essential oils such as peppermint leaf extract or menthol oil to help open up the respiratory passageways.

Echinacea and goldenseal—If a children's herbal cough formula is not available, use this combination.

Homeopathy

It is easiest to use a combination cough formula. Or you can choose the one of the following remedies that best matches your child's symptoms. Unless otherwise indicated, give your child 2 pellets of a 30C potency three times daily. (For infants, crush the pellets into powder and mix it with water.) Improvements should be seen within 24 hours. If there is no improvement within 24 hours, try another remedy. After you first notice improvement, stop giving the remedy unless symptoms begin to return.

Note: Lower potencies (6X, 12X, 6C) may need to be given more often (four times daily).

Aconitum napellus—For a short, dry cough from exposure to dry, cold air; great restlessness, anxiety; hot skin; a cough that gets better when the child lies on his back. The child is thirsty. Useful in the initial stage of a cough—the first 4 hours of symptoms.

Antimonium tartaricum—For a deep, rattling cough. The child has trouble bringing up mucus when he coughs. He may find it hard to breathe at times. He feels better in a cool room with the window open. Used in the more advanced stages of bronchitis.

Arsenicum album—For a cough with burning pain. The cough is worse at night (midnight to 2:00 A.M.). It gets better with warm applications and warm drinks. The child is restless and anxious.

Bryonia alba—For a dry cough that is very painful. It gets worse with any movement or when taking a deep breath. It feels better in the open air. The child has a high thirst for cold drinks and is irritable.

Coccus cacti—For a cough that produces stringy mucus. The child is constantly clearing his throat. The cough leads to vomiting.

Drosera—For a dry, barking cough that may end in gagging. The cough is worse when lying down and tends to come on after midnight.

Hepar sulphuris—For a rattling, barking cough that comes on after exposure to dry, cold air. The child coughs when he is uncovered or gets undressed. There is yellow mucus discharge. The child is irritable.

Ipecacuanha—For a cough with a lot of mucus that makes the child nauseated, gag, or vomit. Mucus may have tinges of blood in it.

Kali bichromicum—Thick, stringy, ropy, yellow or yellowish green mucus is coughed up. The child is worse from eating and drinking.

Phosphorus—For a cold that turns into bronchitis. Dry, tickling cough. The child may have burning in his chest and feels better with cold drinks. The cough is worse when lying on the left side. The child is hoarse. He desires company when sick.

Pulsatilla—For a cough with green or yellow-green mucus. The child is warm and clingy. He feels better when held and with fresh air or in the open air. The cough is often worse at night and while lying down. The child is thirstless.

Rumex crispus—For a dry cough that begins when lying down. There is a tickling sensation in the throat that leads to a cough. The cough gets worse in cold or open air.

Spongia tosta—For a dry, barking cough that is better from warm foods or liquids. The child is hoarse.

Acupressure

Gently press the acupressure point with a thumb for 10 to 15 seconds. Perform on both sides of the body and repeat three times each day.

Pericardium 6—Relaxes the bronchial passageway. Located 2½ finger-widths below the wrist crease, in the middle of the forearm (palm side).

Lung 1—Reduces cough. Located in the front of the shoulder area, in the space below where the collarbone and shoulder meet.

Hydrotherapy

Constitutional hydrotherapy is excellent, as it reduces congestion in the bronchial tubes and brings good immune cells into the infected area. The second option is foot hydrotherapy.

(See Hydrotherapy for Children on page 115 for directions for these treatments.) Perform either treatment one or two times daily.

Also, you can go into the bathroom, turn the shower on, and let steam fill up the room. Then, sit in the bathroom with the child for 5 minutes. This will help him breathe easier.

■ ADVANCED PLAN

Nutritional Supplement

Zinc—Supports the immune system and enhances skin healing. Dosage: children 2 and younger, 5 milligrams; 2 and older, 10 to 15 milligrams. Use for 2 weeks and then stop.

Herbal Remedies

Peppermint tea—Can help reduce irritating coughs.

Ginger tea—For bronchitis where the child is chilly and has mucus production.

Nettle—For a cough due to pollen allergies.

Aromatherapy

Eucalyptus and frankincense—Add equal parts of these to a carrier oil and apply it to the child's chest, or add them to a vaporizer in the child's room. (See Aromatherapy for Children on page 109 for directions.) If the child is taking a homeopathic remedy, use aromatherapy at a different time.

■ WHAT TO EXPECT

Improvement should be noticed within 2 days of treatment. Except where noted, do not discontinue therapy once the child has shown initial signs of improvement; continue until the condition has completely resolved.

Cradle Cap

Common during infancy, this inflammatory skin disease commonly appears as a thick buildup of yellow, greasy scales around a child's scalp and/or the eyebrows, eyelids, ears, and nose. It may also appear around the groin area.

The condition is a type of seborrheic dermatitis, meaning that its cause lies in the overactivity of the sebaceous or oil-secreting glands. Children between the ages of 2 and 12 weeks are prone to cradle cap, which often clears itself by the time a child reaches 8 to 12 months.

The overactivity occurs when initial secretions of oil dry atop and clog the ducts, signaling the glands to produce and secrete more oil as a means of opening their own blocked passageways. The excess oil production creates the chunky crusts or lesions that appear on the surface of the skin. Nutritional deficiencies such as biotin and essential fatty acids are often at the root of this problem.

Washing your baby's head and scalp too gently, even if you do it daily, may not remove the accumulating oils and may increase the likelihood of developing cradle cap. Take care to thoroughly wash your baby's skin with a washcloth. Though the skin is tender and soft, it is rubbery and quite strong.

As with other skin conditions, cradle cap can provide fertile areas for further infections. Conventional treatment focuses on antiseborrheic shampoos and steroid (hydrocortisone) ointments.

■ BASIC PLAN

Diet

Food sensitivities can aggravate this problem. If you are nursing, avoid dairy products, sugar, or other suspected food sensitivities for 2 weeks to see whether it helps. Also increase your intake of essential fatty acids to pass on to the baby. Add ground-up flaxseeds (grind 5 teaspoons daily) to your diet, along with plenty of water, and increase your intake of fresh coldwater fish such as salmon, halibut, and mackerel.

Bottlefed infants may need to switch to a hypoallergenic formula. Also, essential fatty acids should be added to the formula. (See "What If You Are Not Breastfeeding?" on page 131 for more information.)

Nutritional Supplements

The breastfeeding mother should take a combination of an omega-3-rich oil such as flaxseed oil or fish oil, and an omega-6-rich oil such as evening primrose or borage oil. Bottlefed infants should have ¼ teaspoon of flaxseed oil added to their bottles one or two times daily (reduce the amount if diarrhea occurs).

Biotin—Nursing mothers should take 3,000 micrograms twice daily. Infants not being breastfed should be given 300 micrograms daily.

Probiotic—A children's acidophilus supplement that contains bifidus helps to produce biotin in the digestive tract. Give as directed on the container.

Herbal Remedy

Massage your baby's scalp with olive oil. It contains essential fatty acids and helps to loosen the dry flakes of skin. Massage for 10 minutes and then comb away the loosened flakes with a fine-tooth comb. Repeat nightly.

Homeopathy

Pick the following remedy that best matches your child's symptoms. Unless otherwise indicated, give your child 2 pellets of a 30C potency twice daily. (For infants, pellets should be crushed and given in liquid.) Improvements should be seen within 2 weeks. If there is no improvement within 2 weeks, try another remedy. After you first notice improvement, stop giving the remedy unless symptoms begin to return.

Note: Lower potencies (6X, 12X, 6C) may need to be given more often (three times daily).

Calcarea carbonica—The infant is large and flabby, and her head sweats easily. The cradle cap is wet, with a thick yellow or white discharge that forms thick scabs.

Kali sulphuricum—For yellow or yellowish green scaly discharge.

Sulphur—The infant is always warm and kicks her covers off at night. There is profuse perspiration from the head. The cradle cap is dry and red.

Thuja occidentalis—For infants whose cradle cap is unresponsive to an indicated remedy.

■ ADVANCED PLAN

Nutritional Supplement

Infants' multivitamin—Supplies a base of nutrients. Give as directed on the container.

Aromatherapy

Add Roman chamomile and tea tree oil to aloe vera gel or olive oil and rub this onto the child's scalp each night. If the child is taking a homeopathic remedy, use aromatherapy at a different time.

■ WHAT TO EXPECT

Improvements should be noticed within 4 to 6 weeks of treatment. Scales will slough off.

Croup

Known medically as laryngotracheobronchitis, croup is an upper respiratory tract infection that often develops on the heels of another upper respiratory infection such as a sore throat or cold.

Croup is the swelling of the vocal cords and is almost always caused by a respiratory virus that affects and irritates the membranes surrounding the larynx (the voice box).

The inflammation narrows the upper part of the airway, making breathing difficult and coughing expected. Croup is characterized by a hoarse, barking cough combined with difficulty breathing and low-pitched wheezing with each inhalation. Symptoms are usually worse at night.

Croup is common in children ranging from 3 months to 3 years of age. Its symptoms, however, mirror those of choking or a bronchial infection.

Conventional treatment focuses on bronchodilating inhalants, steam, and rest. One easy home remedy is to fill your bathroom up with steam from a hot shower and sit in the room with your child for 5 minutes. This helps to relieve croup symptoms. In addition, a cool, moist humidifier can be used in the child's bedroom at night to soothe the airway. Some children experience symptomatic relief of their coughing with exposure to cold air. Bundle your child up and drive in the car with him with his window rolled down. This can help relieve his cough and help him fall asleep.

You can also help a baby relax by rocking him to soothing music. With an older child, reading him a book while rocking may help. Make sure your child sits upright in your lap.

Caution: Seek immediate medical attention if your child:

- Makes a whistling sound that gets louder with each breath
- Seems to be struggling to get a breath
- Has an unusual amount of drooling
- Cannot bend his neck forward
- Is turning pale, blue, or gray
- Cannot talk or cry

If your child is having trouble breathing or swallowing, do not try to open his mouth to look inside. He may have epiglottitis, in which the throat can close and the child goes into respiratory distress. Instead, go to the emergency room.

■ BASIC PLAN

Diet

Encourage easy-to-digest foods such as soups, stews, and cooked or steamed vegetables. Garlic and onions have antiviral effects; feed them if your child tolerates these foods. Fluids (water, herbal teas) should be consumed regularly throughout the day to prevent dehydration and to help thin and expel bronchial secretions. Omit sugar and dairy products from your child's diet, which can suppress immune function. Fruit juices should be diluted by at least 50 percent.

Nutritional Supplements

Vitamin A—Antiviral and supports the immune system. Daily dosage: infants under 1 year, 1,875 international units (IU); children 1 to 3, 2,000 IU; kids 4 to 6, 2,500 IU; kids 7 to 10, 3,500 IU; males 11 and older, 5,000 IU; females 11 and older, 4,000 IU.

Note: These dosages are for short-term use (up to 10 days). Higher dosages may be used only under a doctor's supervision. Available in liquid drops.

Vitamin C—Helps support the immune system. Dosage: the child's age in years times

Case History

Brian, a 15-month-old, was brought in to our clinic by his mother, a loyal patient of ours. Brian had a history of bronchitis and pneumonia, so she brought him in immediately when he developed a dry cough and looked like he was short of breath. On listening to his lungs, we could hear wheezing as he breathed. By listening to his cough and examining him, it was obvious that he had developed croup. Since his mother said that his coughing improved temporarily after he ate or drank, we prescribed the homeopathic Spongia tosta. We also recommended that his mother give him a hydrotherapy treatment daily. We requested that she call us the next day to report on how he was doing. She did so and joyfully told us that even after the first dose of the Spongia tosta, his coughing calmed down and he got some sleep. In only 12 hours' time, Brian was doing much better. He was totally symptom-free in 4 days.

50 milligrams, twice daily. Reduce the dosage if diarrhea occurs. Consider using a buffered vitamin C powder (nonacidic) or liquid vitamin C. Both work well for infants and children, and can be mixed in juice.

Herbal Remedy

Children's herbal cough formula— Herbs in a formula often include echinacea and/or lomatium, which have an antiviral effect and help stimulate the immune system, combined with herbs that relieve a dry, irritating cough, such as licorice, marshmallow root, plantain, slippery elm, and elecampane. Herbal formulas may also contain essential oils such as peppermint leaf extract or menthol oil to help open up the respiratory passageway. Avoid the herbs goldenseal and wild cherry bark with croup, as they can be too drying to the mucous membranes.

Homeopathy

Give your child a combination homeopathic cough remedy, or pick the one of the following remedies that best matches your child's symptoms. For the remedies below, unless otherwise indicated, give your child 2 pellets of a 30C potency three times daily. (For infants, crush the pellets into powder and mix it with water.) Improvements should be seen within 48 hours. If there is no improvement within 48 hours, try another remedy. After you first notice improvement, stop giving the remedy unless symptoms begin to return.

Note: Lower potencies (6X, 12X, 6C) may need to be given more often (four times daily).

Aconitum napellus—For a dry cough that comes on after the child is exposed to the wind. Intense symptoms come on suddenly. The child has a loud, barking cough and is fearful and anxious. Useful in the initial stages of croup (the first 12 hours).

Hepar sulphuris—The child is sensitive to cold air and drafts of cold air. The cough has become looser. The child is very irritable.

Spongia tosta—For a dry, barking cough that is usually worse before midnight. The cough is better after eating and drinking, especially after warm drinks.

Aromatherapy

Eucalyptus, tea tree oil, and lavender— Add equal amounts of each oil to 40 milliliters of carrier oil (such as grape seed, olive, or sweet almond oil) and apply this mixture to the chest. Or choose one of the oils and add 2 drops to a vaporizer in the child's room. If the child is taking a homeopathic remedy, use aromatherapy at a different time.

Hydrotherapy

Constitutional hydrotherapy helps relieve congestion and stimulates the immune system. Foot hydrotherapy is a second choice. (See Hydrotherapy for Children on page 115 for directions.) Perform either one of these therapies one or two times daily.

■ WHAT TO EXPECT

You should see improvement within 48 hours of beginning natural therapy.

Cuts, Scrapes, and Scratches

A child's skin is fragile and therefore vulnerable to the cuts, scrapes, scratches, and abrasions that accompany the accidents and misadventures of a playful and curious childhood.

Chafing or abrasions may cause the skin to appear pink or irritated. Skinned knees may bring on speckles of blood. But cuts and sharp scrapes upon the more sensitive areas of the head, face, and mouth may bleed profusely with the slightest break because thickets of blood vessels lie closer to the surface of the skin.

Because any wearing in the skin compromises its ability to protect the body from infection, even minor breaks in its surface should be treated aggressively and with care. This is especially the case with younger children, who have had less of a lifetime to develop infection-fighting antibodies to ward away infection.

Also, cuts on the face, feet, and fingers are particularly prone to infection because they are often not covered with clothing and therefore more susceptible to contact with bacteria and other microbes.

See a doctor if a cut:

- Is deeper than ½ inch
- Has dirt or another foreign object that you cannot get out
- Requires stitches
- Is caused by a rusty object or an animal scratch
- Does not stop bleeding in 15 minutes
- Begins to form pus

■ BASIC PLAN

Wash the wound with soap and water immediately after the injury. Keep the wound clean until it heals. Apply an adhesive bandage or gauze to deeper cuts. Mild scratches are best left alone after cleaning to the air, which promotes more efficient healing.

Diet

A whole-foods diet is recommended. (See "Diet" on page 4 for more information.) Sugar products should be avoided while the body is healing.

Nutritional Supplement

Vitamin C—Supports the immune system, promotes tissue healing, and has mild anti-inflammatory effects. The kind with bioflavonoids is preferable. Dosage: the child's age in years times 50 milligrams, twice daily. Reduce the dosage if diarrhea occurs. Consider using a buffered vitamin C powder (nonacidic) or liquid vitamin C. Both work well for infants and children, and can be mixed in juice.

Herbal Remedy

Calendula—An excellent disinfectant that also promotes tissue healing. Apply as a liquid or gel twice daily to cuts or scrapes. Apply before using a bandage.

Homeopathy

Pick the following remedy that best matches your child's symptoms. Unless otherwise indicated, give your child 2 pellets of a 30C potency three times daily. (For infants, crush the pellets into powder and mix it with water.) Improvements should be seen within 48 hours. If there is no improvement within 48 hours, try another remedy. After you first notice improvement, stop giving the remedy unless symptoms begin to return.

Note: Lower potencies (6X, 12X, 6C) may need to be given more often (four times daily).

Arnica montana—Give first for any falls or blows, especially when there is bruising.

Ferrum phosphoricum—For wounds that are bleeding. Give 2 pellets every 15 minutes to help stop bleeding.

Hypericum perforatum—Give for any injuries to nerve tissue.

Ledum—Use for puncture wounds.

Calendula—Helps with tissue healing.

Bach Flower Rescue Remedy—Give to a child who is emotionally upset to help her calm down. Give 2 drops every 30 minutes, for up to three doses.

■ ADVANCED PLAN

Nutritional Supplements

Children's multivitamin—Provides a base of healing nutrients.

Zinc—Supports the immune system and enhances skin healing. Dosage: children 2 and younger, 5 milligrams; 2 and older, 10 to 15 milligrams. Use for 2 weeks and then stop.

Bioflavonoids—Bioflavonoid blends have a natural anti-inflammatory effect, enhance the action of vitamin C, and promote tissue healing. Give 3 milligrams per pound of body weight daily.

Herbal Remedies

Propolis—One of nature's greatest topical disinfectants, and it also promotes healing.

Apply as a liquid or spray to the area of injury.

Tea tree oil—Can be used as a liquid or salve to disinfect the cut and promote healing.

Echinacea and goldenseal combination—Use for immune support for more serious cuts, scrapes, and scratches to prevent infection. Give to the child internally for 5 days.

■ WHAT TO EXPECT

You should see rapid healing of a minor cut within 3 to 7 days.

Cystic Fibrosis

Cystic fibrosis (CF), a genetic condition, causes the body to produce an abnormally viscous and thick mucus. The mucus frequently becomes lodged in the lungs and airways, resulting in shortness of breath and a chronic cough.

Other symptoms include wheezing, recurring bronchitis, fatigue, pneumonia, intestinal obstruction in newborns, salt depletion in hot weather, and salty skin.

CF, the United States' most common fatal genetic disease, occurs when a child inherits a defective gene from each parent. The defect involves the flawed transport of sodium and chloride (salt) with the epithelial cells that line the lungs and pancreas.

Lungs of newborns with CF appear normal at birth and then deteriorate as thick mucus obstructs the airways, leading to progressive respiratory diseases and infections. The mucus also clogs the ducts through which enzymes from the pancreas pass on their way to the small intestine. Without these enzymes, the proper digestion of fats cannot occur, causing chronic diarrhea and malnutrition.

Recent improvements in the diagnosis and treatment of cystic fibrosis has increased the estimated median survival age for those born in the 1990s to 40 years of age. The use of pancreatic enzymes, antibiotic advances, nutritional supplementation, and improvements with diet have contributed to the overall increase in survival frequency. Improved nutritional status has made a positive difference in the pulmonary health of those with cystic fibrosis. The last 2 decades have shown that optimal nutrition is critical to lung health and the subsequent lengthening of the life span of infants, children, and young adults with cystic fibrosis.

Doctors test for CF by determining the amount of chloride in the sweat, taking x-rays of the lungs, analyzing a stool sample, and performing a blood test for the defective gene.

Conventional treatment consists of enzyme support; a high-protein, moderate-fat diet; vitamin supplementation; antibiotics and corticosteroids as needed; ibuprofen; mucus-thinning medications; and physiotherapy. Researchers are working on a cure for cystic fibrosis through gene therapy.

■ BASIC PLAN

Diet

Follow the diet as given by your child's lung specialist. It is important that enough calories be consumed in a day to prevent rapid weight

Vital Study

For a double-blind study published in the *American Journal of Diseases of Children*, 13 cystic fibrosis children with steatorrhea (fat in the stool) of at least 13 grams per day were treated with a taurine dose of 30 milligrams per kilogram of body weight per day. The study continued for two consecutive 4-month durations and involved placebo contrasts as well. Ninety-two percent of the CF children showed decreased fat in the stool while taking taurine—an indicator that their bodies were able to absorb more fat than before.

loss. A high-protein diet with a moderate amount of fat is the general recommendation. Fish, legumes, poultry, nuts, and seeds are all good protein sources.

Reduce or avoid foods that cause mucus for your child. Dairy products are the most common mucus producers, but the offending foods can vary depending on the person.

If yogurt is tolerated, then it is good to eat on a regular basis, as it is a good source of protein. Choose a yogurt that has live cultures so that your child will receive the good bacteria that are destroyed by antibiotics.

Nutritional Supplements

Pancreatic enzymes—Give as prescribed by your child's doctor to help with the digestion and absorption of foods, especially fats. Also, talk to your doctor about the use of plant enzymes, which tend to be more stable and may have better therapeutic activity.

Children's multivitamin—Give a high-potency multivitamin as prescribed by your doctor to increase the body's supply of these nutrients lost from poor absorption.

Vitamin A—Fat-soluble vitamins are often deficient in people with cystic fibrosis, due to the problems with fat absorption. A water-soluble emulsified form of vitamin A is available, and this type should be used due to its superior absorption in this condition. A child's dosage would be 1,000 to 3,000 international units daily; check with your doctor before using.

Vitamin E—Another fat-soluble vitamin that is generally deficient. A water-soluble emulsified form of vitamin E is available and should be used with this condition. A typical child's dosage is 100 international units per 50 pounds of body weight; check with your doctor before using.

Vitamin K—This may be required when long-term antibiotics have been used or if liver disease is present. Check with your doctor to see if this is indicated for your child.

N-acetylcysteine—This supplement can be taken orally or as a spray with an inhaler. It helps to liquefy mucus, acts as an antioxidant, and protects the liver. It is commonly used in both conventional and natural medicine, so talk to your doctor about its use.

Taurine—Improves fat absorption. The recommended dose is 30 milligrams per kilogram of body weight daily. Check with your doctor before using.

Probiotic—Give a children's probiotic supplement containing acidophilus and bifidus to replace good bacteria depleted from antibiotic and steroid use. Consider giving this supplement to your child indefinitely. Follow the directions on the container.

Herbal Remedy

Echinacea, or echinacea and golden-seal—For the acute treatment of infections, particularly viral infections.

Constitutional Hydrotherapy

This is excellent to reduce inflammation and congestion in the lungs, and to prevent and treat respiratory tract infections. Postural drainage should follow the treatment to expel excess mucus: Have the child lean over a bed or a board so that he slants downward. This allows mucus to drain so that it can be coughed up.

■ ADVANCED PLAN

Nutritional Supplements

Lecithin—Helps to break down fats. A typical child's dose is 200 to 400 milligrams every day or every other day. Talk to your doctor about its use.

Coenzyme Q_{10}—Protects against oxidative damage of the cells, which is a problem with CF. A typical child's dosage is 20 to 30 milligrams daily; check with your doctor about using it with your child.

Carnitine—Involved with the cellular metabolism of fatty acids to produce energy. Check with your doctor about using it with your child.

Medium chain triglycerides—These reduce weight gain and failure to thrive. Long-term use actually decreases fatty stools. Check with your doctor about using them with your child.

■ WHAT TO EXPECT

While they are not a cure, natural therapies help to improve the nutritional status of a child with this disease and thus prevent infection. Improvements in the child's overall health should be noticed within 2 months of treatment.

Dandruff

Dandruff is a mild form of dermatitis. It is the condition in which the flakes of dead skin cells on an itching and scaling scalp are shed in a quantity large enough to be unsightly and noticeable.

Infrequent and incomplete shampooing increases the likelihood of a scalp buildup and dandruff. Dirt, sweat, and oil deposits in the child's hair and on the scalp allow the cells of the surface to stick together and promote more frequent shedding of skin cells as flakes that fall to one's shoulders.

Dandruff is more a cosmetic problem than a medical one. Nutritional deficiencies are often involved as underlying causes.

Conventional treatment focuses on anti-dandruff shampoos or antifungal agents.

■ BASIC PLAN

Diet

Essential fatty acid deficiency is often at the root of dandruff. Increase your child's intake of foods that are rich in essential fatty acids, such as fish, seeds and nuts, and ground-up flaxseeds. Breast-feeding mothers should increase their intake of essential fatty acids to pass on to their infants.

Follow a whole-foods diet. (See "Diet" on page 4 for more information.) Food sensitivities may be involved. (See "Food Allergies and Food Sensitivities" on page 298 to learn more.) Yogurt with live cultures helps to increase good bacteria, which destroy fungi that may be involved.

Nutritional Supplements

Give flaxseed oil or fish oil, or better yet, a mixed essential fatty acid formula for infants or children. It should be rich in omega-3 fatty acids and omega-6 fatty acids (especially gamma linoleic acid, or GLA). If using flaxseed oil, give 1 teaspoon daily for children up to age 2, 2 teaspoons for kids 3 to 6, and 2 to 3 teaspoons for children 7 and older. (Start with 1 teaspoon daily, and reduce the dosage if diarrhea occurs.) If using fish oil, give 1 gram per 50 pounds of body weight daily.

Herbal Remedies

Tea tree—Use a 2 to 3 percent tea tree oil shampoo to wash your child's hair.

Olive oil—Rub this into the scalp at night as a moisturizer. It also provides essential fatty acids directly to the scalp.

Homeopathy

Pick the following remedy that best matches your child's symptoms. Unless otherwise indicated, give your child 2 pellets of a 30C potency twice daily. Improvements should be seen within 7 to 10 days. If there is no improvement within 10 days, try another remedy. After you first notice improvement, stop giving the remedy unless symptoms begin to return.

Note: Lower potencies (6X, 12X, 6C) may need to be given more often (three times daily).

Graphites—For scaling with yellow fluid and intense itching. Good for dandruff that is most prevalent at the base of the head.

Kali sulphuricum—Can be helpful especially when there is yellow flaking.

Natrum muriaticum—Can be helpful especially when there is white flaking. The child craves salty foods and desires to be by himself.

Sulphur—For dry, burning, itching dandruff. The child tends to be very warm in general and prone to skin imbalances. He has a high thirst for cold drinks.

■ ADVANCED PLAN

Nutritional Supplements

B complex—Give 25 milligrams daily to children under age 7, or 50 milligrams daily for children 7 and older. Available in liquid form.

Children's multivitamin—Provides a base of nutrients. Give daily. Available in liquid or chewable forms.

Aromatherapy

Add Roman chamomile and tea tree oil to aloe vera gel or olive oil, and rub the mixture onto the scalp each night. If the child is taking a homeopathic remedy, use aromatherapy at a different time.

■ WHAT TO EXPECT

The correct natural treatment should improve the excess dandruff within 4 to 6 weeks.

Depression

It is normal for a child to experience brief periods of sadness or despair for a few hours or even weeks as an emotional response to a difficult, prolonged life experience or traumatic event.

The most general sign is persistent lethargy and loss of interest in the people, activities, and things that used to bring pleasure. Symptoms include frequent fatigue and drowsiness or the inability to sleep; increased irritability; a loss of appetite or overeating; the loss of energy or sociability; the appearance of being worn or unconcerned with him- or herself; frequent and uncontrollable crying spells; the preference to sleep or be alone and reclusive; a marked drop in school performance; and ruminations about death or suicide.

Depression can result from a death of a friend or loved one or from a parental divorce, and it can linger for 2 to 3 months. Depression can stem from a child's experience of constant social anxiety, such as from being involved in fights or being alienated from desired groups in school.

Also, depression may call for the evaluation of a child psychologist or psychiatrist, especially in cases where a triggering event is not evident. Biochemical imbalance can be at the root of depression. Sometimes, depression could be the first sign of serious medical, even mental, illness.

■ BASIC PLAN

The treatment of depression in a child depends on the cause. Psychological, emotional, and spiritual issues need to be looked into and addressed. Natural therapies can help augment the healing process. In some cases, biochemical imbalances due to nutritional deficiencies are at the root of the problem and can be resolved with proper treatment. A multifaceted approach makes sense. It is important to resolve a child's susceptibility to depression so that it is not a lifelong problem.

Diet

A whole-foods diet is recommended. (See "Diet" on page 4 for more information.) Essential fatty acids are important for brain health and have been shown to be effective in alleviating depression. In particular, the essential fatty acid docosahexaenoic acid (DHA) appears to be helpful with depression. Coldwater fish

Vital Fact

The use of a class of pharmaceutical anti-depressant medications known as selective serotonin re-uptake inhibitors (SSRIs) increased tenfold in a recent 4-year period for children. These types of medications have not been well-studied in young children.

such as salmon, mackerel, herring, and halibut are good sources.

Fluctuating blood sugar levels can lead to a depressive state. Make sure that your child is eating regular meals and have snacks available during the day. Simple sugars and refined carbohydrates (as found in breads and pastas) should be limited.

Nutritional Supplements

DHA—This fatty acid is available by itself as a liquid or as part of essential fatty acid formulas. It is a necessary essential fatty acid found in brain cells. Daily dosages: 100 milligrams for children up to age 5, and 100 to 200 milligrams for children 5 and older.

Phosphatidylserine—This is a normal component of brain cells and is shown to help with depression in clinical studies. Daily dosages: 100 milligrams for children from 25 to 75 pounds, 200 milligrams for kids 75 to 100 pounds, and 300 milligrams for kids 100 pounds or more.

Herbal Remedy

St. John's wort—We do not typically recommend St. John's wort for children unless other natural therapies are not working. The dosage depends on the child's body weight. St. John's wort is best used under the guidance of a holistic doctor.

Homeopathy

Pick the following remedy that best matches your child's symptoms. Unless otherwise indicated, give your child 2 pellets of a 30C potency twice daily. Improvements should be seen within 7 to 10 days. If there is no improvement within 10 days, try another remedy. After you first notice improvement, stop giving the remedy unless symptoms begin to return.

Note: Lower potencies (6X, 12X, 6C) may need to be given more often (three times daily).

Aurum metallicum—For serious depression that can lead to suicidal thoughts. The child feels no joy in life and may feel that life is not worth living. She feels better in the sun.

Note: Suicidal tendencies should *always* be discussed with a doctor.

Ignatia—For acute emotional trauma that leads to sadness and grief. The child has trouble relaxing, is uptight, and cries uncontrollably. She has tense muscles.

Kali phosphoricum 6X—The child feels depressed from overstudy or stress. She has trouble concentrating.

Natrum muriaticum—The child feels depressed and wants to be by herself. She is very sensitive to criticism and craves salty foods. There is a history of suppressed grief. She feels worse in the sun.

Pulsatilla—The child is weepy and desires constant attention. She cries easily and is comforted when held. Her mood is changeable and she has low thirst. She feels better in the fresh air.

■ ADVANCED PLAN

Nutritional Supplements

SAMe—This is a normal compound found in the body that is used in the process of manufacturing the neurotransmitters that help regulate mood. Its full name is S-adenosylmethionine. We are unaware of any studies looking at SAMe and childhood depression. However, it is nontoxic, and there are many studies showing it to be effective for adult depression. Use SAMe with the guidance of a holistic doctor; 200 milligrams daily may be helpful for a child.

Children's multivitamin—Provides a base of nutrients. Give daily. Available in liquid or chewable forms.

B complex—Give 25 milligrams daily for children under age 7, or 50 milligrams daily for children 7 and older. Available in liquid form.

Aromatherapy

Orange and lavender—Apply these to the child's bedsheets, or mix them in a carrier oil and apply them to the skin. If the child is taking a homeopathic remedy, use aromatherapy at a different time.

Case History

Kyle, a third grade student, was brought to our clinic for chronic depression. His parents told us that he was susceptible to depression and did not seem to be a happy child. When asked why they thought he was having this problem, they said that Kyle had had an incident where a friend did not want to play with him anymore, which really bothered him. He did not laugh or play like he used to. This had been going on for more than 6 months. Previously, Kyle was a happy-go-lucky child. Based on all his symptoms, we prescribed the homeopathic remedy Natrum muriaticum and recommended that his parents get him counseling. Over the course of 2 months, Kyle's parents felt that the remedy had a dramatic effect on his mood and helped to alleviate his depression. He was happier, more playful, and less serious about everything. We still recommended counseling to address underlying emotional issues.

Acupressure

Four Gates—Helps to release tension. This is a combination of Liver 3, located on top of the foot in the hollow between the big toe and second toe, and Large Intestine 4, located in the webbing between the thumb and index finger. Two people should push gently on all four points at the same time for 15 seconds. Repeat three times. Do this once daily.

■ WHAT TO EXPECT

Improvements should be noticed within 3 to 4 weeks with the correct natural therapy. It is advised that a health professional supervise and evaluate your child's depression.

Diabetes

Diabetes is a condition characterized by blood sugar imbalance. Blood sugar, known as glucose, cannot enter the cells effectively to be burned as fuel. Complications of untreated and undiagnosed diabetes include episodes of extremely high or low blood sugar because of the body's inability to balance its glucose levels. High blood sugar could prompt hyperactivity and lead to diabetic ketoacidosis, which, if untreated, can cause loss of consciousness, coma, and death. Low blood sugar is evident in sudden dizziness, lethargy, paleness, sweating, and a loss of coordination. Digestion breaks carbohydrates such as breads and pastas into their basic components— among them, glucose, which is a simple sugar and fuel for the body. Insulin allows the body's cells to let glucose in, giving cells (and the body) energy.

There are two types of diabetes: type 1 and type 2. Type 1, insulin-dependent diabetes mellitus or juvenile-onset diabetes, is usually diagnosed in childhood and involves such insufficient insulin production that insulin must be taken by injection every day. Type 1 diabetes accounts for about 5 to 10 percent of diagnosed diabetes in the United States.

Type 1 is a chronic condition thought to be an autoimmune disorder in which the body's own immune system attacks the insulin-manufacturing cells in the pancreas, leading to the insufficient production of insulin. Why this happens has yet to be discovered. Some researchers believe that there is a connection between vaccines and type 1 diabetes in children. The use of insulin is required.

Type 2 can be generally managed with diet and supplementation. It accounts for 90 to 95 percent of all diagnosed cases of diabetes in adults.

The first signs that a child has developed diabetes generally appear over a period of 1 to 3 weeks. Symptoms include a noticeable and seemingly unquenchable thirst; a significant increase in the frequency and volume of urination; frequent bedwetting from a child who didn't previously wet the bed; and increased appetite in combination with weight loss.

Conventional treatment of type 1 diabetes (juvenile diabetes) focuses on the use of insulin, diet, and exercise.

Type 2 diabetes is on the rise in children and adolescents as a result of the average American childhood diet and lack of exercise. Obesity is the biggest risk factor for type 2 diabetes. Since exercise helps to regulate blood sugar levels, find aerobic activities that your child likes and have him participate in these on a daily basis. Conventional treatment focuses on diet and exercise, and in some cases, drug therapy.

■ BASIC PLAN

Consult with your child's doctor before following these recommendations. The use of these supplements may require your doctor to reduce your child's medication dosage.

Diet

A diabetic child's diet should be rich in complex carbohydrates, which are found in whole grains, legumes, and root vegetables. Moderate amounts of quality protein sources such as coldwater fish (for example, salmon), lean poultry, and soy are recommended. High-fiber vegetables such as green leafy vegetables, cauliflower, carrots, and broccoli are also recommended. They help to slow the release of blood sugar from the intestines. Fruit can be eaten in moderation and is best consumed with meals. The child's diet should be low in sugars and saturated fat.

Cow's milk should be avoided for the first year of life. Although controversial, some studies find that infants who consume cow's milk have an increased risk of developing type 1 diabetes.

Nutritional Supplements

The following are involved with blood sugar metabolism. Use them under the supervision of a doctor.

Chromium—Daily dosages: 1 to 3 years, 20 to 80 micrograms; 4 to 6 years, 30 to 120 micrograms; 7 years and older, 50 to 200 micrograms.

Vital Fact

According to the Juvenile Diabetes Foundation, 35 American children are diagnosed with type 1 diabetes every day.

Vanadium—A typical dosage is 5 to 20 micrograms daily.

Alpha lipoic acid—A typical dosage is 5 to 25 milligrams daily.

Herbal Remedies

The following herbs support blood sugar metabolism. They can be taken individually or in formulas. The most widely used is gymnema (*Gymnema sylvestre*). (For all of these herbs, follow the herbal dosage information for chronic conditions on page 140.) Maximum dosages are listed below.

Gymnema (25 percent gymneic acid)—Up to 400 milligrams daily.

Bitter melon (*Momordica charantia*)—Up to 400 milligrams daily.

Fenugreek—Up to 300 milligrams daily.

■ ADVANCED PLAN

Nutritional Supplements

Children's multivitamin—Supplies many of the vitamins and minerals required for blood sugar control. Give as directed on the container.

Vitamin C—Required for proper insulin

Vital Fact

The number of children with type 2 diabetes tripled from 1995 to 2000.

action. Dosage: the child's age in years times 50 milligrams, daily. Reduce the dosage if diarrhea occurs. Consider using a buffered vitamin C powder (nonacidic) or liquid vitamin C. Both work well for infants and children, and can be mixed in juice.

Essential fatty acids—Help with insulin balance and can help prevent complications of high blood sugar levels. Give a children's complex containing omega-3 and omega-6 fatty acids, and follow the directions on the label. Or give flaxseed oil at the following daily dosages: children 2 and under, 1 teaspoon; kids 3 to 6, 2 teaspoons; kids 7 and older, 2 to 3 teaspoons (reduce the amount if diarrhea occurs). Another alternative is fish oil; give 1 gram per 50 pounds of body weight daily.

Homeopathy

A specific constitutional treatment from a homeopathic practitioner can be effective.

■ WHAT TO EXPECT

Children with both types of diabetes need to be monitored by a doctor when following the recommendations in this chapter. Children with type 1 diabetes may need to have their insulin requirements lowered, as may children on med-

ication for type 2 diabetes. The recommendations in this chapter are even more effective for those children who are borderline diabetic. Changes in blood sugar levels are usually seen within 1 to 2 weeks of starting treatment.

Diaper Rash

At one time or another during infancy, most babies develop diaper rash—inflammation and irritation of the skin surrounding the buttocks, genitals, or any area covered by the diaper.

The rash may indicate a skin irritation, which could be a result of a yeast infection, bacterial infection, or skin inflammation.

The most common type of diaper rash is chafing dermatitis, which appears as toughened, pink skin where there is friction between the tender skin and a diaper. The skin becomes dry and rigid to avoid a break. A contact rash, another type, is the reaction to the combination of a diaper's chronic moisture, body heat, and the presence of strong chemicals and enzymes in urine and stool forming a noxious mixture around a baby's bottom. A contact rash leaves the area sore, tender, red, dry, and scaling.

Also, there is a fungal diaper rash, which is caused by the presence of *Candida albicans* in the intestinal tract. The skin may be smooth, glossy, and red.

Dry skin from constant cleansing with soap and water, a tight diaper, and diarrhea all increase the chances of a baby developing diaper rash.

Conventional treatment focuses on creams. In the case of fungus, an antifungal cream is used, and with bacteria, an antibacterial cream is used. Barrier creams may be recommended to prevent friction rubs.

■ BASIC PLAN

Change your baby's diapers more frequently, and change a diaper as soon as possible after it has been wet or soiled. Dry the area thoroughly before putting on a new diaper. A hair dryer works well; hold it far enough back that the baby's skin is not burned.

Try a different brand of diaper. Your child may be sensitive to the material of the current diaper, or it may not fit well.

Avoid diapers that are too tight. The diaper needs to "breathe" to avoid moisture buildup.

Leave your child's bottom uncovered and exposed to air for 10 minutes each day.

Diet

Food sensitivities may be at the root of the diaper rash. If your child is solely breastfed, examine the mother's diet. Caffeine, spicy foods, or other foods may be irritating to the child. If the child is given formula, it may need to be switched to a different brand or a hypoallergenic type. If the child is eating foods, see "Food Allergies and Food Sensitivities" on page 298 to figure out what foods may be causing a problem.

Nutritional Supplement

Probiotic—Contains good bacteria that prevents yeast overgrowth. Purchase a children's formula that contains bifidus and acidophilus, and give as directed on the container.

Vital Study

For a controlled study published in the *Journal of Ethnopharmacology,* a standardized gymnema extract was given to 27 people with type 1 diabetes at a dose of 400 milligrams daily for 6 to 30 months. Thirty-seven others continued on insulin therapy alone and were tracked for 10 to 12 months. Insulin requirements were decreased by about one-half and the average blood glucose decreased from 232 milligrams per deciliter to 152 milligrams per deciliter in the gymnema group. The control group showed no significant decrease in blood sugar or insulin requirement.

Herbal Remedy

Calendula gel can work wonders to relieve the irritation of diaper rash. Apply twice daily.

Homeopathy

Pick the following remedy that best matches your child's symptoms. Unless otherwise indicated, give your child 2 pellets of a 30C potency twice daily. (Crush the pellets into powder and mix it with water.) Improvements should be seen within 48 hours. If there is no improvement within 48 hours, try another remedy. After you first notice improvement, stop giving the remedy unless symptoms begin to return.

Note: Lower potencies (6X, 12X, 6C) may need to be given more often (three times daily).

Calcarea carbonica—The child fits the Calcarea carbonica constitution: large, flabby, sweats easily on her head.

Graphites—For diaper rash with a honeylike discharge. Red, dry, cracked skin.

Hepar sulphuris—For an infected rash that smells like rotten cheese. There is pus discharge. The area is very sensitive to touch.

Medorrhinum—For long-standing anal rash, ever since birth. The child prefers to lie on her tummy with her knees drawn up. She is restless and craves orange juice and/or ice.

Sulphur—The most common remedy for diaper rash. The skin is red, irritated, itchy, and may have some yeast growth. The child scratches the rash until it bleeds. Symptoms are worse at night in the warmth of the bed.

■ WHAT TO EXPECT

Improvements should be seen within 48 to 72 hours.

Diarrhea

Diarrhea is the frequent, urgent, and sometimes uncontrollable elimination of loose, watery stools, which often have more volume than typical, compacted stools.

This is a natural mechanism in which the body tries to rid itself of foreign substances and toxins. It can by triggered by microorganisms such as bacteria, viruses, parasites, fungi, and protozoa—all of which children can come in contact with by touching or playing with contaminated playing areas or other children, or by ingesting tainted food or drinking water.

Often, diarrhea is caused by a virus that invades the digestive tract, irritating and inflaming the intestinal walls so that they secrete excess fluids. The fluids increase the frequent wavelike contractions (peristalsis) that move digested food and substances through the digestive tract. This creates intestinal cramping and the loose, watery stools of rapid digestion. Contaminated food and water are the most common source.

Reactions to medication, particularly antibiotics; dietary problems, such as the drinking of too much fruit juice; a milk allergy; a food sensitivity; or food poisoning can lead to diarrhea. Less common causes include irritable bowel disease, celiac disease, pancreatitis, hepatitis, and cystic fibrosis.

Because diarrhea indicates that the body is trying to flush itself of an undesired toxin, it is common in the case of a healthy child to let it run its 1- or 2-day course while guarding against dehydration.

Take care to watch babies who have diarrhea, for dehydration can occur in infants after only a few hours. One simple test you can do is to pinch your baby's skin on his arm. See if the skin bounces back (like your own arm) or returns back slowly and laxly. A slow return may indicate dehydration. Observe your child between bouts of diarrhea and support him with adequate fluids. Chronic bouts of diarrhea may indicate problems with food allergies.

Teething is a common cause of diarrhea in infants.

See your doctor if:

- The stool contains blood
- There is severe abdominal pain
- Vomiting accompanies the diarrhea
- The diarrhea lasts longer than 2 days
- A high fever accompanies the diarrhea
- Your newborn has diarrhea
- There are signs of dehydration—no urination, crying without tears, dry mouth, listlessness

Conventional treatment focuses on rehydration, antidiarrheal medications, and antibiotic use (for bacterial infections that induce diarrhea).

■ BASIC PLAN

Diet

A breastfeeding mother may be eating foods that are causing her infant to have diarrhea. Think about what you have been eating and whether there are any new foods or drinks that may be causing the diarrhea. If so, stop ingesting them and see if your infant improves.

A breastfeeding mother should continue to regularly breastfeed an infant with diarrhea, to prevent dehydration. Breast milk contains immune factors that will help the infant get over the diarrhea quicker.

If your baby is bottlefed, think about whether your baby has been on a new formula since the diarrhea began. If so, switch the formula, which may be irritating him. Nondairy formulas are best. Some infants also react to soy formulas. We recommend starting out with a hypoallergenic formula.

For older children, the BRAT diet (bananas, rice, applesauce, and toast) is one of the best ways to help calm down diarrhea. Bananas should be ripe, with the central core removed; the rice should be white and well-cooked; and the toast should be made from white bread.

Soups, broths, and steamed and cooked vegetables are also good to eat, as they are easily digested.

Sugar and grain products should be avoided until the diarrhea clears. Juice should be avoided, as it can contribute to increased bowel movements. Some infants and children get loose stools from consuming too much juice in one day, especially juices that contain sorbitol.

An oral electrolyte solution helps to prevent dehydration. Pedialyte and Naturalyte are examples; they're available at your local pharmacy or supermarket. Use unflavored versions in order to avoid the sugar substitute aspartame, which we do not recommend. Use as directed on the container or as instructed by your doctor. Research has shown that homemade electrolyte solutions are not as effective as commercial children's electrolyte solutions and should not be relied upon to prevent dehydration. Older kids can use electrolyte drinks such as Gatorade and Recharge.

Chronic diarrhea can be the result of food

sensitivities. (See "Food Allergies and Food Sensitivities" on page 298 for more information.)

Nutritional Supplement

Probiotic—Look for a children's acidophilus and bifidus supplement. These good bacteria have been shown to be helpful in treating infectious diarrhea. Give as directed on the container.

Herbal Remedies

Ginger tea—Helps to soothe an irritated digestive tract and reduce diarrhea.

Echinacea and goldenseal—This combination is used when the diarrhea is caused by an infection.

Homeopathy

Use a combination diarrhea formula, or pick the one of the following remedies that best matches your child's symptoms. For the remedies below, unless otherwise indicated, give your child 2 pellets of a 30C potency three times daily. (For infants, crush the pellets into powder and mix it with water.) Improvements should be seen within 48 hours. If there is no improvement within 48 hours, try another remedy. After you first notice improvement, stop giving the remedy unless symptoms begin to return.

Note: Lower potencies (6X, 12X, 6C) may need to be given more often (four times daily).

Aloe socotrina—Yellowish, mucus-filled stool with lots of gas. The child's rectum burns after passing stool. There is rumbling and gurgling in the abdomen, with a sudden urge to move bowels.

Arsenicum album—For watery stool and burning anus. The child has nausea. Vomiting may occur at the same time as diarrhea. Symptoms are worse from midnight to 2:00 A.M. The child is anxious and restless and feels chilly. For diarrhea caused by food poisoning or the flu. The child feels better with warm drinks. He is thirsty for sips of warm water.

Chamomilla—For diarrhea that accompanies teething. Green diarrhea and lots of gas. The child is very irritable.

China officinalis—For diarrhea that has led to exhaustion and weakness. Useful to take during or after an acute bout where lots of fluids have been lost, to regain strength.

Ipecacuanha—For diarrhea that is accompanied by constant nausea.

Mercurius solubilis or vivus—For severe burning diarrhea with bloody stools. Symptoms are worse at night. The child alternates between chills and sweating.

Nux vomica—For diarrhea from food poisoning or eating spicy foods. The child is chilly and irritable.

Phosphorus—For watery stool that is usually painless. The child craves and feels better with cold drinks or food.

Podophyllum—For watery, profuse diarrhea with a yellow, pasty stool. There is rumbling and gurgling of the abdomen before diarrhea. Lots of gas passes with the diarrhea. The child feels weak and faint after passing stool. Symptoms are often worse in the morning.

Pulsatilla—For diarrhea from eating fruit or greasy foods. Symptoms are worse at night and stools are changeable. The child wants to be held.

Sulphur—For burning diarrhea that smells like rotten eggs. Diarrhea is worse in the morning and gets the child out of bed. The rectum is red and burning. Stool burns when passing out.

Veratrum album—For odorless, profuse diarrhea that looks like rice water. Vomiting occurs at the same time. The child is very chilly and desires cold drinks with ice.

■ ADVANCED PLAN

Nutritional Supplement

Activated charcoal—One teaspoon given twice daily to children 3 years and older helps to stop diarrhea. Do not use for more than 2 days. Use under the guidance of a doctor.

Herbal Remedies

Slippery elm—Soothing and helps to treat diarrhea. Use it as a powder at 1 teaspoon per 50 pounds of body weight daily, mixed into applesauce or other food. Children who are old enough to swallow a pill can take the capsule form, at 1 capsule three times daily.

Marshmallow root—A soothing herb for the digestive tract.

Raspberry or blackberry tea—Helps to reduce diarrhea by acting as an astringent. Give the child ½ cup three times daily.

Acupressure

Gently press the acupressure point with a thumb for 10 to 15 seconds. Perform on both sides of the body and repeat three times each day.

Stomach 36—Located four finger-widths below the kneecap and one finger-width toward the outside of the leg (outside of the shinbone, on the muscle).

Large Intestine 4—Located in the webbing between the thumb and index finger.

Aromatherapy

If the child is taking a homeopathic remedy, use aromatherapy at a different time.

For diarrhea caused by a viral infection, add lavender and tea tree oil to a carrier oil and rub it over the child's abdomen.

For diarrhea caused by food poisoning, add 2 drops of German chamomile and 3 drops of peppermint to a carrier oil and rub it over the child's abdomen.

For diarrhea caused by stress, add 1 drop of Roman chamomile and 3 drops of lavender to a carrier oil and rub it over the child's abdomen.

■ WHAT TO EXPECT

You should see improvements within 24 to 48 hours.

Dizziness

Fumbling footsteps and spinning falls toward the ground indicate the loss of coordination and balance common to a child feeling dizzy. Dizziness is a common symptom of many conditions, including acute allergic reactions, viral infection, low blood sugar, bee stings, concussions, dehydration, and exhaustion. Middle ear infections or serous otitis media (fluid in the middle ear) can also cause dizziness.

See your doctor if:

- The episode lasts more than 30 minutes
- There are reoccurring episodes
- The dizziness occurs after the child bangs her head
- You suspect that your child has an ear infection
- You suspect that the dizziness is from an acute allergic reaction

■ BASIC PLAN

Diet

Make sure that your child is getting regular meals throughout the day. Low blood sugar can be a cause of dizziness. Meals containing only carbohydrates (pastas, breads, fruits, and sugars) may create further blood sugar problems. For a more balanced blood sugar level, feed your child meals that contain quality protein sources and fiber from vegetables.

Dehydration can also cause dizziness. Make sure that your child is drinking enough fluids during the day.

Food sensitivities may be a factor and should be identified and treated. (See "Food Allergies and Food Sensitivites" on page 298 for more information.) Chiropractic or cra-

niosacral therapy may also be helpful (see pages 502 and 503 for more information).

Herbal Remedy

Ginkgo biloba—For dizziness related to poor circulation.

Homeopathy

Pick the following remedy that best matches your child's symptoms. Unless otherwise indicated, give your child 2 pellets of a 30C potency every 2 hours. Improvements should be seen within 6 hours. If there is no improvement within 6 hours, try another remedy. After you first notice improvement, stop giving the remedy unless symptoms begin to return.

Note: Lower potencies (6X, 12X, 6C) may need to be given more often (every hour).

Aconitum napellus—For dizziness that is the result of fright or anxiety. The child is also restless and fearful. For dizziness that accompanies panic attacks.

Cocculus—For dizziness that occurs with motion sickness, such as looking out the car window. The child must lie down because she is so dizzy.

Kali phosphoricum 6X—For dizziness related to stress or anxiety.

Gelsemium—For dizziness related to the flu. Give 2 pellets twice daily for up to 3 days.

Aromatherapy

Peppermint—Add 1 drop to a carrier oil or put 1 drop on a tissue and put it under the child's pillow. If the child is taking a homeopathic remedy, use aromatherapy at a different time.

■ WHAT TO EXPECT

Improvement will occur only if the cause of the dizziness is treated. Work with a doctor to find the cause, and then incorporate the natural therapies in this section.

Dry Skin

Healthy skin is constantly being coated by sebum (oil generated by the body) and moisture from outside humidity. When skin loses some water to the environment through evaporation or due to an insufficient supply of its own natural oils, it can become dry, chapped, flaking, itchy, and cracked.

The skin constantly loses water from body cells; the water slowly migrates to the skin surface and evaporates. The incidence of dry skin increases for children who live in dry climates because the arid air speeds up the evaporation process. Children who live in cold climates and who spend winters inside homes that are warmed by dry heat are also susceptible to dry skin.

Well-hydrated skin helps protect a child. Dry skin can create tiny cracks or scratches that make the child vulnerable to soap and clothing irritations, or to bacterial or viral infections.

Low thyroid function can also result in dry skin. Although it is uncommon in children, it should be ruled out.

Nutritionally speaking, essential fatty acid deficiency is often an underlying cause of dry and cracked skin.

Conventional treatment focuses on moisturizing creams and lotions.

■ BASIC PLAN

Diet

Sources of essential fatty acids are important. Ground-up fresh flaxseeds provide a rich source of omega-3 fatty acids: You can grind 1 teaspoon per 50 pounds of body weight (children weighing 30 to 50 pounds may also use 1 teaspoon) and give this amount daily, with 8 ounces of water.

Seeds and nuts are also good sources, as is fresh fish. (See "Essential Fatty Acids" on page 8 for more information.) Margarine and hydrogenated oils should be avoided, as they create fatty acid imbalance.

Food sensitivities may be a contributing factor and should be identified and treated. (See "Food Allergies and Food Sensitivities" on page 298 for more information.)

Nutritional Supplements

Choose one of the following three supplements.

Essential fatty acid complex—Choose a children's blend that contains omega-3 fatty acids and omega-6 fatty acids (especially GLA, or gamma linolenic acid). Give as directed on the container.

Flaxseed oil—Daily dosages: children up to 2 years, 1 teaspoon; kids 3 to 6, 2 teaspoons;

kids 7 and older, 2 to 3 teaspoons. Reduce the dosage if diarrhea occurs.

Fish oil—Daily dosage: 1 gram per 50 pounds of body weight.

Herbal Remedy

Calendula gel or cream—Apply this to dry patches of skin. Best applied after a bath or shower to lock in moisture.

Homeopathy

Pick the following remedy that best matches your child's symptoms. Unless otherwise indicated, give your child 2 pellets of a 30C potency twice daily. (For infants, crush the pellets into powder and mix it with water.) Improvements should be seen within 2 weeks. If there is no improvement within 2 weeks, try another remedy. After you first notice improvement, stop giving the remedy unless symptoms begin to return.

Note: Lower potencies (6X, 12X, 6C) may need to be given more often (three times daily).

Natrum muriaticum—For dry skin, cracked fingernails. The child feels worse in the sun and wants to be alone. He craves salty foods.

Petroleum—For dry, deep-cracking skin that may bleed. Dryness is worse in the winter and better in the summer.

Rhus toxicodendron—For dry, itchy skin that is worse in cold weather. The child is very restless and craves milk.

Sulphur—For dry, burning skin. The child is very warm in general and has a high thirst for cold drinks. The child has itchy skin. He is restless.

Aromatherapy

Add Roman chamomile to a carrier oil such as aloe vera gel and rub it over the area of dry skin. Repeat daily. If the child is taking a homeopathic remedy, use aromatherapy at a different time.

■ WHAT TO EXPECT

Dry skin can take time to improve with nutritional therapy. Underlying deficiencies such as essential fatty acid deficiency can take 1 to 2 months before skin dryness improves.

Ear Infection

Swelling, inflammation, or infection of the ear (especially the middle ear) results in ear pain. The medical term is otitis media, but most parents just know it and dread it as an earache. Most children suffer from one or more acute ear infections in their childhoods. A baby is often more fussy and cries more than usual (especially at night), may seem off-balance, and pulls at one or both of his ears. A fever is usually present.

Statistics show that acute ear infections affect two-thirds of American children under age 2, while chronic ear infections affect two-thirds of children under age 6. More than 50 percent of all pediatrician visits are for ear infections. Most ear infections are associated with an upper respiratory infection or allergy. The most common bacterial cause (40 percent of the time) is *Streptococcus pneumoniae.*

Chronic middle ear infections refer to chronic swelling of the eardrum as a result of fluid accumulation. One of the reasons infants are more susceptible to ear infections is because the eustachian tube (which drains fluid from the middle ear) is more horizontal and does not drain as efficiently. This tube becomes more vertical and drains better as children get older. The key is to prevent the buildup of this fluid so that germs do not have an environment in which to grow. A healthy immune system is also key. The techniques to do this are addressed in the Basic Plan on page 279.

Conventional treatment of acute ear infections includes antibiotics and pain/fever relievers such as acetaminophen. Antibiotics are a common first-line treatment, but many experts are concerned about the overprescribing of antibiotics for conditions such as ear infections and colds. This practice has contributed to antibiotic-resistant bacterial infections and to the development of conditions such as candida. (See "Candida" on page 217 for more information.) Studies show that children treated with antibiotics have a greater risk of becoming carriers of *Streptococcus pneumoniae,* the bacteria known to cause most ear infections. As well, the chances of this bacteria being resistant to antibiotics is increased.

The usefulness of antibiotics for ear infections is questionable. Studies show that ap-proximately 80 percent of untreated children have clinical resolution by 7 to 14 days, as compared with approximately 95 percent of those treated with antibiotics. We find that most children with acute ear infections experience rapid improvement within 24 hours when given proper natural therapy, and do not require antibiotics.

The biggest controversy with conventional treatment is the prescription of antibiotics for otitis media with effusion. This is simply the presence of fluid in the middle ear in the absence of signs or symptoms of acute infection. Antibiotics may appropriately be deferred in this group of children, as recommended in the clinical guidelines published by the U.S. Agency for Health Care Policy and Research, as most cases of otitis media with effusion resolve spontaneously. It must also be recognized that fluid left in the middle ear after antibiotic treatment is normal. Approximately 70 percent of children have fluid in the middle ear 2 weeks after appropriate antibiotic therapy, 50 percent have fluid at 1 month after, 20 percent have fluid at 2 months after, and 10 percent have fluid at 3 months after. According to studies, this fluid that remains does not need to be treated with antibiotics as is typically done.

It must also be noted that if antibiotics are used, a shorter duration of 5 to 7 days is sufficient if there are no complications (such as perforation of the tympanic membrane, or a child with a compromised immune system) instead of the typical 10-day course. We do realize and acknowledge that certain cases of otitis media require antibiotics, and that this needs to be decided on an individual basis.

For chronic ear infections or fluid, surgery may be recommended. A tube is inserted through the eardrum to assist drainage of fluid into the throat; this is known as tympanostomy. The benefits of this procedure are controversial as well, and in many cases (most cases, in our experience) it can be avoided with the following natural approaches.

Here are some of the common causes of ear infections:

- Exposure to secondhand smoke. Smoke causes fluid buildup in the ears and suppression of the immune system. It is one of the most preventable causes of ear infections.
- Food allergies. Reactions to foods create fluid buildup and wear down the immune system. Studies have confirmed food allergies as a major cause of ear infections. Common trigger foods are dairy foods (cow's milk and cheese), sugar, wheat, citrus fruit, soy, eggs, corn, and apples. These foods should be omitted for a period of time or rotated in the child's diet to see if she improves. Cow's milk is the most common food allergy contributing to ear infections, but specific testing by a practitioner can identify reactive foods. (See "Food Allergies and Food Sensitivities" on page 298 for more information.)

   Also, many middle ear problems begin after a baby begins to eat solid foods. The earlier solid foods are introduced, the greater the chances of developing ear infections. (See "Introducing Food to Your Baby" on page 19 for more on how to introduce solid foods properly.)

- Environmental allergies. Common ones include molds, dust, animal dander, and pollen (as in hay fever). An air purifier is recommended.
- Day care. Kids who go to day care get exposure to other kids with infections and increased exposure to "bad bugs."
- Not being breastfed. Breastfeeding allows for the transport of immune factors from the mother to the child, and it matures the digestive tract so that the child is less susceptible to food allergies. Bottle formulas tend to be cow's milk–based, which can cause an allergy problem.

Other ear infection risk factors include:

- The season. The incidence of earaches is highest in the winter. In northern climates, ear infections increase in frequency beginning in September.
- Fetal alcohol syndrome. More than 90 percent of children with fetal alcohol syndrome have problems with ear infections. Fetal alcohol syndrome is caused by the mother drinking alcohol during the pregnancy.
- Genetics. Nearly 60 percent of children with Down's syndrome experience problems with otitis media.
- Nutritional deficiencies. Deficiencies of vitamins A and C and essential fatty acid imbalance can contribute to ear infection risk.

• Injuries. Children who suffer a trauma at birth (such as from a forceps delivery or vacuum extraction) and children with neck and head injuries are more susceptible. These children may be helped by chiropractic, osteopathic, or craniosacral therapy. (See Natural Health Care Modalities and Resource Guide on page 499 for more on these therapies.)

■ BASIC PLAN

Diet

For bottlefed babies, switch to a nondairy formula. If your baby is already on a nondairy formula and having ear problems, switch to a hypoallergenic formula. Do not bottlefeed while your child is lying on her back. This leads to fluid accumulation in the middle ear. Hold your baby so that she points 30 degrees or more upward.

If you breastfeed your baby, you should avoid (or at least rotate) the common food allergens mentioned above so that you do not pass allergenic portions to your baby. Also, when breastfeeding at night, hold your infant up and allow burping and swallowing to help keep milk from accumulating in the eustachian tube.

Children should avoid sugar and dairy products. Try to identify potential food allergens. (See "Food Allergies and Food Sensitivities" on page 298 for more information.) Keep your child well-hydrated with purified water, diluted fruit juice, herbal teas, and soups and broths.

Nutritional Supplement

Vitamin C—Provides support to the immune system. Dosage: the child's age in years times 100 milligrams, twice daily. Reduce the dosage if diarrhea occurs. Consider using a buffered vitamin C powder (nonacidic) or liquid vitamin C. Both work well for infants and children, and can be mixed in juice.

Herbal Remedy

Mullein drops or mullein/garlic oil drops—Put 2 warm drops in the affected ear three times daily. Do not use if your child's eardrum is perforated or if fluid is draining from the ear. Always have your child's ear checked before you put these drops in the ear, to make sure it is not perforated or draining fluid.

Homeopathy

Pick the following remedy that best matches your child's symptoms. Unless otherwise indicated, give your child 2 pellets of a 30C potency every hour. (For infants, crush the pellets into powder and mix it with water.) Improvements should be seen within 3 hours. If there is no improvement within 3 hours, try another remedy. After you first notice improvement, stop giving the remedy unless symptoms begin to return.

Note: Lower potencies (6X, 12X, 6C) may need to be given more often (every 30 minutes).

Aconitum napellus—Helpful for an acute earache that comes on very quickly. The child experiences violent pain and restlessness. The child has high thirst and a high fever. Often occurs after being out in the cold, dry wind. Only helpful if used during the first few hours of the ear infection.

Belladonna—For a sudden onset of earache with a high fever. The child's face and eardrum are red. Right ear infection is more common than left side. Pupils may be dilated, and the child looks and feels hot, but the feet can feel cold. There is throbbing pain.

Chamomilla—The child is very irritable, angry, and hard to console. She appears to be in a lot of pain, often screaming and crying. She wants to be carried, but it helps for only a short period of time. One cheek is often red, the other one pale. A great remedy for earaches that occur at the same time as teething.

Ferrum phosphoricum—Recommended for a child who has a fever and feels warm. The face and affected ear are red, as is indicated for Belladonna, but the child does not act sick.

Hepar sulphuris—The ears are very sensitive to touch and cold and to drafts of air. The child is irritable. There is sharp pain in the ear. The ear feels better with warm applications. There can be discharge from the ear that smells like rotten cheese.

Lachesis—Best when the left ear is affected or when the infection starts in the left ear and moves to the right. The earache is worse with warm applications and at night.

Lycopodium—For right-sided ear infections. Symptoms are worse from 4:00 to 8:00 P.M. They are better with warm applications to the ear.

Mercurius solubilis or vivus—The top choice for an earache that often has pus discharge. Sweating is common. The tongue often has a thick coating. The child has bad breath and increased salivation. Symptoms are worse at night. The child is sensitive to hot and cold temperatures. There can be a smelly discharge from the ear.

Pulsatilla—Given for a child who has a fever, cries a lot, is clingy and wants to be held for comfort. The ear feels full and plugged up. Ear pain feels better with cold applications or in the open air, and worse with warmth or in a warm, stuffy room. The child is not thirsty. Fever and ear infection often develop at night.

Silica—For chronic ear infection and fluid buildup that leads to hearing loss and chronic pain. Cold and wind bothers the child. Lymph nodes are swollen. A ruptured ear drum has offensive discharge.

If you are uncertain about which choice to select, you can also purchase a combination homeopathic earache formula.

Hydrotherapy

Alternate a hot and cold cloth over the affected ear to help reduce pain and congestion. Follow this sequence of 30 seconds hot, then 30 seconds cold, and repeat.

■ ADVANCED PLAN

Nutritional Supplements

The following are dosages for an acute ear infection. They all work to support the immune system.

Vitamin A— Daily dosage: infants under 1 year, 1,875 international units (IU); children 1 to 3, 2,000 IU; kids 4 to 6, 2,500 IU; kids 7 to 10, 3,500 IU; males 11 and older, 5,000 IU; females 11 and older, 4,000 IU.

Note: These dosages are for short-term use (up to 10 days). Higher dosages may be used only under a doctor's supervision. Available in liquid drops.

Zinc—Also enhances skin healing. Dosage: children 2 and younger, 5 milligrams; 2 and older, 10 to 15 milligrams. Use for 2 weeks and then stop.

Thymus glandular extract—Give one to two 250-milligram tablets or capsules daily.

Herbal Remedies

Echinacea or echinacea/goldenseal combination—Supports the immune system to help the child get over an infection.

Larix—Easy to add to a baby's formula for immune system enhancement. If breastfeeding, have baby suck the herb from your finger.

Aromatherapy

Mix equal parts Roman chamomile (for its anti-inflammatory effects) and tea tree (which stimulates the immune system and is antibacterial and antiviral) essential oils in a full teaspoon of olive oil. Rub this mixture all around the ear, including the hairline, and down the sides of the neck (to improve lymphatic drainage). If the child is taking a homeopathic remedy, use aromatherapy at a different time.

Case History

Fourteen-month-old Jessica was brought to our office by her mother for an acute ear infection. She was screaming and obviously in a lot of discomfort. Her fever was 103°F and her face was bright red. She had been tugging at her right ear the past evening and woke up at 5:00 A.M. with a raging ear infection. Her ear canal was a deep red color and slightly swollen. Her mother said that this was the fourth ear infection in 3 months, and she did not want Jessica to receive another round of antibiotics if possible. We gave Jessica a dose of the homeopathic remedy Belladonna in our office and left mother and daughter alone for 30 minutes while consulting with other patients. When we came back, Jessica was asleep in her mother's arms. Her temperature had dropped to 101°F. Her mother stated that about 5 minutes after taking the remedy, Jessica had calmed down and stopped screaming and crying. We recommended that Jessica's mom give her the Belladonna a few more times at home that day, as well as giving children's echinacea. The next day, Jessica was still doing fine, and on visual examination of the ear, no redness or inflammation was present. With continued natural treatment, she never experienced another ear infection.

Vital Study

K. H. Friese, M.D., and his colleagues divided 131 young children (average age 5) into two groups. One group of 28 children received conventional treatment such as decongestants, antibiotics, and fever-reducing medicines (12 different drugs in all) for ear infections. Another group of 103 children was treated with one or more of 12 homeopathic remedies. Children receiving homeopathic treatment, on average, experienced 2 days of ear pain and required 3 days of therapy. Nearly 71 percent had not had another ear infection after 1 year, and nearly 30 percent had had a maximum of three recurrences. In contrast, children treated with conventional medicine, on average, experienced 3 days of ear pain and required 10 days of therapy. Nearly 57 percent did not have a recurrence after 1 year, while 43 percent experienced a maximum of six recurrences.

Acupressure

Gently press each of the following acupressure points with a thumb for 10 to 15 seconds. Perform on both sides of the body and repeat three times each day.

Gallbladder 20—Located at the base of the skull on both sides of the spine, where there is a depression beside the neck muscle.

Triple Warmer 17—Located directly below the bottom portion of the ear in the space where the jaw connects.

Large Intestine 4—Located in the webbing between the thumb and index finger. Helpful when fever is involved with the ear infection.

■ FOR LONG-TERM IMMUNE SUPPORT

Diet

Children's multivitamin—Follow the dosage directions on the label.

Vitamin C—Supports the immune system. Dosage: the child's age in years times 50 milligrams, daily. Reduce the dosage if diarrhea occurs. Consider using a buffered vitamin C powder (nonacidic) or liquid vitamin C. Both work well for infants and children, and can be mixed in juice.

Essential fatty acids—These reduce allergic reactions and inflammation. The best examples are flaxseed oil, fish oil, and mixed essential fatty acid complexes. Choose a children's complex that contains omega-3 and omega-6 fatty acids, and give it daily, as directed on the container. Or give 1 gram of fish oil per 50 pounds of body weight daily. Or give flaxseed oil at the following daily dosages: children up to age 2, 1 teaspoon; kids 3 to 6, 2 teaspoons; kids 7 and older, 2 to 3 teaspoons. Reduce the flaxseed oil dosage if diarrhea occurs.

Probiotic—Contains *Lactobacillus acidophilus* and *bifidus* to restore the "good bacteria" that normally inhabit the ear. Especially important to give if your child has been on antibiotics. Choose a formula made for children. Give for 2 months or longer and as directed on the container.

Homeopathy

For chronic ear infections, a constitutional homeopathic medicine can be quite helpful. Consult a homeopathic practitioner. Spinal work treatment by a chiropractor or craniosacral practitioner can be very helpful. (See pages 502 and 503 for more information.)

■ WHAT TO EXPECT

With acute ear infections, improvement should be seen within 24 hours. Our experience with using homeopathic remedies is that improvement is often seen within 30 minutes to 3 hours after taking the correct remedy. Have your child monitored by a doctor. For chronic ear infections, natural therapy equals (and in some cases, surpasses) the effectiveness of conventional medicine. Work with a holistic physician such as a naturopathic doctor to address the cause of the ear infections. The vast majority of chronic cases can be resolved with natural therapies. Regular testing with a tympanogram is recommended, to measure the ability of the eardrum to vibrate and make sure that there is not a fluid buildup.

Earwax Buildup

On the outer side of the ear canal are skin glands that manufacture a protective wax. This wax traps foreign particles and lubricates the ear canal. But when an excess amount of earwax accumulates, it can block the ear canal.

When blockage occurs due to wax buildup, children may complain of muffled hearing, especially after showering or swimming. That's because sound waves are unable to pass to the eardrum. In severe cases, they may develop fever or pain if there is blood or pus present.

Cotton swabs pushed too deeply into the ear canal can cause earwax buildup. Food sensitivities and nutritional deficiencies are often the root cause in the overproduction of earwax.

Conventional treatment focuses on irrigating the wax out of the ear. This procedure should be done at your doctor's office. Apply 2 drops of warm olive oil into your child's ears the night before the cleaning to help loosen up the wax. (Do not apply oil in the ear if there has been a recent perforation.)

■ BASIC PLAN

Diet

A whole-foods diet is recommended. (See "Diet" on page 4 for more information.) Sources of essential fatty acids are important. Ground-up, fresh flaxseeds provide a rich source of omega-3 fatty acids. Grind 1 teaspoon per 50 pounds of body weight (children weighing 30 to 50 pounds may also use 1 teaspoon) and give this amount daily, with 8 ounces of water.

Seeds and nuts are also good sources, as is fresh fish. Margarine and hydrogenated oils should be avoided, as they create fatty acid imbalance.

Food sensitivities may also be a contributing cause and should be identified and treated. (See "Food Allergies and Food Sensitivities" on page 298 for more information.)

Nutritional Supplements

Choose one of the following three supplements.

Essential fatty acid complex—Choose a children's blend that contains omega-3 fatty acids and omega-6 fatty acids (especially GLA, or gamma linolenic acid). Give as directed on the container.

Flaxseed oil—Daily dosages: children up to 2 years, 1 teaspoon; kids 3 to 6, 2 teaspoons; kids 7 and older, 2 to 3 teaspoons. Reduce the dosage if diarrhea occurs.

Fish oil—Daily dosage: 1 gram per 50 pounds of body weight.

■ ADVANCED PLAN

Nutritional Supplements

Children's multivitamin—Provides all the nutrients involved with tissue healing. Give as directed, daily.

Grape seed extract or pycnogenol—Has a natural anti-allergy effect that may be related to the earwax buildup. Give 1 milligram per pound of body weight daily.

■ WHAT TO EXPECT

Improving the nutritional status of a child can help prevent wax buildup. This can take 6 weeks or longer.

Eczema

Known medically as atopic dermatitis, eczema is a chronic skin inflammation disease characterized by patches of dry, itchy skin. It can develop in infants but tends to first appear by age 5.

In infants, the symptoms include a rash on the entire body, including the face. Soon, flaky red patches emerge that itch and cause the baby to scratch. The scratching can lead to seeping, crusting, and infection.

In children, the symptoms include a red, itchy, weepy rash on the face and neck, behind the ears, in the bends of the elbows, behind the knees, on the hands, and (less commonly) on other areas. The rash can itch, swell, and ooze.

Food sensitivities, poor digestive function, and essential fatty acid deficiencies are the main causes of eczema. Exposure to animal dander or emotional stress can also play a role. A child diagnosed with eczema is more susceptible to developing asthma or hay fever.

See a doctor if there are signs of infection (pus or red streaks) from the skin being scratched.

We do not recommend that children use topical creams, whether natural or pharmaceutical, on a long-term basis. They are best used during times of intolerable itching to provide relief. The natural approach in this chapter works to treat the cause of eczema. Sometimes, at the beginning of natural treatment (the first couple of weeks), the eczema gets worse and then clears. This is the body detoxifying and should not be suppressed. It is important that children who have been on long-term hydrocortisone cream treatment do not discontinue this medicine all at once. This can lead to a rebound effect where the eczema gets even worse, as the skin is used to the suppressive effect of the cortisone. Instead, gradually reduce the amount and frequency of the cortisone cream over time while using the natural therapies to treat the real cause.

Conventional treatment focuses on antihistamine medications, moisturizing creams, and topical hydrocortisone (steroid) ointment. Double-rinse your child's clothes to prevent reactions from detergent, or use a hypoallergenic detergent. Also, dress your child in cotton clothes; they are more comfortable for children with eczema than clothes made from wool or the harsher synthetics.

■ BASIC PLAN

Diet

Food sensitivities are often the underlying factor that brings on eczema. Common ones include dairy, wheat, citrus fruit, sugar, and soy. A child's food sensitivities must be identified and treated. (See "Food Allergies and Food Sensitivities" on page 298 for more information.) Breastfeeding mothers whose infants have eczema also need to be wary of food sensitivities that they could be passing on to their children. Bottlefed children may be sensitive to the formula they are using. Try switching to a non-cow's-milk formula. Some children do fine with soy-based formulas, and some are sensitive to it. Predigested hypoallergenic formulas are available for infants and children who are sensitive to both cow's milk and soy formulas.

Improve your child's essential fatty acid balance. Omega-3 sources of essential fatty acids need to be increased. Examples include flaxseeds, flaxseed oil, fish, nuts, and seeds. (See "Essential Fatty Acids" on page 8 for more information.) Breastfeeding mothers should increase these foods in their diets or take essential fatty acid supplements.

Reduce your child's intake of saturated fats that promote skin inflammation. Food sources of saturated fats include red meat and dairy products.

Spicy foods can cause eczema flare-ups and should be used sparingly.

Nutritional Supplements

Vitamin C—Supports the immune system and has mild anti-inflammatory effects. The type with bioflavonoids is preferable. Dosage: the child's age in years times 50 milligrams, twice daily. Reduce the dosage if diarrhea occurs. Consider using a buffered vitamin C powder (nonacidic) or liquid vitamin C. Both work well for infants and children, and can be mixed in juice. Ester C works well for children with a citrus sensitivity.

Choose one of the following three supplements.

Essential fatty acid complex—Choose a children's blend that contains omega-3 fatty acids and omega-6 fatty acids (especially GLA, or gamma linolenic acid). Give as directed on the container.

Flaxseed oil—Start with 1 teaspoon and increase if necessary using the following dosages: children 3 to 6, 2 teaspoons; kids 7 and older, 2 to 3 teaspoons. Reduce the dosage if diarrhea occurs.

Fish oil—Daily dosage: 1 gram per 50 pounds of body weight.

Herbal Remedies

Burdock root—A liver and skin detoxifier. Give the tincture twice daily for at least 8 weeks.

Chickweed *(Stellaria media)*, calendula, and chamomile are each available in creams. Any one of them can ease symptoms but should only be used short-term—1 to 2 weeks—while the eczema is calming down. However, we do feel that these are a better option than cortisone cream. Creams are better for wet, weeping eczema rashes, while salves are better for dry, scaling eczema.

Oatmeal bath—Add a cup of oatmeal powder such as Aveeno to a warm bath. Or, put regular oatmeal (such as Quaker Oats) into a cheesecloth bag, tie it with a string, and hang it under the faucet or float it in the tub. Have the child soak in the warm bath for 5 to 15 minutes. When done, pat the child dry so that a film of oatmeal is left on the skin. This film contains the anti-itch properties of the oatmeal.

Herbal soap—Calendula and oatmeal soaps are available and should be used instead of commercial soaps, which often contain irritating perfumes.

Homeopathy

Pick the following remedy that best matches your child's symptoms. Unless otherwise indicated, give your child 2 pellets of a 30C potency twice daily. (For infants, crush the pellets into powder and mix it with water.) Improvements should be seen within 5 days. If there is no improvement within 5 days, try another remedy. After you first notice improvement, stop giving the remedy unless symptoms begin to return.

Note: Lower potencies (6X, 12X, 6C) may need to be given more often (three times daily).

Arsenicum album—For burning pains that occur with the itching. The child is very restless.

Graphites—For thick, dry skin with deep cracks. A honeylike discharge oozes from the skin.

Medorrhinum—For eczema since birth. The child often has asthma as well. The child is very warm.

Petroleum—For extremely dry skin that is worse in the winter.

Psorinum—For symptoms similar to Sulphur (see next page), but the child is not generally as warm. For eczema that causes great discomfort and does not respond to indicated remedies.

Pulsatilla—For eczema that feels better in the open air. The child has characteristic Pulsatilla symptoms—he is shy and clingy.

Rhus toxicodendron—For eczema that begins as small watery vesicles that break open when scratched. The skin feels better with hot water. The child is restless.

Sulphur—The most common remedy for eczema. Symptoms include burning and tremendous itching. The child may scratch the skin until it bleeds. Symptoms are usually worse at night and from bathing. The child has a high thirst for cold drinks.

■ ADVANCED PLAN

Nutritional Supplements

Children's multivitamin—Provides all the nutrients involved with skin healing. Give as directed daily.

Zinc—Supports the immune system and enhances skin healing. Dosage: children 2 and younger, 5 milligrams; 2 and older, 10 to 15 milligrams. Can be used long-term under the supervision of a natural doctor.

Quercitin—Daily dosage: 3 milligrams per pound of body weight.

Vitamin E oil applied topically can help with skin healing and prevent infection.

Herbal Remedy

Formulas containing detoxifying herbs such as dandelion root, nettle, red clover (*Trifolium pratense*), and licorice root can be helpful. Use

Case History

Patricia was a 5-year-old who had eczema on her face, elbows, and back for 4 years. Her mother stated that she would scratch her skin every night until it bled. When Patricia's mother brought her in, she had been on hydrocortisone cream on and off for the past 2 years. It did not seem to be helping much anymore, and her mother was concerned because Patricia was so uncomfortable. We put Patricia on a diet free of milk and sugar products. We also prescribed an essential fatty acid formula to take every day. In addition, we prescribed homeopathic Sulphur to be taken daily. We slowly weaned her off the hydrocortisone cream by having her use it every other day for a couple of weeks, then every 2 days, and so on until she was off it. Her skin was completely clear after 2 months of natural treatment, and it has been a few years since she has needed any creams to help her skin.

under the guidance of a natural health care practitioner.

Aromatherapy

Add equal parts lavender, Roman or German chamomile, and geranium to 40 milliliters of a carrier oil such as grape seed, olive, or sweet almond. Apply to the affected area before bedtime. If the child is taking a homeopathic remedy, use aromatherapy at a different time.

■ WHAT TO EXPECT

The correct natural therapy should alleviate chronic eczema. If a child is not on hydrocortisone cream, then improvements are usually noticed within 2 to 4 weeks. Longstanding cases may take many months to totally clear. Be patient if your child is on hydrocortisone cream; work with a holistic doctor to slowly wean him off of this suppressive medication.

Eye Problems

Often unexpectedly, and in less time than it takes to blink, foreign bodies can lodge in a child's eye. Foreign bodies come from many sources, including chemical particles in the air, dirt, smog, cosmetics, yard debris, and even eyelashes.

When a foreign body enters the eye, the eye reacts with a flow of tears to attempt to flush away this offending substance. The eye is naturally wet, more porous and sensitive than skin.

When the substance is chemical, it can cause a burning sensation of the eye, swelling in the cornea, and possibly, temporary or permanent vision loss. Common chemical sources of eye problems are ammonia, bleach, cosmetics, detergents, disinfectants, drain cleaners, solvents, oven cleaners, and other household liquids, as well as liquid fertilizer or pesticides.

Reacting to the foreign body by rubbing the eyes worsens the condition. Unfortunately, eye rubbing is a natural reaction by babies and children who do not understand the consequences.

■ IMMEDIATE PLAN

For chemicals in the eye—Immediately flush the eye with water. Repeat several times and take the child to the emergency room.

For a foreign body in the eye—If a large particle in the eye will not come out through tearing or flushing with water, call your pediatrician. If an object appears to be embedded in the eye, seek emergency care.

Homeopathy

Symphytum 30C—For trauma to the eyeball. Give 2 pellets twice, as soon as possible after the eye injury. For infants, crush the pellets into powder and mix it with water.

Bach Flower Rescue Remedy—To help calm a child down after the injury. Give 2 drops to relieve anxiety. (For infants, put the drops in ¼ cup of water, then give ¼ teaspoon of the water.)

■ WHAT TO EXPECT

Following the proper procedure can provide quick relief of eye discomfort and damage. Work with a doctor to get the correct treatment.

Fatigue

Children are usually bundles of energy. When they constantly say, "I'm tired," parents need to pay special attention.

Fatigue can range from mild yawning to severe lethargy, intermittent or continuous. The causes may be related to lifestyle changes, stress, nutritional deficiencies, poor digestive function, or an underlying disease.

Temporary fatigue can be linked to a disruption in a child's sleep routine, taking up a new sport, staying up late with friends, or being involved in too many activities.

Fatigue can also be linked to a medical condition, including depression, chronic fatigue syndrome, mononucleosis, hypothyroidism, leukemia, iron deficiency anemia, or a viral or bacterial infection.

Have your child examined by a doctor if she displays any of these symptoms:

- Fatigue that lasts more than 2 weeks
- Longer or more frequent naps
- Difficulty sleeping
- Constant crying and sadness
- Dark circles under the eyes
- Bad breath

If no underlying disease is detected, the typical conventional treatment is rest. Adequate sleep is key to improving your child's energy levels. If your child's fatigue is related to emotional stress, then take time to be with your child and talk about what is bothering her. Give encouragement and support. Seek counseling if necessary. (See "Depression" on page 263 for more information.)

The natural treatment of fatigue depends on the cause. For example, if a child has iron deficiency anemia, then diet and supplements that focus on the anemia are indicated. Likewise, low-grade infections or depression would have different treatments to resolve the fatigue. This treatment section focuses on natural approaches to fatigue when no underlying cause is identifiable.

■ BASIC PLAN

Diet

Increase the amount of energy-producing foods your child eats. A whole-foods diet is recommended. (See "Diet" on page 4 for more information.) Too much sugar (soft drinks, table sugar, candy) in the diet may seem to energize a child, but only for short bursts, and a steady diet of high-sugar foods only leads to long-term fatigue as well as to food sensitivities. Regular meals and snacks throughout the day are important to keep blood sugar levels from getting too low.

Adequate protein is also important to maintain energy. It is important that your child eats breakfast; otherwise, the body's blood sugar levels can be thrown off for the rest of the day. If your child experiences fatigue at school in the afternoon, pack her lunch to make sure that it is nutritious. Make sure that your child is drinking enough water throughout the day. Dehydration, even in a minor state, can cause fatigue.

Nutritional Supplements

Children's multivitamin—Provides nutrients involved with energy production. Give as directed on the container daily.

Essential fatty acid complex or flaxseed oil—Give daily to increase essential fatty acids in the diet. If using an essential fatty acid complex, choose a children's blend that contains omega-3's and omega-6's, and follow the directions on the label. If using flaxseed oil, give the following dosages: children up to age 2, 1 teaspoon; kids 3 to 6, 2 teaspoons; kids 7 and older, 2 to 3 teaspoons. Reduce the dosage if diarrhea occurs.

Herbal Remedies

Siberian ginseng—Helps the body adapt to physical and mental stress. For children over age 10, you can have them take a dose twice daily for 4 weeks, then take a 1-week break, and repeat if necessary for one more cycle of 4 weeks. Siberian ginseng is used to help the body adapt to stress and gently increase energy levels over time. It is not as stimulating as Chinese ginseng.

Nettle—This is a very nutritive herb that younger children can take. It is rich in energy-producing minerals.

Homeopathy

Pick the following remedy that best matches your child's symptoms. Unless otherwise indicated, give your child 2 pellets of a 30C potency twice daily. Improvements should be seen within 7 days. If there is no improvement within 7 days, try another remedy. After you first notice improvement, stop giving the remedy unless symptoms begin to return.

Note: Lower potencies (6X, 12X, 6C) may need to be given more often (three times daily).

Gelsemium—For fatigue that includes drowsiness, weakness, and possibly muscle soreness.

Kali phosphoricum 6X—Good to use if the child is fatigued from mental stress. Give 2 pellets twice daily.

Phosphoric acid—The child is extremely fatigued and has an unusually strong craving for carbonated drinks.

Silica 6X—For chronic bouts of fatigue where the child is always coming down with colds and other infections. Give 2 pellets twice daily.

■ ADVANCED PLAN

Nutritional Supplements

B complex—A liquid dose daily can help improve energy levels. For children under age 7, give 25 milligrams daily; for kids 7 and older, give 50 milligrams daily.

Bee pollen or royal jelly—Supports energy production. For children under age 7, give 1 capsule daily; for kids 7 and older, give 1 to 2 capsules daily.

Aromatherapy

Peppermint—Add 1 drop to a vaporizer and leave it on in areas of the house where the child plays during the day. Do not use peppermint in the evening, as it may cause insomnia.

If the child is taking a homeopathic remedy, use aromatherapy at a different time.

Acupressure

Gently press the following acupressure points with a thumb for 10 to 15 seconds. Perform on both sides of the body and repeat three times each day.

Stomach 36—Located four finger-widths below the kneecap and one finger-width toward the outside of the leg (outside of the shinbone on the muscle).

Liver 3—Located on top of the foot in the hollow between the big toe and second toe.

■ WHAT TO EXPECT

When the cause of the fatigue is treated, energy improvements should be seen within 10 days.

Fever

A fever is a symptom of an underlying illness and the body's way of stimulating the immune system. Anyone with an elevated body temperature at least 1° above 98.6°F is said to have a fever. However, in babies, the healthy body temperature can vary from 97° to 100°F because the body temperature is not yet developed. In healthy children, body temperatures can fluctuate by 2° above or below 98.6°F.

Taking your child's temperature regularly—when he isn't sick—can help you pinpoint his normal range.

Often, a fever is accompanied by facial flushing and beads of sweat on the forehead.

Fevers are a source of worries for parents, but they can often be as much a friend as a foe. When a child has a mild fever, it could be a signal that his natural defense system is waging a war against an invading microbe. As the army of white blood cells battle, they release substances called pyrogens. These pyrogens activate the hypothalamus, a part of the brain that serves as the body's thermostat regulator, to turn on the internal heat and raise the body temperature to fight off invaders. When this occurs, heat is lost through the skin, and blood vessels dilate.

The onset of a high fever may lead to a febrile seizure in some children. Their muscles become rigid and they experience convulsions, even loss of consciousness for up to 15 minutes. This is an emergency situation that requires immediate medical attention. Upon recovering, a child may sleep for a long time. As horrific as they are to witness, febrile seizures rarely develop into epilepsy or cause permanent harm to the child.

Children with temperatures above 102°F may require medical intervention. If your child is less than 3 months of age, notify your doctor about any fever. Be sure to have your child checked by a doctor if he shows any of these symptoms:

- Acts confused, lethargic, or delirious
- Experiences a seizure
- Vomits or has diarrhea
- Complains of a stiff neck or has dilated pupils

- Has had the fever for more than 72 hours
- Cries continuously
- Is difficult to awaken
- Has a significant decrease in urine output or appears dehydrated
- Has trouble breathing

Conventional treatment focuses on fever-reducing medications such as acetaminophen.

Caution: Never give aspirin to a child who has a fever. This can cause an immune reaction leading to the development of Reye's syndrome, a potentially fatal illness. Also avoid the herbal painkiller white willow, as it contains ingredients similar to aspirin.

■ BASIC PLAN

Diet

Do not force your child to eat if he is not hungry. Instead, offer light, easy-to-digest soups and broths.

Regular water intake is important to prevent dehydration. Herbal teas and highly diluted fruit juices can also be given. Frozen fruit juice pops are popular with kids. Sugar products should be avoided because of sugar's suppressive effect on the immune system.

Breastfeeding should be maintained for nursing infants.

Nutritional Supplements

Vitamin C—Supports the immune system and has mild anti-inflammatory effects. The type with bioflavonoids is preferable. Dosage: the child's age in years times 50 milligrams, twice daily. Reduce the dosage if diarrhea occurs. Consider using a buffered vitamin C powder (nonacidic) or liquid vitamin C. Both work well for infants and children, and can be mixed in juice.

Calcium—May help to prevent febrile seizures. Give 250 to 500 milligrams daily.

Herbal Remedies

Echinacea—Has fever-reducing properties and helps stimulate immune cells to fight an infection.

Yarrow, chamomile, or elder flower (or a combination of these herbs) in tea or tincture form helps to reduce a fever and make a child more comfortable. Peppermint is also cooling and adds a pleasant taste.

Homeopathy

Combination fever remedies are available. Or pick the one of the following remedies that best matches your child's symptoms. For the remedies on the next page, unless otherwise indicated, give 2 pellets of a 30C potency every 2 hours. (For infants, crush the pellets into powder and mix it with water.) Improvements should be seen within 6 hours. If there is no improvement within 6 hours, try another remedy. After you first notice improvement, stop giving the remedy unless symptoms begin to return. For very high fevers (104°F), take the indicated remedy every 15 minutes and seek immediate medical attention.

Note: Lower potencies (6X, 12X, 6C) may need to be given more often (every 1 to 2 hours).

Aconitum napellus—Useful at the very beginning of a fever (the first 4 hours) when there is sudden onset. This often occurs after the child has been exposed to the cold or wind. The child is restless and fearful, and may be crying. One cheek may be red and the other pale.

Arsenicum album—For fever that occurs or increases between 12:00 and 2:00 A.M. The child is chilly along with the fever. Anxiety and restlessness are usually present. The child feels better with sips of warm water.

Belladonna—For a sudden, intense fever. The child's body feels very hot (especially his face) but his feet are cold. The child does not usually get any chills. The pupils may be dilated, and the cheeks and face are often bright red. The child may be sensitive to light and have a throbbing headache. He may be delirious and hallucinate from the fever.

Bryonia alba—The child has a fever and a tremendous thirst. His face is flushed. He is very irritable and does not want to move.

Chamomilla—For a fever that accompanies teething. One cheek is red while the other is pale. The child is very irritable.

China officinalis—The fever is periodic—it comes and goes. For a fever with chills, tremendous sweating, and weakness.

Ferrum phosphoricum—The child has a fever but does not act sick. His face is red and his body is warm. Use this remedy if you do not know which remedy to use.

Pulsatilla—The child has a fever with low thirst. He wants to be held and is very clingy. He feels better with an open window or in the open air. The symptoms change a lot during the fever.

Pyrogen or pyrogenium—The fever is high and the child appears very sick. His body feels bruised and aching. The child's pulse does not match up to the fever (for instance, he has a high fever but a low pulse). This is not a common remedy in stores, so you may need to see a homeopathic practitioner.

Sulphur—For acute or long-lasting fevers where the child's whole body is warm. He has a high thirst for cold drinks. His feet get really hot, and he wants them and the rest of his body uncovered. The top of the child's head gets very hot, and his body sweats easily.

Hydrotherapy

Constitutional or foot hydrotherapy works very well in helping to control fevers and fight infections. (See Hydrotherapy for Children on page 115 for directions.) Perform either of these techniques one or two times daily.

Acupressure

Large Intestine 4—Located in the webbing between the thumb and index finger. Gently press the acupressure point with a thumb for 10 to 15 seconds. Perform on both sides of the body and repeat three times each day.

■ WHAT TO EXPECT

Natural therapies help to manage a fever and keep the child comfortable. Improvement should be seen within 12 to 24 hours. If the child does not improve within 24 hours or seems to be getting worse, be sure to consult with a doctor.

Fifth Disease

This acute viral infection usually starts with a couple days of fever, headaches, nausea, and muscle aches. Within a week to 10 days, the child develops a fiery red blotchy or flat, lacelike rash on her cheeks (it looks like the cheeks have been slapped) that spreads to her legs, arms, and torso as delicate-looking, bumpy rashes.

The incubation period during which the infected child is contagious is 4 to 14 days. Once the child has a rash, she is usually no longer contagious to others.

Fifth disease outbreaks usually occur during the spring. The disease can be transmitted from the mother to the fetus during pregnancy, sometimes resulting in stillbirth or the baby being born with fetal anemia.

Conventional treatment focuses on symptom relief with pain- and fever-reducing medications. Aspirin should never be used with a viral condition, as it can lead to Reye's syndrome.

■ BASIC PLAN

Diet

Make sure that your child gets plenty of fluids to prevent dehydration. Stay consistent with breastfeeding or bottlefeeding for infants. Older children should drink at least six glasses of water throughout the day. Fruit juices, if used, should be diluted with water by at least 50 percent, as simple sugars can weaken the immune system. Homemade warm broths and soups are best; they are easy to digest and moisten the respiratory tract. Fresh garlic added to the soup is helpful as long as your child is not sensitive to it. Do not give fried foods, as they are hard to digest. Avoid giving your child dairy products; they can contribute to mucus formation.

Nutritional Supplements

Vitamin C—Supports the immune system and has mild anti-inflammatory effects. The type with bioflavonoids is preferable. Dosage: the child's age in years times 50 milligrams, twice daily. Reduce the dosage if diarrhea occurs. Consider using a buffered vitamin C powder (nonacidic) or liquid vitamin C. Both work well for infants and children, and can be mixed in juice.

Vitamin A—Supports the immune system. Daily dosage: infants under 1 year, 1,875 international units (IU); children 1 to 3, 2,000 IU; kids 4 to 6, 2,500 IU; kids 7 to 10, 3,500 IU; males 11 and older, 5,000 IU; females 11 and older, 4,000 IU.

Note: These dosages are for short-term use (up to 10 days). Higher dosages may be used only under a doctor's supervision. Available in liquid drops.

Herbal Remedy

Echinacea—Stimulates immune function and has antiviral activity. Look for a flavored children's glycerin-based formula.

Homeopathy

Pick the following remedy that best matches your child's symptoms. Unless otherwise indicated, give your child 2 pellets of a 30C potency three times daily. (For infants, crush the pellets into powder and mix it with water.) Improvements should be seen within 48 hours. If there is no improvement within 48 hours, try another remedy. After you first notice improvement, stop giving the remedy unless symptoms begin to return.

Note: Lower potencies (6X, 12X, 6C) may need to be given more often (four times daily).

Ferrum phosphoricum—The child has a fever but does not act sick. Her face is flushed.

Pulsatilla—The child is feverish. She becomes clingier than normal and does not want an adult to leave her side. She is weepy and has low thirst. She may develop yellow or green mucus from the sinus.

Acupressure

Large Intestine 4—Relieves head congestion and fever. Located in the webbing between the thumb and index finger. Gently press the acupressure point with a thumb for 10 to 15 seconds. Perform on both sides of the body and repeat three times each day.

■ ADVANCED PLAN

Herbal Remedies

Astragalus—Supports the immune system and tonifies the lungs.

Lomatium—A potent antiviral herb that inhibits the replication of viruses.

Larix—A good immune system enhancer. It is available in a powder form that blends into water and juice, sometimes with a mild, sweet taste.

Aromatherapy

German chamomile—Add to the child's bath, swish it around, and place the child in the bath for 15 to 20 minutes. If the child is taking a homeopathic remedy, use aromatherapy at a different time.

■ WHAT TO EXPECT

The child should be more comfortable after natural therapy and have gradual improvement over 5 to 7 days.

Flu

The flu, or influenza, is a highly contagious viral infection of the respiratory tract.

The three types of influenza viruses are known as A, B, and C. Each features a different strain of viruses. Strains are also typically named after the region where they were first identified, such as the Hong Kong flu.

Flu viruses are spread by airborne particles released from an infected person's respiratory tract. Outbreaks tend to occur during the winter months, when more people are indoors and the humidity is low.

Although a child becomes contagious within 2 days of contracting the virus, he usually doesn't display any outward symptoms for about 5 days. Common flu symptoms include fever, headache, chills, muscle aches, sneezing, sore throat, fatigue, chest pain, dry cough, and loss of appetite.

The flu usually lasts 5 to 6 days. If symptoms persist or worsen, the child is at risk of developing pneumonia, croup, seizures, or encephalitis.

See your doctor if your child has:

- A high fever
- A seizure
- Breathing problems
- A stiff neck or dilated pupils

Conventional treatment focuses on increased fluids, rest, and fever and pain reducers.

The flu vaccine is commonly recommended for children and adults. We do not advocate the general use of the flu vaccine but instead recommend strengthening one's immune system to be more resistant to the flu and to many other viruses and other pathogens. However, for children with heart conditions, diabetes, respiratory problems, or immune system deficiencies (such as HIV), it is worth considering the flu vaccine.

Caution: Do not give your child aspirin with the flu, as it can lead to Reye's syndrome, a serious condition that can affect the brain and liver.

■ BASIC PLAN

Diet

Make sure that your child gets plenty of fluids to prevent dehydration. Stay consistent with breastfeeding or bottlefeeding for infants. Older children should drink at least six glasses of water throughout the day. Fruit juices, if used, should be diluted with water by at least 50 percent, as simple sugars can weaken the immune system. Homemade warm broths and soups are best; they are easy to digest and moisten the respiratory tract. Fresh garlic added to the soup is helpful as long as your child is not sensitive to it. Do not give fried foods, as they are hard to digest. Avoid giving your child dairy products as they can contribute to mucus formation.

Nutritional Supplement

Vitamin C—Supports the immune system and has mild anti-inflammatory effects. The type with bioflavonoids is preferable. Dosage: the child's age in years times 50 milligrams, twice daily. Reduce the dosage if diarrhea occurs. Consider using a buffered vitamin C powder (nonacidic) or liquid vitamin C. Both work well for infants and children, and can be mixed in juice.

Herbal Remedies

There are several herbs that can be used to treat viral infections such as the flu. Choose one of the following or a formula that contains a combination of them.

For children over 2, we frequently recommend a formula that we call the virus cocktail. It includes echinacea (10 drops), astragalus (10 drops), lomatium (10 drops), reishi (5 drops), and licorice root (5 drops). Add each of these herbs to 2 ounces of warm water or diluted juice. Give every 2 to 3 waking hours for 2 days, and then every 4 hours until complete recovery.

Children under 2 can be given one or more of the following herbs based on weight.

Echinacea—Stimulates immune function and has antiviral activity. Look for a children's glycerin-based formula. A great herb to start with.

Elderberry—Some studies have shown this to be an excellent flu fighter.

Astragalus—Supports the immune system and tonifies the lungs.

Lomatium—A potent antiviral herb that inhibits the replication of viruses.

Larix—A good immune system enhancer. It is available in a powder form that blends into water and juice, sometimes with a mild, sweet taste.

Homeopathy

Use a combination flu formula, or pick the one of the following remedies that best matches your child's symptoms. For the remedies below, unless otherwise indicated, give your child 2 pellets of a 30C potency three times daily. (For infants, crush the pellets into powder and mix it with water.) Improvements should be seen within 24 hours. If there is no improvement within 24 hours, try another remedy. After you first notice improvement, stop giving the remedy unless symptoms begin to return.

Note: Lower potencies (6X, 12X, 6C) may need to be given more often (four times daily).

Aconitum napellus—For the initial stages of a flu. The child is chilly and spikes a fever. His face is flushed. Symptoms come on rapidly.

Anas barbariae—A specific remedy for the flu. Most useful in the beginning stages. If you do not know what remedy to use, you can give this one. Oscillococcinum and Flu Solution are retail names for this remedy.

Arsenicum album—The child has flu symptoms along with diarrhea and vomiting. He is very restless, anxious, and thirsty for small sips of water. Fever is present, but the child feels chilled.

Bryonia alba—For flu with severe aching of the joints. The child feels worse from the slightest motion and has a very high thirst. He may have a headache and prefers a cool room and open air. He is irritable.

Belladonna—For flu with a rapid onset of a high fever. The child's face flushes and his pupils dilate, and he may complain of a headache. His body is hot, but his hands and feet are cold.

Eupatorium perfoliatum—For a high fever and severe aching of the bones. The child is thirsty for cold drinks.

Ferrum phosphoricum—For the initial stage of the flu. The child has a flushed face but does not act very sick.

Gelsemium—The most common remedy for the flu. The child feels very weak, sleepy, and sometimes dizzy. His muscles ache and feel like they are bruised. He may feel chills in the spinal area. There is a headache at the back of the head.

Nux vomica—The child is very chilly and irritable with the flu.

Rhus toxicodendron—The child is very restless and has aching and stiffness, especially in his back and neck. He feels better with constant movement. It is hard to find a comfortable position.

■ ADVANCED PLAN

Nutritional Supplements

Vitamin A—Supports the immune system. Daily dosage: infants under 1 year, 1,875 international units (IU); children 1 to 3, 2,000 IU; kids 4 to 6, 2,500 IU; kids 7 to 10, 3,500 IU; males 11 and older, 5,000 IU; females 11 and older, 4,000 IU.

Note: These dosages are for short-term use (up to 10 days). Higher dosages may be used only under a doctor's supervision. Available in liquid drops.

Zinc—Helps to support immune function. Zinc gluconate lozenges should be used only in children who are old enough to suck on them without choking—age 5 and older. They should not exceed 30 milligrams daily of elemental zinc for more than 5 days.

Thymus glandular extract—Give one to two 250-milligram tablets or capsules daily. Or use a homeopathic liquid preparation (give 5 drops twice daily).

Herbal Remedies

Ginger root tea—Helpful to reduce flu symptoms such as chills, nausea, and digestive upset. Give the child ½ cup to 1 cup twice daily.

Yarrow tea or tincture can be used if a high fever accompanies the cold.

Homeopathy

Influenzinum—An excellent remedy to give preventively if a flu epidemic is in the area. Give a 30C potency twice daily for 2 days as a preventative. Also helpful to take to get over the flu more quickly, or you can use it if other indicated remedies are not working. In addition, it is helpful for children who do not seem to fully recover from a bout with the flu.

Aromatherapy

Eucalyptus and peppermint—Add 1 drop of each to a vaporizer in the child's room. For his nighttime bath, use ginger instead of the peppermint, since peppermint can stimulate and make it harder to fall asleep. If the child is taking a homeopathic remedy, use aromatherapy at a different time.

Acupressure

Gently push on the following points for 15 seconds. Do this on both sides of the body. Repeat three times. Perform this treatment once daily.

Liver 3—Located on top of the foot, in the hollow between the big toe and second toe.

Large Intestine 4—Located in the webbing between the thumb and index finger.

■ WHAT TO EXPECT

Improvements should be noticed within 24 to 48 hours.

Food Allergies and Food Sensitivities

Often mistaken as one and the same, food allergies and food sensitivities are two different conditions although the terms are often used interchangeably.

Technically speaking, a food allergy is a measurable immune response to a normally harmless substance: food. Symptoms include itchy hives, lip swelling, nausea, vomiting, diarrhea, wheezing, and difficulty breathing.

Common food allergies, not surprisingly, are popular foods such as milk, eggs, chocolate, citrus fruits, soy, peanuts, and wheat. Preservatives, additives, and coloring agents in foods can also trigger an allergic reaction.

Food sensitivities are reactions to food where there is not necessarily an immune response (measurable by standard lab tests), but the child still experiences an adverse reaction. Symptoms include but are not limited to cramps, bloating, headache, mood changes, reoccurring infections, runny nose, and skin rashes. Food sensitivities are uncomfortable but milder and not life-threatening, as food allergy reactions can be. Symptoms may occur immediately or up to 36 hours after ingesting the offending food.

Most food sensitivities (80 to 90 percent) are acquired as opposed to genetic. We believe that a lack of variety in the diet can lead to the development of food sensitivities. Most kids eat the same 25 foods all the time. Thus, they run the risk of developing intolerances to these foods in addition to an increased risk of nutritional deficiencies. Interestingly, children often crave the very foods to which they are sensitive.

Poor digestive function can also lead to the development of food sensitivities. In the phenomenon known as leaky gut syndrome, damage to the intestinal lining allows larger than normal particles (proteins) to get into the bloodstream, causing an immune response.

Many children with food sensitivities develop dark circles under the eyes, as well as lines under the eyelids that are known as Denny's lines.

Many cases of food sensitivities can be improved or desensitized with the natural therapies discussed below.

The conventional approach is to use the skin scratch test or a blood test to identify the offending food or foods. Unfortunately, these tests are not very accurate when it comes to food sensitivities, because they pick up only food allergies, which are measurable immune responses. (Most reactions to food are food sensitivities.) So, unless your child has had a serious allergic reaction, such as hives or her throat closing off, the standard tests won't pick much up. The natural testing approaches are subtler and pick up sensitivities much more effectively.

Once tests have identified the food at the root of the problem, avoidance of the food is recommended. Severe food allergy reactions are treated with epinephrine and/or antihistamines such as Benadryl.

Caution: If your child has a severe allergic reaction to a food, seek emergency medical attention immediately. Symptoms to watch for include difficulty breathing, hives, or vomiting.

■ BASIC PLAN

Diet
The first step is to identify your child's food sensitivities. There are various ways to do this.

Case History

Ten-year-old Steven had major problems with many food sensitivities. His mother said that he would react to wheat, dairy, apples, corn, sugar, broccoli, carrots, and onions. As a result, he would suffer from gas and bloating, fatigue, sinusitis, and mood swings. Our testing confirmed that he reacted to these foods plus a few more. We had Steven focus on grain products that were easier on his system, such as kamut, spelt, and amaranth. We also had his mother rotate all his other foods so that he was not eating the same foods all the time. We prescribed food sensitivity homeopathic drops of the foods to which he was sensitive, as well as an herbal formula to improve his digestion. Since he had a history of repeated antibiotics, we also recommended a probiotic supplement (containing the friendly bacteria acidophilus and bifidus). We retested him 1 month later and found that his sensitivities had decreased. He was having fewer reactions to foods. On retesting 3 months later, only a few sensitivities remained. His mother found that the dark circles under his eyes had cleared up, his mood and energy had improved, and he was having less digestive upset. Steven still had to limit the amount of wheat products that he ate, but otherwise he had a much less restricted diet and better vitality.

Following are the four most common ways that holistic practitioners identify food sensitivities:

1. Elimination/reintroduction diet. The most common food sensitivities are eliminated from the child's diet and then reintroduced one at a time to see whether any adverse reactions occur. (For example, if your child is on the elimination diet and her chronic runny nose stops, you can assume that it was due to one or more of the foods that was eliminated. If the runny nose comes back when a particular food is reintroduced, you can correlate it with the reintroduced food.) The most common food sensitivities include wheat, dairy, sugar, soy, citrus fruit, peanuts, chocolate, and eggs. Pick a few of the foods from this list, eliminate them for 2 weeks, and then reintroduce them one at a time. Repeat this technique with a few more foods until you have tested them all (as well as any other foods that you suspect).

2. Applied kinesiology. In this technique, a holistic practitioner tests for food sensitivities by having the food contact the child while the strength of a muscle is tested. A weakened muscle response indicates an offending food. Infants can also be tested with a modification of this technique.

3. Electrodermal testing. An electro-acupuncture machine runs a current through the food being tested as the practitioner measures the electrical potential on an acupuncture point on the child's skin. A food to which the child is sensitive will show up as a lower reading, due to electrical and/or acupuncture meridian interference from the offending food.

This type of testing is also known as a Vega test. Studies have shown it to be accurate compared with other types of testing.

4. Antibody-antigen blood test. This type of test measures antibodies in the blood to certain foods. The most comprehensive test is IgE and IgG4 done together.

Note: To prevent food sensitivities, rotate different foods throughout the week in your child's diet. Try not to give the same food all the time.

Breastfeeding mothers need to be careful about eating foods to which they or their infants are sensitive. Eating such foods can result in symptoms for the infants.

Nutritional Supplements

Plant- or microbial-derived enzymes— Help to digest foods more efficiently. Give a digestive enzyme complex with meals or add it to an infant's formula for enhanced digestion. A breastfeeding mother can also take such a complex to digest foods more efficiently and cause fewer problems for her child (such as colic, ear infections, digestive upset, and rashes).

Probiotic—Choose one that contains children's acidophilus and bifidus. These optimize good bacteria in the digestive tract, which helps to break down food. Especially important if there is a history of antibiotic use. Give as directed on the container.

Herbal Remedies

Ginger root, fennel, peppermint, and anise are all good digestive herbs that can be used as

Vital Fact

A child has a 67 percent chance of developing food allergies if both of his parents have food allergies.

teas, tinctures, or in capsule form if reactions to foods occur.

Homeopathy

Once you know what your child is sensitive to, desensitization by giving homeopathic doses of the offending food can be helpful. For example, a child sensitive to apples is given 2 pellets of homeopathic Apple 6X twice daily for 1 to 2 months. This appears to reduce the body's reaction to the offending food in many cases.

■ ADVANCED PLAN

Nutritional Supplements

Quercitin—Has a natural antihistamine effect. Daily dosage is 3 milligrams per pound of body weight. Best taken between meals.

L-glutamine—Helps to improve intestinal cell health. Give 3 milligrams per pound of body weight daily. Use under the direction of a practitioner.

Homeopathy

Constitutional homeopathy from a practitioner is helpful for the long-term treatment of food sensitivities, especially if the child suffers from multiple sensitivities.

NAET (Nambudripad's Allergy Elimination Techniques) is a popular approach among holistic practitioners that appears to work well to desensitize people against food sensitivities. It involves the principles of homeopathy and acupuncture. Consult with a practitioner who is trained in this technique.

■ WHAT TO EXPECT

The number of foods to which a child is sensitive and the severity of the reaction usually improves within 4 to 6 weeks of natural treatment. Do not try to self-treat severe food allergies. Consult with practitioners who specialize in food sensitivity treatment.

Food Craving

Food craving is the strong, sometimes uncontrollable desire for a certain type of food. Sweets, fats, and carbohydrates top the list of desired foods among children.

There are body signals that might urge children to take the next bite. Research has shown that the hypothalamus in the brain plays a major role in appetite.

Medical conditions such as iron deficiency anemia can lead to strange cravings for inedible materials, such as chalk and dirt. This condition, known as pica, warrants a doctor's attention.

Often, emotions can fuel a child's appetite.

Some seek food when they are bored, tired, angry, lonely, or stressed. Food cravings can also be the result of a nutritional deficiency or a signal of blood sugar imbalance.

■ BASIC PLAN

Diet

Food sensitivities may be at the root of food cravings. (See "Food Allergies and Food Sensitivities" on page 298 for more information.) Although this phenomenon is not well understood, children often strongly crave the foods to which they are sensitive.

Increasing variety in the diet may help in the long run to decrease food cravings. The craving for sweets may be the result of low blood sugar (hypoglycemia) or a need for more protein in the diet.

Nutritional Supplements

Chromium and vanadium—These two minerals may be helpful if sweet cravings are strong. Give as part of a high-potency children's multivitamin or as separate supplements. Chromium daily dosages are as follows: children ages 1 to 3 years, 20 to 80 micrograms; 4 to 6 years, 30 to 120 micrograms; ages 7 and older, 50 to 200 micrograms. Consult a practitioner for a more exact dosage. Vanadium dosages range from 5 to 20 micrograms daily; see a practitioner for a dosage tailored to your child.

Magnesium—A daily dose of 250 to 500 milligrams can be helpful for some children who have strong sweet cravings.

Homeopathy

Constitutional homeopathy can be helpful for strong food cravings. Following are some common remedies and the food cravings for which they can be helpful. Pick the one that best matches your child's symptoms. Unless otherwise indicated, give your child 2 pellets of a 30C potency twice daily. Improvements should be seen within 7 days. If there is no improvement within 7 days, try another remedy. After you first notice improvement, stop giving the remedy unless symptoms begin to return.

Note: Lower potencies (6X, 12X, 6C) may need to be given more often (three times daily).

Lycopodium—For a strong craving for sweets.

Natrum muriaticum—For a strong craving for salty foods.

Pulsatilla—For a strong craving for sweets and creamy foods.

Sulphur—For a strong craving for spicy foods.

■ ADVANCED PLAN

Nutritional Supplement

Children's multivitamin—Provides a base of nutrients to help protect against nutritional deficiencies.

■ WHAT TO EXPECT

You should see an improvement within 4 weeks of treatment. The cravings may not completely go away, but they can often be reduced.

Food Poisoning

One of the most unpleasant and potentially dangerous conditions is food poisoning. A child's body reacts to toxins produced by bacteria that contaminate food. The most common food bacteria are salmonella and staphylococcus.

Symptoms range from nausea, overall body weakness, fever, and abdominal cramps to violent episodes of vomiting and diarrhea as the body tries to rid itself of the contaminated food.

Most cases of food poisoning can be avoided. Food poisoning occurs as a result of improper handling, storing, or cooking of food. That's why it's important to teach your children to always wash their hands thoroughly with soap before eating and especially before helping you prepare a meal.

Teach your children to immediately refrigerate foods such as mayonnaise, egg salad, potato salad, rice pudding, and fried rice. These foods can be easily contaminated. Encourage your kids to follow the old adage in deciding whether or not to eat leftovers: "When in doubt, throw it out."

Food poisoning can also occur from a child eating plants that contain toxic chemicals (certain types of mushrooms) or foods contaminated with chemicals (for instance, heavy metals such as lead). If you suspect that your child has eaten a poisonous plant or a chemical-contaminated food, seek medical attention immediately.

Fortunately, most cases of food poisoning

are short-lived and a child's appetite will return within 1 to 2 days. However, head to the emergency room if your child has a medical condition that impairs his immune system, or if he displays any of these severe symptoms:

- Violent vomiting
- A fever exceeding 102°F
- Vision problems
- Severe diarrhea that last more than 1 day or that contains blood
- Trouble breathing or talking
- Headache and dizziness
- Suspected dehydration

Here are some of the more common types of food poisoning.

Staphylococcus: Foods that have been handled by people with skin infections can be contaminated when left at room temperature. The classic example is a potato salad left out for a long time at a picnic. Symptoms usually come on very quickly (within 2 to 8 hours) and usually begin to resolve within 12 hours. They may include severe nausea and vomiting, abdominal cramps, diarrhea, headache, and fever.

Salmonella: This is an infection caused by one of the many types of salmonella bacteria. The most common contaminated foods include unpasteurized milk and undercooked poultry and eggs. This infection causes acute intestinal distress with sudden onset of headache, fever, abdominal pain, diarrhea, nausea, and sometimes vomiting. Dehydration in infants can be severe. Symptoms start 16 to 48 hours after eating and can last up to 7 days.

Botulism: This can be a very severe and potentially fatal poisoning. Home-canned foods are the most common source of the spores that cause toxicity to the nervous system. Commercially prepared foods can also be at fault. Botulinum spores are very resistant to heat. It is recommended that canned foods be exposed to moist heat at 248°F for 30 minutes to kill the spores. The toxins that are produced by the spores can be killed through heat by cooking the food at 176°F for 30 minutes. Symptoms usually come on 18 to 36 hours after ingestion of the botulinum toxin. They can include nausea, vomiting, and abdominal cramps, followed by neurological symptoms such as vision changes, muscle weakness, difficulty breathing, and constipation.

Note: Infant botulism occurs most often in children less than 6 months old. Botulinum spores may be present in honey, and children under 1 year old should not be given honey—their immune systems may not be able to handle it.

E. coli: This infection usually occurs as the result of undercooked beef or unpasteurized milk, or through fecal-oral contamination. The *Escherichia coli* bacterium infects the digestive tract and typically leads to bloody diarrhea (and, possibly, kidney failure). Children less than 5 years old and the elderly are most susceptible to the damaging effects of this infection. Symptoms usually include severe abdominal cramps, and watery diarrhea followed by bloody diarrhea. The entire range of diarrhea usually lasts 1 to 8 days. Fever is usually absent or low-grade.

Clostridium perfringens: This bacterium is found in feces, water, soil, and the air. Contaminated meat left at room temperature is the main source of infection. Symptoms usually begin after 6 to 24 hours after ingestion. They usually resolve within 24 hours. Common symptoms include watery diarrhea and abdominal cramps.

Traveler's diarrhea: This infection is caused by a bacterium endemic to the local water. It can also be caused by other bacteria or by viruses. It occurs in areas that lack adequate water purification. Common symptoms include nausea and vomiting, loud gurgling noises of the abdomen, abdominal cramps, and diarrhea beginning 12 to 72 hours after the contaminated water or food is ingested.

Parasitic infections: *Giardia* is the most common example. This parasite is transmitted through the fecal-oral route, mainly through water contamination. In most cases, there are no symptoms. When there are symptoms, they usually take 1 to 3 weeks after exposure to appear. Common symptoms are watery, malodorous diarrhea; abdominal cramps and distention; flatulence and burping; nausea; low-grade fever; and fatigue.

Chemical food poisoning: Plants or animals that contain a naturally occurring poison fall under the heading of chemical food poisoning. So do those that contain environmental poisons. Common examples include wild mushrooms, such as *Amanita phalloides;* wild and domestic plants, including yew, nightshade, castor bean, morning glory, and many others; fish; and shellfish. Fruits and vegetables sprayed with insecticides or other chemicals can also lead to chemical poisoning if they are not washed before they are eaten.

Conventional treatment for food poisoning focuses on identifying the type of organism causing the infection and then prescribing an antimicrobial medicine (for instance, antibiotics for bacterial infections). For non-microbial food poisoning, treatment varies; it may include inducing vomiting and giving intravenous fluids or other medications. Meanwhile, activated charcoal capsules taken internally can help to absorb toxins from food poisoning. They should be used under the guidance of a practitioner, and only on a short-term basis. (See the Advanced Plan.)

■ BASIC PLAN

Diet

The most important thing is to keep your child hydrated with water and electrolyte drinks such as Pedialyte. Easy-to-digest foods such as soups, broths, and steamed vegetables are recommended.

Nutritional Supplement

Probiotic—Choose a children's probiotic that contains acidophilus and bifidus. Helps to fight infectious bacteria and replaces destroyed good bacteria if antibiotics are needed. Give the maximum dosage for your child's age that is listed on the container. If antibiotics are used, then supplement for at least 2 months. It is wise to give this to your child preventively if you are traveling to countries with suspect water.

Herbal Remedies

Ginger root or peppermint leaf—Helps to relieve diarrhea, nausea, and vomiting. Give to your child as a fresh tea or in the tincture or capsule form.

Echinacea and goldenseal—This combination is a good general approach for immune support and antiviral/antibacterial effects.

Homeopathy

Use a combination diarrhea formula and/or nausea formula. Or pick the one of the following remedies that best matches your child's symptoms. For the remedies below, unless otherwise indicated, give your child 2 pellets of a 30C potency every hour for up to four doses. If there is no improvement within 4 hours, try another remedy. After you first notice improvement, stop giving the remedy unless symptoms begin to return.

Aloe socotrina—For acute diarrhea with gas and jellylike mucus in the stool.

Arsenicum album—The most common remedy for food poisoning. Symptoms include diarrhea (especially burning diarrhea), burning pains in the abdomen, vomiting, chilliness, anxiety, and restlessness. Symptoms tend to be worse between midnight and 2:00 A.M. The child feels better with warm drinks.

China officinalis—For diarrhea that has led to exhaustion and weakness. There is undigested food in the stool. Useful to take after an acute bout of food poisoning to regain strength.

Mercurius corrosivus—For bloody, burning diarrhea. The child may alternate between being chilly and sweaty.

Nux vomica—For cramping and painful diarrhea that feels better temporarily from passing stool or with warm applications. The child is chilly and irritable. This is also a good general remedy to use for ill effects from food, such as spicy or rich foods.

Phosphorus—For burning diarrhea or abdominal pain that is better with cold drinks or cold food.

Podophyllum—For profuse, watery diarrhea with gas. Stool may contain yellow mucus.

Veratrum album—For profuse, stools that look like rice water and that occur simultaneously with forceful vomiting.

■ ADVANCED PLAN

Nutritional Supplement

Activated charcoal capsules—Taken internally, these can help to absorb toxins from the food poisoning. Use under the guidance of a practitioner and only on a short-term basis. Works best when taken in the first stages of food poisoning (when you first realize that your child has food poisoning).

Herbal Remedies

For parasitic infections, herbs such as garlic, black walnut, wormwood (*Artemisia absinthium*), and grapefruit extract are effective. However, they should be used only under the guidance of a herbalist or doctor who has experience using herbs to treat parasitic infections. The herbs listed can have side effects and need to be used in very small amounts with children.

Acupressure

Stomach 36—Located four finger-widths below the kneecap and one finger-width toward the outside of the leg (outside of the shinbone on the muscle). Gently press the acupressure point with a thumb for 10 to 15 seconds. Perform on both sides of the body and repeat three times each day.

Aromatherapy

German chamomile and black pepper—Add these to a carrier oil and rub it over the child's abdomen. If the child is taking a homeopathic remedy, use aromatherapy at a different time.

■ WHAT TO EXPECT

Improvement should take place within 24 to 48 hours. If your child appears dehydrated, see a doctor immediately.

Foot Odor

Surprisingly, children's feet sweat more than most adults' feet. When this perspiration smells like rotten cheese, it is medically referred to as bromhidrosis. We know it better as stinky feet.

The soles of the feet, like the rest of the body, contain sweat glands. Perspiration is a normal body function to regulate temperature and expel toxins through skin pores. When normal perspiration is unable to be released, foot odor builds and intensifies.

Fetid bacteria coupled with the normal shedding of skin cells frequently cause foot odor. Children who wear the same shoes every day without allowing them to air out and dry run the risk of worsening foot odor.

General toxicity from poor digestion and elimination can be a contributing factor to smelly feet.

For extremely pungent foot odor that doesn't seem to respond to home treatment, the cause may be a fungus or other infection that requires medical attention to correct.

Conventional treatment focuses on deodorant creams, topical antifungal ointments (for fungal infections), soaks in Epsom salts or vinegar (diluted), and proper hygiene.

Choose shoes that are made from material that breathes, such as leather. Sandals are a good option in warm climates. Have two pairs of running shoes so that you can alternate their use, making for drier shoes. Wet shoes cause the skin on the feet to break down, leading to a bad smell. Change your child's socks two or three times daily, especially after playing or sports, to prevent perspiration buildup. Cotton socks that are blended with acrylic are best. Pure cotton socks tend to hold in moisture. Regular washing of the feet with soap and water makes good hygienic sense and prevents bacteria buildup.

■ BASIC PLAN

Diet

A whole-foods diet is recommended. (See "Diet" on page 4 for more information.) Increasing green vegetables in the diet helps with detoxification and supplies more fiber for proper elimination. Plenty of water to assist detoxification in the cells is important. Foods that help detoxify the liver, such as carrots and beets, are indicated. Food sensitivities are a problem for some children with smelly feet. (See "Food Allergies and Food Sensitivities" on page 298 for more information.)

Nutritional Supplement

Chlorophyll—Available in liquid form. Give your child 1 teaspoon daily for internal detoxification.

Homeopathy

Pick the following remedy that best matches your child's symptoms. Unless otherwise indicated, give your child 2 pellets of a 30C potency twice daily. Improvements should be seen within 7 days. If there is no improvement within 7 days, try another remedy. After you first notice improvement, stop giving the remedy unless symptoms begin to return.

Note: Lower potencies (6X, 12X, 6C) may need to be given more often (three times daily).

Calcarea carbonica—The child's feet and head sweat easily and have a musty odor. The child has characteristic Calcarea carbonica symptoms: large and flabby. (See "Constitutional Homeopathic Remedies for Children" on page 60 for more about constitutional types and remedies.)

Sulphur—Indicated for children who are prone to stinky feet and bad odor from their bodies in general. The child tends to be very warm and sweats easily. Skin problems are common for children requiring Sulphur.

Silica—For the child who tends to be thin and chilly but whose feet sweat profusely.

Aromatherapy

Tea tree oil— Have your child soak her feet nightly in a bowl of warm water that has 5 drops of tea tree oil added to it. This will help to destroy bacteria or fungi causing the foot odor. Likewise, you can add 1 drop to each of your child's shoes to act as a disinfectant and improve the smell. And you can add 2 drops to the washing machine when you wash the shoes.

■ WHAT TO EXPECT

Once you have implemented the recommendations in this chapter, you should notice improvement within 2 weeks.

Frostbite

Many children love to play in snow, making snowmen, creating snow angels, and engaging in friendly snowball battles. Often, they bound into the house sporting rosy cheeks.

In their desire to have fun, they may forget to come inside occasionally and warm up. If they are physically active, their clothing can become wet from snow and perspiration and become damp. Exposure to severe cold temperatures and wind chill can also lead to frostbite. Although all parts of the body can be affected, the nose, ears, fingers, and toes are most susceptible.

Frostnip is a related term that refers to a reversible injury due to exposure to subfreezing conditions. Cold, white areas on the skin can occur.

Frostbite is characterized by progressive symptomatic stages. Skin exposed to cold temperatures may first turn red and be painful. During the second stage, the skin turns waxy white and becomes numb. Ice crystals actually form within or between tissue cells. Frostbite can advance to become hard and frozen and, finally, turn black—a sign of dead tissues.

Caution: If your child appears to be in the second stage of frostbite or worse, take him immediately to the emergency room after putting on warm clothes. Emergency treatment at the hospital focuses on warming the frostbitten area with water, warming the entire body, giving antibiotics to prevent infection, and doing studies to assess the damage and circulation.

■ IMMEDIATE TREATMENT

First, get your child indoors and change him into warm clothes. Do not rub your child's skin, as this can cause more damage. If the frostbite is serious (the second stage or worse, as defined previously), get your child to an emergency room immediately for treatment. Do not try to warm the frostbitten area first before going to the emergency room. Other-

wise, minorly frostbitten areas should be warmed in water that is tolerable to your hand (not warmer than 105°F) to avoid scalding the child. The child's whole body should be kept warm. Plenty of water and electrolyte solutions should be given to prevent dehydration.

■ BASIC PLAN

Herbal Remedies

Ginger root or cinnamon tea—These teas have a warming effect and also promote circulation. Give 1 to 2 cups.

Ginkgo biloba and cinnamon help to promote circulation to the extremities.

Homeopathy

Pick the following remedy that best matches your child's symptoms. Unless otherwise indicated, give your child 2 pellets of a 30C potency every 15 minutes for up to three doses. If there is no improvement within 2 hours, try another remedy. After you first notice improvement, stop giving the remedy unless symptoms begin to return.

Note: Lower potencies (6X, 12X, 6C) may need to be given more often (every 10 minutes).

Agaricus muscarius 30C—For redness, burning, and swelling from frostbite. The first remedy to try for frostbite.

Nitric acid—Used for more mild cases of frostbite, where the child feels splinterlike pains.

Pulsatilla—For bluish discoloration and pain, especially of the legs.

Zincum metallicum—The child experiences restless legs.

■ WHAT TO EXPECT

The recommendations in this section should rapidly improve first-stage frostbite within 15 to 30 minutes. If there is no improvement, seek medical attention as you would for more severe frostbite.

Gas

Gas doesn't discriminate when it comes to age. In fact, babies under age 6 months commonly experience gas. From birth to 6 months, a baby doubles his body weight and needs a large amount of food to support this time of accelerated growth.

Babies can develop gas when breastfeeding, sucking on a bottle, or during crying episodes. In all three scenarios, the baby accidentally swallows excess air, which causes gas pain in the intestinal tract. This buildup of gas as well as bacteria in the digestive system leads to flatulence. What the mother eats can create gas in a breastfed infant.

Younger children may also experience gas-related stomachaches that can last up to 2 or more minutes. Like babies, children can swallow air while eating. Gas can also be triggered by certain foods, such as beans or green peppers, or by food sensitivities, as well as by certain conditions that disrupt the body's natural ability to absorb and digest food.

An imbalance of the intestinal flora can lead to excessive gas. This is usually the result of antibiotic use.

■ BASIC PLAN

Diet

The breastfeeding mother needs to pay attention to what she eats, since there may be a correlation between her diet and the digestive irritation of her child. Common foods that can aggravate the breastfed infant can include coffee, chocolate, dairy products (milk and cheese), spicy foods, nutritional brewer's yeast, and citrus fruits. Experiment with these foods by avoiding one at a time and see whether your child improves. Drug medications and nutritional supplements can also be the cause of the problem and should be ruled out.

Besides the typical gas-forming foods such as beans, foods that trigger sensitivities can be at the root of excessive gas with older children as well. (See "Food Allergies and Food Sensitivities" on page 298 to see what foods might be causing the problem.) Dairy products are a common problem, especially for kids who are lactose intolerant. Spicy foods are common irritants as well.

Nutritional Supplements

Probiotic—A children's acidophilus and bifidus supplement can be helpful to improve elimination. It is especially important for infants who have been on antibiotics. Give as directed on the container for 8 weeks or longer.

Herbal Remedies

Fennel, anise, cardamom, ginger root, peppermint, and chamomile, either alone or in combination, can help to reduce intestinal gas and spasms. They can be given to children or infants as a fresh tea or in liquid form.

Homeopathy

Use a combination indigestion formula, or pick the one of the following remedies that best matches your child's symptoms. For the remedies below, unless otherwise indicated, give your child 2 pellets of a 30C potency every 30 minutes for up to three doses. (For infants, crush the pellets into powder and mix it with water.) If there is no improvement within 2 hours, try another remedy. After you first notice improvement, stop giving the remedy unless symptoms begin to return.

Note: Lower potencies (6X, 12X, 6C) may need to be given more often (every 15 minutes).

Carbo vegetabilis—For tremendous gas and bloating. The child may feel faint and feels better from belching, cold air, and from being fanned.

Colocynthis—For abdominal gas that makes the child bend over from pain or pull her legs up to her waist. Gas pains feel better from pressure and lying face downward, as well as from warmth.

Lycopodium—For bloating and distended abdomen that feels better with warm drinks or warm applications and rubbing of the abdomen. The gas often occurs in the evening (4:00 to 8:00 P.M.).

Magnesia phosphorica—For gas pains that feel better with warm drinks or warm applications to the abdomen. If you are unsure of which remedy to use, pick this one. Works well when taken with warm water.

Nux vomica—For gas pains that make the child irritable. She strains to pass gas. There may be abdominal pain from spicy foods. The child feels better with warm applications or warm drinks and wants her clothes to be loosened around the abdomen.

Pulsatilla—For gas after eating rich or fatty foods such as ice cream. Symptoms are worse in the evening. The child wants to be held.

■ ADVANCED PLAN

Aromatherapy

German chamomile and ginger—Dilute this combination in 40 milliliters of a carrier oil such as grape seed, olive, or sweet almond, and rub it on the child's abdomen. If the child is taking a homeopathic remedy, use aromatherapy at a different time.

Acupressure

Gently press each of the following acupressure points with a thumb for 10 to 15 seconds. Perform on both sides of the body and repeat three times each day.

Large Intestine 4—Located in the webbing between the thumb and index finger.

Stomach 36—Located four finger-widths below the kneecap and one finger-width toward the outside of the leg (outside of the shinbone on the muscle).

■ WHAT TO EXPECT

Acute relief of intestinal gas is usually achieved within 5 to 15 minutes. Dietary changes and balancing of digestive flora (good bacteria) are often required to alleviate chronic intestinal gas.

German Measles

This is a milder form of measles as compared with regular measles (rubeola). German measles is also referred to as 3-day measles or rubella. This contagious childhood viral infection usually occurs in the spring. It is spread through respiratory droplets. The rash is similar to that of measles but is less extensive and has a fine, dark pink, blotchy appearance. It generally begins on the face and neck and spreads to the trunk, legs, and arms. Swollen glands around the head are common, and the throat is often red but not always sore to the child. The face may be flushed at the beginning of the rash, and rose-colored spots appear in the mouth, which disappear in 3 days. The child may feel fatigued and have some joint pain, but in general, symptoms are mild. A child with German measles is contagious for approximately 7 days before the rash appears to 5 days after the rash appears.

Caution: It is very important that a pregnant woman not be exposed to German measles, as it can adversely affect her developing baby. If your child develops German measles, notify anyone who was exposed to your child in the week before the rash appeared (this includes parents of playmates, and any other adults too) so that they, too, are kept away from pregnant mothers.

Conventional treatment focuses on prevention with vaccination (part of the MMR vaccine) and fever/pain medications (such as acetaminophen) as needed. Make sure that your child is not given aspirin. As with any viral illness, the use of aspirin can lead to a potentially dangerous condition known as Reye's syndrome.

■ BASIC PLAN

Diet

Make sure that your child gets plenty of fluids to prevent dehydration. Stay consistent with breastfeeding or bottlefeeding for infants. Older children should drink at least six glasses of water throughout the day. Fruit juices, if used, should be diluted with water by at least 50 percent, as simple sugars can weaken the immune system. Homemade warm broths and soups are best; they are easy to digest and moisten the respiratory tract. Fresh garlic added to the soup is helpful as long as your child is not sensitive to it. Do not give fried foods, as they are hard to digest. Avoid giving your child dairy products as they can contribute to mucus formation.

Nutritional Supplement

Vitamin C—Supports the immune system and has mild anti-inflammatory effects. The type with bioflavonoids is preferable. Dosage: the child's age in years times 50 milligrams, twice daily. Reduce the dosage if diarrhea occurs. Consider using a buffered vitamin C powder (nonacidic) or liquid vitamin C. Both work well for infants and children, and can be mixed in juice.

Herbal Remedy

Echinacea—Look for a flavored children's glycerin-based formula. In addition, the combination of echinacea and goldenseal works well to prevent secondary infections of the skin.

Homeopathy

Pick the following remedy that best matches your child's symptoms. Unless otherwise indicated, give your child 2 pellets of a 30C potency three times daily. (For infants, crush the pellets into powder and mix it with water.) Improvements should be seen within 2 days. If there is no improvement within 2 days, try another remedy. After you first notice improvement, stop giving the remedy unless symptoms begin to return.

Note: Lower potencies (6X, 12X, 6C) may need to be given more often (four times daily).

Aconitum napellus—For the initial onset of a high fever and a rash. The child is very thirsty.

Belladonna—For a sudden onset of a high fever accompanied by a red face. The head and face feel very hot, while the feet are cold.

Ferrum phosphoricum—The child does not feel or act sick but has a fever and flushing of the face. Useful in the first 24 hours of the disease.

Pulsatilla—The child is feverish, whiny,

and wants to be held. She has low thirst. She feels better in the open air and worse in a warm room.

Sulphur—The child is very hot and sweaty, and may be itchy. She has a high thirst for cold drinks.

Rubella nosode—This homeopathic dilution of German measles can be given to reduce the length and severity of the disease. Give your child a 30C potency twice daily for 2 days after exposure to the illness or when it is first diagnosed.

■ ADVANCED PLAN

Nutritional Supplements

Vitamin A—Supports the immune system. Daily dosage: infants under 1 year, 1,875 international units (IU); children 1 to 3, 2,000 IU; kids 4 to 6, 2,500 IU; kids 7 to 10, 3,500 IU; males 11 and older, 5,000 IU; females 11 and older, 4,000 IU.

Note: These dosages are for short-term use (up to 10 days). Higher dosages may be used only under a doctor's supervision. Available in liquid drops.

Zinc—Supports the immune system. Dosage: children 2 and younger, 5 milligrams; 2 and older, 10 to 15 milligrams. Use for 2 weeks and then stop.

Herbal Remedies

Lomatium—A potent antiviral herb that inhibits the replication of viruses.

Larix—A good immune system enhancer. It is available in a powder form that blends into water and juice, sometimes with a mild, sweet taste.

Aromatherapy

Add equal parts lavender, bergamot, and tea tree oil to 1 teaspoon of vegetable oil and mix into a bath. Swish the water around before the child gets in. If there is a high fever, add ginger. If the child is taking a homeopathic remedy, use aromatherapy at a different time.

Hydrotherapy

Constitutional or foot hydrotherapy stimulates the immune system. (See Hydrotherapy for Children on page 115 for more on these therapies.) Perform the therapy one or two times a day until the illness resolves.

■ WHAT TO EXPECT

Natural therapy will help make the child more comfortable within 24 to 48 hours and prevent complications, such as secondary infections.

Gingivitis

Gingivitis is a gum disease that develops over time. In the early stages, there are few or no symptoms. But as time passes, the gums become red and swollen and tend to bleed easily. The gum line begins to separate from the tooth. Without intervention, gingivitis can lead to tooth decay and tooth loss.

At the root of the problem is plaque, which, if not removed, can harden into mineral deposits known as tartar. Working together, plaque and tartar trap food particles between teeth that attract bacteria.

The message here is to develop proper oral hygiene habits for your children as soon as they are born. Don't wait until your baby has a mouthful of teeth to care for his gums. Routinely examine your baby's teeth, gums, and tongue for any signs of trouble.

Once your toddler has teeth, make sure that his teeth and tongue are brushed and flossed daily. Once your child is older and better coordinated, teach him how to floss using a fun-flavored waxed dental floss.

Diet and nutritional status are important for healthy gums. Various vitamin deficiencies can adversely affect gum health. Mercury fillings may also contribute to gingivitis. Consult with your child's dentist for an evaluation.

■ BASIC PLAN

Start brushing your baby's teeth when the first teeth appear, around 6 to 7 months of age. Use a baby toothbrush, a piece of gauze, or a piece of rubber on your finger to clean the gums and teeth. You can use a dab of a natural children's toothpaste, but don't use a toothpaste containing fluoride until your child is 2 years old.

Diet

Avoid food and drinks that are high in refined sugars and starches. Avoid sodas and other sweetened carbonated beverages, as well as acidic foods.

Breastfed infants may have fewer problems with gingivitis.

For the best gum health, a child's diet should focus on vegetables, legumes, and whole grains. (See "Diet" on page 4 for more on creating a healthful diet for your child.)

Do not let your baby sleep with a bottle of juice or milk. Bacteria build up faster with these fluids in the mouth.

Nutritional Supplement

Vitamin C—Supports the immune system and has mild anti-inflammatory effects. The type with bioflavonoids is preferable. Dosage: the child's age in years times 50 milligrams, daily. Reduce the dosage if diarrhea occurs. Consider using a buffered vitamin C powder (nonacidic) or liquid vitamin C. Both work well for infants and children, and can be mixed in juice. Make sure to rinse with water after using the vitamin C.

Herbal Remedy

A mouth rinse containing myrrh (3 drops) combined with either Oregon grape or goldenseal (3 drops) in an ounce of water helps to cleanse and reduce gingivitis. Have your child gargle and swish this solution in his mouth twice daily. Another option is to add 5 drops of calendula to an ounce of water and have your child swish it in his mouth and then spit it out.

Homeopathy

Pick the following remedy that best matches your child's symptoms. Unless otherwise indicated, give your child 2 pellets of a 30C potency two times daily. (For infants, crush the pellets into powder and mix it with water.) Im-

provements should be seen within 7 days. If there is no improvement within 7 days, try another remedy. After you first notice improvement, stop giving the remedy unless symptoms begin to return.

Note: Lower potencies (6X, 12X, 6C) may need to be given more often (three times daily).

Kreosotum—For inflamed gums that are spongy and bleed easy. The child often has decaying teeth as well.

Mercurius solubilis or vivus—The gums are swollen, the child has bad breath, and there may be increased salivation, especially at night.

Phosphorus—The gums are soft and spongy and bleed easily. The child's mouth feels better with cold drinks.

Silica—Gum boils or abscesses develop slowly and heal slowly. The gums are sensitive to cold.

■ ADVANCED PLAN

Nutritional Supplements

Coenzyme Q$_{10}$—One of the best supplements for chronic gingivitis. An average child's dosage is 10 to 20 milligrams. Use under a doctor's supervision. Toothpastes containing coenzyme Q$_{10}$ are now available and may be helpful for gingivitis.

Folic acid oral rinse—Studies have shown that this treatment heals gingivitis. Use as prescribed by a doctor.

Children's multivitamin—Provides a base of vitamins and minerals for gum tissue health.

Probiotic—If your child has a history of antibiotic use, give him a children's acidophilus and bifidus supplement. These good bacteria are part of the normal flora of the mouth that keep harmful bacteria from overgrowing. Give as directed on the container.

Acupressure

Large Intestine 4—Can help relieve gum soreness and tooth pain. Located in the webbing between the thumb and index finger. Gently press the acupressure point with a thumb for 10 to 15 seconds. Perform on both sides of the body and repeat three times each day.

■ WHAT TO EXPECT

Over the course of 6 to 8 weeks, the gingivitis should be improved with natural therapies as long as oral hygiene is maintained.

Growing Pains

Children grow at different rates. Some seem to grow out of their clothes and shoes faster than others. But generally, the growth rate for all children should follow a steady course. Whatever the speed, when the body grows, children can develop pain associated with it.

Problems develop usually between ages 4 and 9, a peak growth period, when some children develop unexplained leg pain. The pain typically occurs at night and can last a few minutes to hours before disappearing. For some children, the pain registers in the bones. In others, it lodges in the muscles.

Most growing pains are associated with sore, overtaxed, tight muscles. They hurt more at night when the child is relaxed. Don't confuse growing pains with muscle cramps. Cramps always come with muscle spasms, usually in the calf muscles. Growing pains do not include muscle spasms. In either case, massage can help, as can many of the remedies outlined here.

In our experience, nutritional deficiencies are often at the root of growing pains. Diet, nutritional supplements, and homeopathy work extremely well for this condition.

Conventional therapy focuses on pain medications such as acetaminophen and aspirin.

■ BASIC PLAN

Diet

Feed your child a whole-foods diet. (See "Diet" on page 4 for more information.) Quality protein sources are important, such as fish, legumes, nuts, and lean poultry.

Increasing the sources of calcium, magnesium, and potassium is especially important. Many children who drink cow's milk still get growing pains. They most likely are sensitive to the cow's milk and are not getting much use from the calcium in it. The other problem may be that there is more of a magnesium deficiency occurring, which the cow's milk won't correct. Calcium-rich food sources include carrots and broccoli. Calcium-enriched nondairy milks are recommended, too. Magnesium-rich foods include whole grains, nuts, legumes, soy, and green leafy vegetables. Potassium-rich foods include fruits and vegetables, especially apples, bananas, carrots, oranges, potatoes, tomatoes, cantaloupe, peaches, plums, and strawberries.

Vitamin D is important and is found in green leafy vegetables, eggs, and dairy products. Sunlight exposure also helps in the production of vitamin D.

Boron, found in nuts and seeds, is involved in bone development. Silica can be helpful and can be found in rolled oat cereals, such as porridge or Swiss muesli; in almonds; and in pumpkin seeds.

Decrease the consumption of sugars and soft drinks, which leach minerals out of the body.

Nutritional Supplements

Calcium and magnesium—Give 500 milligrams of calcium and 250 to 500 milligrams of magnesium daily. Available together in a blend.

Children's multivitamin—Ensures that all the vitamins and minerals for bone health are present. Also contains vitamin D required for proper bone growth. Give as directed on the container.

Homeopathy

Pick the following remedy that best matches your child's symptoms. Unless otherwise indicated, give your child 2 pellets of a 30C potency two times daily. Improvements should be seen within 7 days. If there is no improvement within 7 days, try another remedy. After you first notice improvement, stop giving the remedy unless symptoms begin to return.

Note: Lower potencies (6X, 12X, 6C) may need to be given more often (three times daily).

Calcarea carbonica—The child for whom this constitutional remedy is prescribed is usually plump and sweats easily on the back of her head. She often gets leg cramps and pain at night. (See "Constitutional Homeopathic Remedies for Children" on page 60 for more on constitutional remedies.)

Calcarea phosphorica 3X or 6X—The best remedy for growing pains in children, especially when they occur at night. Give 2 pellets two or three times daily.

Causticum—For growing pains accompanied by muscle and joint stiffness.

Magnesia phosphorica 3X or 6X—Helps to reduce muscle spasms and cramps. Works well in combination with Calcarea phosphorica. Give 2 pellets two or three times daily.

■ ADVANCED PLAN

Herbal Remedy

Nettle—Contains silica and other minerals involved in bone formation. Give twice daily.

Aromatherapy

German chamomile—Add it to a carrier oil and rub it onto the painful area once daily. If the child is taking a homeopathic remedy, use aromatherapy at a different time.

■ WHAT TO EXPECT

Nutritional supplements and the correct homeopathic remedies usually provide relief within 5 to 7 days. Continued supplementation may be required to prevent the growing pains from returning.

Hair Loss

In the medical condition called alopecia, the hair follicles that normally develop hair become dormant, and hair loss occurs. Alopecia can be limited to certain patches of hair loss on the scalp, or it can cause a total loss of body hair. A child can lose his eyebrows and eyelashes.

The early signs are one or two coin-size patches on the scalp that are void of any hair. You may notice it while brushing your child's hair. Often, hair stylists are the first to discover these hairless patches.

Alopecia should not be mistaken for major hair fallout that is caused by scalp ringworm.

What causes alopecia is still unknown. However, researchers theorize that the body's immune system somehow disrupts and attacks hair follicle growth. This condition may also be genetic. Systemic diseases and certain medications can also cause hair loss. Nutritional deficiencies must also be suspected.

■ BASIC PLAN

Diet

Feed a whole-foods diet (see "Diet" on page 4). Quality protein sources are important, such as fish, legumes, nuts, and lean poultry. Silica is needed for proper hair development and is available in rolled oat cereals such as porridge or Swiss muesli, in almonds, and in pumpkin seeds. Decrease the consumption of sugars and soft drinks, which leach minerals out of the body.

Food sources of essential fatty acids are very important for hair health. Fish such as salmon, halibut, trout, and mackerel are good sources. Fresh fish two or three times weekly is recommended. Flaxseeds are an excellent source of the important alpha linolenic acid. They can be ground up and sprinkled on salads or added to shakes. Grind 1 teaspoon per 50 pounds of body weight (children weighing 30 to 50 pounds may also use 1 teaspoon) and give this amount daily, with 8 ounces of water.

Food sensitivities may also be a culprit in hair loss. (See "Food Allergies and Food Sensitivities" on page 298.)

Nutritional Supplements

Children's multivitamin—Provides a base of the essential vitamins and minerals.

Choose one of the following three supplements.

Essential fatty acid complex—Choose a children's blend that contains omega-3's and omega-6's, especially alpha linolenic acid (ALA) and GLA (gamma linolenic acid). Give as directed on the container.

Flaxseed oil—Daily dosages: children up to 2 years, 1 teaspoon; kids 3 to 6, 2 teaspoons; kids 7 and older, 2 to 3 teaspoons. Reduce the dosage if diarrhea occurs.

Fish oil—Daily dosage: 1 gram per 50 pounds of body weight.

Herbal Remedy

Nettle—Contains silica and other minerals required for healthy hair. Give 10 drops of the tincture form twice daily.

Homeopathy

Pick the following remedy that best matches your child's symptoms. Give 2 pellets two or three times daily for at least 6 weeks. If improvement is noted, then continue for an additional 6 weeks.

Silica 3X or 6X—Strengthens brittle hair.

Natrum muriaticum 6X—For hair loss that accompanies grief. The child wants to be by herself, may crave salt, and is sensitive to the sun.

■ ADVANCED PLAN

Nutritional Supplements

B complex—Give daily in addition to a multivitamin, especially if the hair loss is due to extreme stress. Daily dosages: children under age 7, 25 milligrams; children 7 and older, 50 milligrams.

Methylsulfonylmethane (MSM)—Contains the mineral sulfur, which helps hair development. Give 5 milligrams per pound of body weight daily.

Herbal Remedy

Rosemary—Increases scalp circulation. Add 3 drops of rosemary essential oil to 1 ounce of your child's shampoo and apply daily.

■ WHAT TO EXPECT

If the hair loss is due to nutritional deficiencies, then improvement should be seen within 2 months of treatment. Work with a holistic doctor to find the root cause of the hair loss.

Vital Fact

On average, the head contains more than 100,000 hair follicles. Each person normally sheds 50 to 100 hairs a day.

Hair, Oily

Heredity has a major say in the health of your hair. Considered more of a trait than a condition, oily hair tends to run in families. And brunettes are more apt to have oily hair than blondes or redheads.

To be precise, the oil doesn't actually come from your hair but from your scalp, which contains sebaceous glands. These glands secrete sebum, a blend of fatty acids designed to keep your scalp from becoming dry or flaky.

Hormones control sebum production. These hormones tend to go into overdrive during puberty. As a result, excess sebum is produced, coating each hair shaft and weighing it down. The hair looks greasy, matted, and flat.

■ BASIC PLAN

Diet

Follow a whole-foods diet. (See "Diet" on page 4 for more information.) Decrease the consumption of sugars and soft drinks, which leach minerals out of the body.

Foods that contain essential fatty acids are

very important for preventing oily hair. Fish such as salmon, halibut, trout, and mackerel are good sources, as are nuts such as walnuts. Fresh fish two or three times weekly is recommended. Flaxseeds are an excellent source of the important alpha linolenic acid (ALA). They can be ground up and sprinkled on salads or added to shakes. Grind 1 teaspoon of flaxseeds per 50 pounds of body weight (children weighing 30 to 50 pounds may also use 1 teaspoon) and give this amount daily along with 8 ounces of water.

Nutritional Supplements

Choose one of the following three supplements.

Essential fatty acid complex—Choose a children's blend that contains omega-3's and omega-6's, especially alpha linolenic acid (ALA) and GLA (gamma linolenic acid). Give as directed on the container.

Flaxseed oil—Daily dosages: children up to 2 years, 1 teaspoon; kids 3 to 6, 2 teaspoons; kids 7 and older, 2 to 3 teaspoons. Reduce the dosage if diarrhea occurs.

Fish oil—Daily dosage: 1 gram per 50 pounds of body weight.

Herbal Remedies

Try herbal shampoos, such as chamomile, that are specially designed for oily hair. Use as directed on the container.

■ WHAT TO EXPECT

Nutritional therapy and an effective shampoo can improve this condition within 2 to 3 weeks.

Hand, Foot, and Mouth Disease

Small, firm, but painful red spots or blisters that appear on the palms of the hands, soles of the feet, and inside the mouth indicate that a child has hand, foot, and mouth disease. In addition, a child usually has a sore throat and a fever.

The condition, caused by the Coxsackievirus, can progress to create blisters on the gums, palate, and lips and red, painful sores between the fingers and toes. Although the fever usually subsides within 4 days, the sores and blisters can last a week or longer.

Conventional treatment is bed rest and fever-reducing medications.

Caution: Do not give aspirin with this condition because of the risk of Reye's syndrome, a potentially fatal illness where liver and brain damage can occur.

■ BASIC PLAN

Diet

Make sure that your child gets plenty of fluids to prevent dehydration. Stay consistent with breastfeeding or bottlefeeding for infants. Older children should drink at least six glasses of water throughout the day. Fruit juices, if used, should be diluted with water by at least 50 percent, as simple sugars can weaken the immune system. Homemade warm broths and soups are best; they are easy to digest and moisten the respiratory tract. Fresh garlic added to the soup is helpful as long as your child is not sensitive to it.

Do not give fried foods, as they are hard to digest. Avoid giving your child dairy products as they can contribute to mucus formation and reduce the effectiveness of the immune system.

Nutritional Supplement

Vitamin C—Supports the immune system. Dosage: the child's age in years times 50 milligrams, twice daily. Reduce the dosage if diarrhea occurs. Consider using a buffered vitamin C powder (nonacidic) or liquid vitamin C. Both work well for infants and children, and can be mixed in juice.

Herbal Remedies

Echinacea—Stimulates the immune system to fight a viral infection.

Larix—A good immune system enhancer. It is available in a powder form that blends into water and juice, and may have a mild, sweet taste.

Homeopathy

Pick the following remedy that best matches your child's symptoms. Unless otherwise indicated, give your child 2 pellets of a 30C potency twice daily. (For infants, crush the pellets into powder and mix it with water.) Improvements should be seen within 48 hours. If there is no improvement within 48 hours, try another remedy. After you first notice improvement, stop giving the remedy unless symptoms begin to return.

Note: Lower potencies (6X, 12X, 6C) may need to be given more often (three times daily).

Arsenicum album—For profuse, clear, watery discharge from the nose that causes the upper lip to be red. Symptoms are worse between 12:00 and 3:00 A.M., when the child wakes up. The child is anxious, restless, and fearful.

Ferrum phosphoricum—The child is feverish but does not act very sick. His face is flushed.

Gelsemium—The child feels droopy and drowsy and perhaps dizzy. He has chills up and down his back and body, he feels very tired, and his muscles ache. He has a headache at the base of his neck.

Pulsatilla—The child is feverish. He becomes more clingy than normal and does not want an adult to leave his side. He is weepy and has low thirst. He may develop yellow or green mucus from the sinus.

Hydrotherapy

Constitutional or foot hydrotherapy stimulates the immune system and relieves congestion of upper respiratory passageways and sinus. (See Hydrotherapy for Children on page 115 for directions.) Perform either therapy one or two times daily.

■ ADVANCED PLAN

Nutritional Supplements

Vitamin A—Supports the immune system. Daily dosage: infants under 1 year, 1,875 international units (IU); children 1 to 3, 2,000 IU; kids 4 to 6, 2,500 IU; kids 7 to 10, 3,500 IU; males 11 and older, 5,000 IU; females 11 and older, 4,000 IU.

Note: These dosages are for short-term use

(up to 10 days). Higher dosages may be used only under a doctor's supervision. Available in liquid drops.

Zinc—Supports the immune system and enhances skin healing. Dosage: children 2 and younger, 5 milligrams; 2 and older, 10 to 15 milligrams. Use for 2 weeks and then stop.

Thymus glandular extract—Give one to two 250-milligram tablets or capsules daily. Also available in a homeopathic liquid preparation (give 5 drops twice daily).

Herbal Remedies

Astragalus—Supports the immune system.

Lomatium—A potent antiviral herb that inhibits the replication of viruses.

Fresh **ginger tea** can help relieve chills that accompany an infection. Have your child sip a cup of warm ginger tea during the day. If using fresh ginger root, make a decoction. If using a tea bag, make an infusion. (See "Herbal Preparations" on page 30 for more on tea decoctions and infusions.)

Yarrow can be used if a high fever accompanies the infection.

Acupressure

Large Intestine 4—Helps to relieve fever and head congestion. Located in the webbing between the thumb and index finger. Gently press the acupressure point with a thumb for 10 to 15 seconds. Perform on both sides of the body and repeat three times each day.

■ WHAT TO EXPECT

Natural therapy helps to keep your child more comfortable and prevents secondary infec-tions. The child should feel better within 2 to 3 days of natural therapy.

Headaches

Headaches aren't limited to stress-filled, al-ways-on-the-go adults. Children can develop some irritating head throbbers, too.

The first step is to distinguish between ten-sion and migraine headaches. Tension headaches refer to dull but steady pain felt on both sides of the head or at the base of the neck. These head-aches are primarily caused by tense neck and head muscles. Poor posture, jaw clenching, emo-tional stress, fatigue, and loud noises or bright lights can bring on tension headaches.

Most tension headaches are run-of-the-mill kinds that can be easily treated. But contact your doctor if the headaches are particularly severe or frequent, or if they are accompanied by vomiting. These could be symptoms of more serious conditions such as allergies, eye problems, or sinus infections.

Migraine headaches are more serious. Usu-ally, a child about to have a migraine will see sparkling lights in her vision just prior to an onset—a phenomenon called an aura. This is followed by pounding pain on one or both sides of the head—pain so strong that it inter-feres with her normal routine, causes light and sound sensitivities, and even causes nausea and vomiting. However, symptoms vary from child to child.

Experts suspect that certain foods such as chocolate, aged cheeses, processed meats, caf-feinated drinks, and monosodium glutamate

(MSG) trigger migraines. Like other nutrition-oriented doctors, we have found that various food sensitivities and nutritional deficiencies can induce migraines. Blood sugar imbalance can be a root cause as well. Constipation needs to be addressed if it is a problem with your child. Depression, sleep disruption, barometric pressure changes, perfumes, carbon monoxide, stress, and bright lights have also been linked to migraines.

There are two main theories as to what happens during a migraine headache. One is that there is an initial constriction of blood vessels reducing bloodflow, followed by a compensating dilation of the blood vessels. The second is that there is an abnormality of function of the nerve cells in the brain. In any event, the underlying trigger needs to be addressed.

Conventional treatment of headaches focuses on pain relievers such as ibuprofen or acetaminophen. Diagnostic scans such as a CT scan or MRI may be ordered to rule out more serious causes. Also, make sure that your child is not exposed to toxic chemicals. (See "Environment" on page 25 for more information.) Spinal and soft tissue treatment from a massage therapist, naturopathic physician, chiropractor, osteopath, or craniosacral therapist can be helpful. (See the Natural Health Care Modalities and Resource Guide on page 499 for more on these therapies.) Stress reduction is important, and counseling may be required.

■ BASIC PLAN

Diet

Food sensitivities contribute to many cases of headaches in children, especially with migraines. Dairy (cow's milk and cheese) is the first category of foods that should be omitted from the diet for a week or two to see if there is an improvement. Other common food sensitivities include wheat, chocolate, citrus fruits, sugar, and soy. (See "Food Allergies and Food Sensitivities" on page 298 for more information.) Artificial sweeteners and preservatives should be avoided by focusing on a whole-foods diet. (See "Diet" on page 4.)

Essential fatty acids are important to prevent chemical imbalances that can lead to headaches. Fish such as salmon, halibut, trout, and mackerel are good sources, as are nuts, such as walnuts. Fresh fish two or three times weekly is recommended. Flaxseeds are an excellent source of the important alpha linolenic acid (ALA). They can be ground up and sprinkled on salads or added to shakes. Grind 1 teaspoon per 50 pounds of body weight (children weighing 30 to 50 pounds may also use 1 teaspoon) and give this amount daily along with 8 ounces of water.

In general, make sure your child is getting plenty of water, as dehydration can lead to headaches. Fruits and especially vegetables are important to provide adequate amounts of fiber in your child's diet so that her bowels stay regular. Constipation is an undertreated cause of headaches. If your child is not having at least one complete bowel movement daily, then she likely is not getting enough fiber or fluids.

Nutritional Supplements

Calcium and magnesium—These are important to keep the nervous system, muscles, and blood vessels relaxed to prevent headaches. Studies show that magnesium defi-

Case History

Sherry, a 7-year-old girl, was brought to our office for the treatment of chronic migraine headaches. Her migraines were so severe that pain medications helped only slightly. When we asked Sherry's parents about her digestive health, her mother commented that she had a bowel movement every 4 to 5 days. In addition, she craved milk and cheese products. We had Sherry's parents increase the fiber in her diet with steamed vegetables and 2 teaspoons of ground-up flaxseeds daily. In addition, we had Sherry alternate between rice, oat, and almond milk instead of cow's milk. Within 1 week, her bowels started to move more regularly. In 2 weeks, her bowels were moving daily, and she had not had a headache. Ten months later, Sherry's mother reported that her migraine headaches were no longer a problem as long as she avoided cow's milk and took in enough fiber for her bowels to move regularly.

ciency is associated with migraine headaches. We recommend 500 milligrams of calcium and 250 milligrams of magnesium daily. They are available together in a formula.

Herbal Remedies

Feverfew is a popular treatment for migraine headaches. It does not treat the cause of the headaches but can be used for symptomatic re-

lief. It is safer than pain relievers such as aspirin.

Chamomile can be helpful for tension headaches. Have your child drink a fresh cup of chamomile tea or take the liquid (glycerin-based or tincture form) if she feels a headache starting.

Homeopathy

For the acute relief of a headache, use a combination headache formula, or pick the one of the following remedies that best matches your child's symptoms. For the remedies below, unless otherwise indicated, give your child 2 pellets of a 30C potency every 30 minutes for up to four doses. If there is no improvement within 2 hours, try another remedy. After you first notice improvement, stop giving the remedy unless symptoms begin to return.

Note: Lower potencies (6X, 12X, 6C) may need to be given to your child more often (every 15 minutes).

Belladonna—For a right-sided headache that starts on the back of the head (the right side) and extends to the right eye or forehead. The child has throbbing pain, as if her head will burst. She feels better lying down in a dark, quiet room.

Bryonia alba—For pain in the left eye or forehead that extends to the whole head. Symptoms are worse with any movement and feel better with pressure and stillness. Constipation may be associated with the headache. The child is irritable with the headache and wants to be alone.

Calcarea phosphorica—For schoolchildren who get chronic headaches and stomachaches. There is pain at the back of the head.

Gelsemium—Dull, heavy pain at the back of the neck starts to feel like a tight band is around the head. The child feels tired and dizzy and has blurred vision. The headache improves after urination.

Glonoinum—For a pounding, bursting headache, especially when it starts after sun exposure.

Iris versicolor—For right-sided migraine headaches that feel like the head is constricted. Nausea and vomiting occur with the headache.

Lachesis—For left-sided headaches with a burning feeling. The child wakes up with the headache. Heat and touch worsen the headache, and open air makes it feel better.

Lycopodium—For a right-sided headache in the temple area. Worse 4:00 to 8:00 P.M.

Natrum muriaticum—A good remedy for headaches from being in the sun. Also a good preventive remedy for migraine headaches. The child wakes up with a migraine headache. Headaches come on from stress or grief. The child feels better lying down in a dark, cool room.

Nux vomica—For headaches from stress, overwork, and bad reactions to food. The headache feels better with cold applications. There is stomachache and nausea along with the headache. The child is irritable. Worse with noise, light, and opening the eyes. For headaches caused by constipation.

Sanguinaria—The headache begins in the right side of the neck or shoulder and radiates to the right eye. The child feels better after vomiting.

Spigelia—For a stitching, sharp, or burning

Vital Fact

The brain itself cannot feel pain because it does not contain sensory nerves. The pain experienced from a headache actually takes place in the meninges (the membranes covering the brain) and in the skin and muscles covering the skull.

pain around the left eye, or pain that feels like it is going into the left eye.

Hydrotherapy

Place an ice pack (wrapped in a thin towel) on the back of the child's neck and put her feet in a bucket of warm water for 10 minutes.

■ ADVANCED PLAN

Homeopathy

Constitutional homeopathy from a practitioner works well to prevent headaches.

Aromatherapy

Lavender—Add to a carrier oil or cream and rub it along the hairline. Make sure not to get any in the eyes. If the child is taking a homeopathic remedy, use aromatherapy at a different time.

Acupressure

Try the following points and then choose the one or combination that provides the greatest

Vital Fact

By age 15, 5 percent of all adolescents will have experienced a migraine attack.

relief for your child. Gently press each of the acupressure points with a thumb for 10 to 15 seconds. Perform on both sides of the body and repeat three times each day.

Gallbladder 20—Located below the base of the skull, in the space between the two vertical neck muscles.

Large Intestine 4—Located in the webbing between the thumb and index finger.

Liver 3—Located on top of the foot, in the hollow between the big toe and second toe.

Yuyao—The indentation in the middle of the eyebrow (directly up from the pupil).

■ WHAT TO EXPECT

You should see relief of the headache within 15 minutes to an hour. While natural therapies can be helpful to relieve acute headaches, they are best used to treat the underlying cause so that headaches do not occur in the first place.

Heart Arrhythmia

This condition is the disruption of the heart's normal, steady beating or pacing mechanism. It disturbs the pattern of impulses that stimu-late the contractions of the heart's upper chambers (atria) and/or the lower chambers (ventricles), creating rhythm abnormalities. Heart arrhythmias and murmurs are often benign, although only your child's doctor can determine this.

Some of the more serious rhythm abnormalities arise from a variety of causes: aging; heart attack or heart damage; hormonal alterations, particularly thyroid disorders; or external triggers, such as food, alcohol, tobacco, caffeine, and medications.

There are three types of rhythm disturbances: tachycardia (racing heartbeat), bradycardia (sluggish heartbeat), and palpitation (skipping, fibrillating, or fluttering heartbeat). Symptoms of arrhythmia can range from none at all to dizziness and fainting, fluttering in the chest, and even sudden death.

Tachycardia describes rapid beating at a rate above 100 beats per minute. It can occur normally—as a response to exercise, heightened emotion, pain, or fever. But beating too quickly, such as at a rate above 150 beats per minute, prevents the adequate filling of the heart chambers with blood, bringing on dizziness, light-headedness, and fainting.

A heartbeat of less than 60 times per minute, which is classified as bradycardia, can describe the normal endurance athlete's resting heartbeat. But beating fewer than 30 or 40 times per minute leads to a lack of sufficient bloodflow to the brain. That can cause weakness, confusion, and fainting.

Skipping, flipping, or fluttering heartbeats describe the type of arrhythmia called palpitations. The most common arrhythmia is atrial fibrillation, when the upper chambers' electrical signals are totally uncoordinated, resulting in quivering contractions of 400 to even 600 times per minute. The results are an irregularly spaced heartbeat of 80 to 180 times per minute and a risk that pools of blood will form clots in the upper chambers.

Infants sometimes experience heart murmurs—extra heart sounds—that are often not dangerous arrhythmia and that can disappear with time.

Conventional treatment focuses on identifying any mechanical or anatomical defect and correcting it with medication and/or surgery. Heart conditions that are deemed insignificant may not be treated and are monitored over time.

■ BASIC PLAN

If your child is on medication for a heart arrhythmia, it is critical that you do not stop or alter the medication while using the following natural approaches. You must work closely with a doctor to properly monitor and evaluate your child's condition. Consult with your doctor before using any of these therapies.

Diet

Follow a whole-foods diet. (See "Diet" on page 4 for more information.) Food sensitivities may occasionally play a role in heart arrhythmias and should be investigated. Also, food preservatives should be avoided as well. (See "Food Allergies and Food Sensitivities" on page 298.)

Keeping blood sugar levels even may be helpful for heart rhythm abnormalities. This involves your child eating regular meals with balanced proportions of proteins, carbohydrates, and fiber. (See "Diabetes" on page 266 for more about this diet.) Essential fatty acids from coldwater fish such as salmon, mackerel, and herring are important for heart function, as are oils such as olive oil.

Nutritional Supplements

These supplements should be used under the guidance of a knowledgeable physician.

Calcium and magnesium—Required for proper electrical conduction of the heart. Typical dosages are 500 milligrams of calcium and 250 to 500 milligrams of magnesium daily.

Coenzyme Q$_{10}$—Required for the heart muscle cells to contract efficiently. Typical dosages are 15 to 30 milligrams daily.

Taurine—Helps the heart contract stronger and more efficiently. Typical dosages are 250 to 500 milligrams daily.

L-carnitine—Works to strengthen heart contractions. Typical dosages are 50 to 100 milligrams daily.

Herbal Remedy

Hawthorn berry—Improves bloodflow to the heart and increases the heart's pumping ability. Can be helpful for mild cases of irregular heartbeats. Use under the direction of a health professional.

■ WHAT TO EXPECT

Work with your doctor to incorporate natural therapies. Cases deemed not serious enough to require conventional medications may respond to natural therapies.

Heartburn

Irritating stomach acids are sometimes regurgitated into a child's esophagus, causing a condition known as gastroesophageal reflux disorder (GERD) and a pain that most adults describe as heartburn.

When a child experiences heartburn, the discomfort of indigestion often creeps from the abdomen to the chest area surrounding the heart and may radiate to the neck, throat, and face.

Heartburn is common after meals or when the child is lying down. It may be accompanied by regurgitation of digestive juices and excessive salivation.

A child may be having heartburn if he is having chest pain or discomfort when lying down or bending over and it is accompanied by an acid taste in his mouth and throat and a bloated feeling. Heartburn is said to be among the hidden causes of colicky and night-waking babies.

The valve between the esophagus and stomach may not be closing properly, allowing for stomach acid to irritate the esophagus. Food sensitivities are a common cause of heartburn. A less common cause of heartburn and ulcers in children is an overgrowth of the bacterium *Helicobacter pylori*. Also, a condition called hiatal hernia can lead to heartburnlike symptoms.

Conventional treatment focuses on antacid medications that neutralize or reduce stomach acid. If *H. pylori* is present, antibiotics are given.

Note: Peppermint can worsen symptoms of heartburn. Avoid it in food and as an herbal remedy if your child is suffering from indigestion.

■ BASIC PLAN

Diet
Food sensitivities are the most common reason for heartburn. Different foods can be a trigger depending on the child. Common ones we see with children include dairy (cow's milk and cheese), citrus fruits (especially oranges), tomatoes, spicy foods such as garlic, and wheat. See "Food Allergies and Food Sensitivities" on page 298 to learn how to identify potential sensitivity reactions in your child.

Herbal Remedy
Slippery elm—Soothing to the lining of the esophagus and stomach. For children over age 5, give a slippery elm lozenge twice daily (children this old should be able to suck it without choking). For younger children, give the powdered form, at ½ teaspoon in ¼ cup water twice daily.

Homeopathy
Pick the following remedy that best matches your child's symptoms. Unless otherwise indicated, give your child 2 pellets of a 30C potency every 30 minutes for up to three doses. If there is no improvement within 2 hours, try another remedy. After you first notice improvement, stop giving the remedy unless symptoms begin to return.

Note: Lower potencies (6X, 12X, 6C) may need to be given more often (three times daily).

Arsenicum album—For a burning sensation in the esophagus or stomach that is alleviated by drinking milk. The child wants to sip water frequently, which may cause vomiting.

Carbo vegetabilis—For heartburn accompanied by belching.

Lycopodium—For a sour taste in the mouth or belching that burns. The child may feel better with warm drinks. He craves sweets.

Nux vomica—The most common remedy for heartburn. The child may have high levels of stress or react to spicy foods.

Pulsatilla—For heartburn from eating fatty food. The child has a thick-coated, moist, white tongue. He has nausea with little vomiting and an absence of much pain. He has a very distended feeling, so that his clothes must be loosened.

Acupressure

Conception Vessel 12—Located halfway between the lower edge of the breastbone and the navel. Gently press the acupressure point with a thumb for 10 to 15 seconds. Repeat three times each day.

■ ADVANCED PLAN

Nutritional Supplement

Probiotic—Choose a children's acidophilus and bifidus supplement, which replaces the good bacteria required for good digestion. Give as directed on the container.

Herbal Remedies

Licorice, **fennel**, **chamomile**, and **slippery elm** all reduce heartburn symptoms. Use them alone or in combination.

Aromatherapy

Peppermint—Add to a carrier oil and rub it over the chest and abdomen. If the child is taking a homeopathic remedy, use aromatherapy at a different time.

Acupressure

Stomach 36—Located four finger-widths below the kneecap and one finger-width toward the outside of the leg (outside of the shinbone on the muscle). Gently press the acupressure point with a thumb for 10 to 15 seconds. Perform on both sides of the body and repeat three times each day.

■ WHAT TO EXPECT

Relief of acute heartburn should be noticed within 1 to 2 hours, while chronic cases should improve within 10 days of treatment. If there is no improvement, consult with a doctor or natural health care practitioner.

Hemorrhoids

Hemorrhoids are a painful and excessive swelling and bulging of the large veins that lie just beneath the layer of tissue lining the anal canal.

It's common for these veins to swell during a bowel movement, but the pressure of extra weight (as from obesity, chronic constipation with straining, heavy lifting, or pushing and prolonged sitting) can cause these veins to flare up, become irritated, and even bleed. Chronic diarrhea can also be a cause.

In extreme cases, a blood clot called thrombosis forms, causing the blocked vein and surrounding mucous membranes to become dark and appear dead. See your doctor if your child experiences painful rectal bleeding.

Hemorrhoids in children are often caused or aggravated by the painful passing of a sharp, rigid stool, such as those passed by a constipated child. Symptoms include bright, red blood not mixed with the stools during a bowel movement; rectal bleeding; anal itching; and prolapse—a feeling that the rectum is swelling or poking outside after a bowel movement.

Doctors look for a discharge of blood from the irritated veins, skin irritation outside the anus, and edema (fluid swelling) in the rectal lining.

The underlying cause of hemorrhoids in children is usually a low-fiber diet, food sensitivities, lack of exercise, stress, or anxiety.

Conventional treatment focuses on increasing fiber in the diet, giving fiber supplements, and possibly, using a hemorrhoid cream or suppository.

■ BASIC PLAN

Diet

A high-fiber diet is key to preventing and treating hemorrhoids. Insoluble fiber as found in vegetables and whole grains helps to increase the bulk of the stool, thus improving bowel passage. Steamed and cooked vegetables such as broccoli, cauliflower, and carrots are important to serve daily for fiber. Carrot sticks, celery, and cauliflower with dip as snacks between meals are helpful for older children. Whole grains, such as in oatmeal or whole wheat bread, are also a good source of fiber. Bran muffins mixed with fruit such as raisins are popular with children, and they're a good way to increase fiber intake.

Ground-up flaxseeds are another excellent source of fiber. Grind 1 teaspoon of flaxseeds per 50 pounds of body weight (children weighing 30 to 50 pounds may also use 1 teaspoon), and give this amount daily, mixed with food, in a healthy protein or fruit or vegetable shake, or in juice. Always accompany with 8 ounces of water.

Avoid or reduce the intake of bananas and dairy products, which can be constipating. (For more information, see "Constipation" on page 245.)

Food sensitivities can irritate hemorrhoids and worsen symptoms. Tomatoes, nuts, and citrus fruits are common foods that worsen hemorrhoids. (See "Food Allergies and Food Sensitivities" on page 298 for more information.)

Nutritional Supplement

Vitamin C—Promotes tissue healing and has mild anti-inflammatory effects. The type with bioflavonoids is preferable. Daily dosage: the child's age in years times 50 milligrams. Reduce the dosage if diarrhea occurs. Consider using a buffered vitamin C powder (nonacidic) or liquid vitamin C. Both work well for infants and children, and can be mixed in juice.

Herbal Remedy

Witch hazel—Has an astringent effect on hemorrhoids. Apply it as a topical ointment, or use ¼ cup of a witch hazel solution diluted in a sitz bath (a small, warm tub). Witch hazel solutions are available at most pharmacies.

Note: Herbs such as horse chestnut and butcher's broom are commonly used for hemorrhoids. Their effect on children has not been studied. If you use them, do so under the guidance of a knowledgeable practitioner.

Homeopathy

Use a combination hemorrhoid formula, or pick the one of the following remedies that best matches your child's symptoms. For the remedies below, unless otherwise indicated, give your child 2 pellets of a 30C potency two times daily. Improvements should be seen within 3 days. If there is no improvement within 3 days, try another remedy. After you first notice improvement, stop giving the remedy unless symptoms begin to return.

Note: Lower potencies (6X, 12X, 6C) may need to be given more often (three times daily).

Aesculus hippocastanum—The child describes the pain as if her rectum is being poked with sticks. Pain extends to the back.

Aloe—For large, painful hemorrhoids. The doctor states that the hemorrhoids look like a bunch of grapes. Better with cold applications. There is mucus in the stool.

Hamamelis—For bleeding hemorrhoids. Throbbing pain in the rectum lasts hours after a bowel movement.

Nux vomica—For painful hemorrhoids that come on as a result of chronic constipation and straining with bowel movements. The child is irritable and impatient and feels like her bowel movements are never complete.

Ratanhia peruviana—The child experiences a lot of pain after a bowel movement. It is cutting pain that feels like she is sitting on broken glass.

Sulphur—For itching, burning hemorrhoids that tend to be worse at night. Morning diarrhea is another symptom. The child is very warm and sweats easily.

■ ADVANCED PLAN

Nutritional Supplement

Grape seed extract or pycnogenol—Strengthens blood vessels and reduces inflammation. Give 1 milligram per pound of body weight daily.

Aromatherapy

German chamomile—Add it to a lukewarm bath (sitz bath) and have the child sit for 5 to 10 minutes. If the child is taking a homeopathic remedy, use aromatherapy at a different time.

Acupressure

Gently press the following points with a thumb for 15 seconds. Repeat three times. Do this once daily.

Liver 3—Located on top of the foot, in the hollow between the big toe and second toe.

Large Intestine 4—Located in the webbing between the thumb and index finger.

■ WHAT TO EXPECT

Once a child is getting enough fiber and fluids in her diet, her hemorrhoid symptoms will lessen within 1 to 2 weeks. Using the natural therapies in this chapter will quicken the healing and prevent future reoccurrences.

Hepatitis

Hepatitis is the general term for inflammation of the liver—the body's largest internal organ, located beneath the breastbone and extending under the bottom of the right side of the rib cage. Hepatitis can be caused by drugs and chemicals, but it is most commonly caused by a virus.

One of the liver's functions is to produce and metabolize bile, which is necessary to break down fats and expel toxins from the body. With hepatitis, bilirubin, a pigment normally excreted in bile, builds up in the bloodstream and accumulates in the skin. This causes the characteristic yellowish color of the skin and eyes, as well as dark urine. The symptoms of heptatis include nausea, fatigue, loss of appetite, weight loss, clay-colored stools, fever, and diarrhea. Blood tests show an elevation of one or more liver enzymes.

There are different viruses that cause hepatitis. The main three are A, B, and C. Other hepatitis viruses include D, E, and G. Hepatitis A, which has a 15- to 45-day incubation period, is highly contagious and spread by direct contact with an infected person or through feces-tainted food or water.

Hepatitis B has an incubation period of 30 to 180 days. It is spread through transfusions of infected blood, the use of unsterile needles, and sexual contact. This type of hepatitis is associated with liver cancer.

Hepatitis C has an incubation period of 15 to 150 days. This is the most common form of viral hepatitis in adults. In the past, it was contracted through contaminated blood transfusions. Now, intravenous drug use and sexual intercourse are the main modes of infection. Many cases of hepatitis C become chronic, and it is one of the leading causes of liver transplants.

Conventional treatment includes a doctor's evaluation and depends on the severity of the condition. The child may be observed, and if improvement is being made, little intervention may be given. Hepatitis A and E are self-limiting and usually clear up without treatment. For more serious cases, pharmaceutical medications are used to reduce symptoms. The antiviral drug interferon may be used to augment the immune system for viral hepatitis, although its benefit is questionable for long-term use. There are vaccines for hepatitis A and B.

Natural therapies can help to heal the liver after a diagnosis is made.

■ BASIC PLAN

Diet

To promote healing of the liver and to provide a diet that is supportive to the immune system, include lots of vegetables (carrots and beets are excellent) and a moderate amount of fruits, whole grains, and legumes. Steamed artichokes in particular are healing to the liver.

Reduce or eliminate foods that are taxing to the liver, such as fried foods, refined sugar products, foods containing trans fatty acids (such as margarine and vegetable shortening), and saturated fats (found in meat and dairy products).

Make fresh juices from foods such as apples, beets, and carrots. Start with a small amount of juice to see how the child tolerates it. Also give your child six to eight 8-ounce glasses of purified water throughout the day.

Eating smaller more and more frequent meals is recommended. Soups and stews are good, as they are easy to digest.

Nutritional Supplements

Vitamin C—Supports the immune system and has mild anti-inflammatory effects. The type with bioflavonoids is preferable. Dosage: the child's age in years times 50 milligrams, twice daily. Reduce the dosage if diarrhea occurs. Consider using a buffered vitamin C powder (nonacidic) or liquid vitamin C. Both work well for infants and children, and can be mixed in juice.

Phosphatidylcholine—Helps the liver to process fats, and protects the liver cells. Use as directed by your natural health care practitioner. A typical children's dosage is 100 to 500 milligrams.

Note: Avoid the single use of vitamins A, D, and E unless you have been instructed to do so by a physician. These fat-soluble vitamins can build up when liver function is compromised.

Herbal Remedies

Milk thistle (85 percent silymarin)—Protects the liver and promotes liver cell re-generation. This herb can help bring elevated liver enzyme counts down.

If your child has viral hepatitis, herbs such as **echinacea**, **astragalus**, **reishi**, **lomatium**, and **licorice root** are indicated for their antiviral and immune-enhancing effects. Use formulas containing this blend, or start with one of the herbs to support the immune system.

Homeopathy

Pick the following remedy that best matches your child's symptoms. Unless otherwise indicated, give your child 2 pellets of a 30C potency twice daily. Improvements for acute hepatitis (such as hepatitis A) should be noted within 2 to 3 days. For chronic hepatitis (such as B or C), improvements should be seen within 2 to 3 weeks. If there is no improvement in acute hepatitis within 48 hours, or in chronic hepatitis within 3 weeks, try another remedy. After you first notice improvement, stop giving the remedy unless symptoms begin to return.

Note: Lower potencies (6X, 12X, 6C) may need to be given more often (three times daily).

Cardus marianus—For inflammation of the left lobe of the liver. Symptoms are worse lying on the left side.

Chelidonium majus—For pain under the right rib cage that radiates to the right shoulder blade. The child feels better with warm drinks.

China officinalis—The liver is very sensitive to touch. The child has bloating of the abdomen and sweating at night. He belches, with a bitter taste in his mouth.

Lycopodium—For hepatitis where bloat-

Vital Study

For a study in the journal *Acta Physiologica Hungarica,* scientists investigated the use of milk thistle (silymarin) in a group of 21 people who had active liver disease (cirrhosis). People who took 420 milligrams of silymarin had a 15 percent drop in the liver enzyme AST (aspartate aminotransferase) and a 23 percent decrease for the enzyme ALT (alanine aminotransferase). These enzymes are typically elevated in people with cirrhosis.

ing, indigestion, and flatulence are prominent symptoms. The child feels better with warm drinks and with belching.

Mercurius solubilis or vivus—For a sore liver that is tender to pressure. Liver pains extend to the spine. The child has bloody urine and/or greenish stool. Symptoms are worse at night.

Natrum sulphuricum—For jaundice accompanied by watery and yellow diarrhea. The tongue has a greenish coating. The child has pronounced depression.

Nux vomica—For liver disease where constipation is a problem. The child is chilly and irritable.

Phosphorus—For hepatitis that occurs from solvent and toxin exposure. The child feels better with ice-cold drinks. He has a high thirst but may vomit liquids easily. He feels worse lying on his left side.

■ ADVANCED PLAN

Nutritional Supplements

Children's multivitamin—Provides a base of the essential vitamins and minerals. Give as directed on the container.

Selenium—Give 1 microgram per pound of body weight daily for immune system support. Use under the guidance of a practitioner.

Alpha lipoic acid—A potent antioxidant that protects the liver. Give 1 milligram per pound of body weight daily.

Thymus glandular extract—Supportive to the immune system. Give as directed on the container (usually 250 milligrams for a child) or as directed by a practitioner.

Herbal Remedies

Liver-supportive herbs include **dandelion root**, **chicory**, and **Phyllanthus amarus** (especially for hepatitis B).

Find out about a Chinese herbal medicine and acupressure/acupuncture from a practitioner of oriental medicine. There are many good Chinese formulas for hepatitis.

■ WHAT TO EXPECT

Natural therapy helps to prevent liver damage. Chronic hepatitis infection, such as hepatitis C, usually shows improvements in liver enzyme values within 2 to 3 months of natural therapy. Antioxidants and herbs such as milk thistle are highly recommended to protect the liver if conventional therapy such as interferon is used.

Hiccups

When a child eats too quickly, shoveling fork-fuls of food into his or her mouth and swallowing everything—including air—the body reacts with a case of the hiccups. Even a case of the giggles can bring on hiccups. In babies, hiccups can develop when they swallow too much air while nursing or drinking formula.

Hiccups are sudden, involuntary spasms of the diaphragm, which is the partition of thin muscles and tendons separating the chest cavity from the abdominal cavity. The spasms occur because swallowed air has no place to go in the digestive system and must come out as a series of comedic and sometimes frustrating "hic-CUPS!" Irritation of the nerve that serves the diaphragm can also be a cause.

Hiccups are usually more of an annoyance than a cause for alarm. In most children, they disappear within 10 minutes. But if your child's hiccups stubbornly persist beyond a day or so, check with your doctor. The longevity of the hiccups may indicate a symptom of a more serious underlying disease.

The conventional approach for short episodes of hiccups is to let them run their course. Various techniques are used by parents with success, including having the child hold her breath, drinking water with the nostrils pinched, and many other tactics. These techniques increase the blood levels of carbon dioxide, which inhibits hiccups.

Spinal and muscle therapy by a naturopathic physician, chiropractor, osteopath, massage therapist, or craniosacral therapist can be helpful for chronic susceptibility to hiccups. (See the Natural Health Care Modalities and Resource Guide on page 499 for more on these therapies.)

■ BASIC PLAN

Have an adult hold a glass of water while the child drinks and plugs her ears. While this technique is not scientifically tested, it seems to work.

Diet

Hiccups in infants usually passes with time or feeding.

Have your child eat more slowly and chew her food more thoroughly. This will prevent her from swallowing too much air. In chronic cases, food sensitivities may be playing a role. (See "Food Allergies and Food Sensitivities" on page 298 for more information.)

Herbal Remedies

Peppermint or **chamomile** tea can be helpful to relieve hiccups. Give ¼ to ½ cup as needed to relieve hiccups.

Homeopathy

Magnesia phosphorica 6X—If you don't know what to give, try Magnesia phosphorica. It helps to relax the spasming muscles of the diaphragm. Give 2 pellets every 5 minutes, for up to four doses. (For infants, crush homeopathic pellets into powder and mix it with water.)

Nux vomica 30C—For hiccups that are accompanied by digestive irritation. The child may be irritable with the hiccups.

Acupressure

Gently press the following pressure points with a thumb for 10 to 15 seconds. Perform on both hands and repeat three times in a row.

Pericardium 6—Located 2½ finger-widths below the wrist crease, in the middle of the forearm (the palm side).

Heart 9—Located on the inside of the "pinky finger" at the base of the nail.

Aromatherapy

Peppermint—Add 1 drop to a vaporizer, or add it to a carrier oil and rub it on the child's chest. If the child is taking a homeopathic remedy, use aromatherapy at a different time.

High Blood Pressure

The pumping of the heart and the degree of constriction or dilation of the arteries determines the force exerted against the walls of the arteries—which is the measure known as blood pressure.

Blood pressure varies with a child's activity. Factors that play a role include physical activity, emotion, weight, and nutritional status. But sometimes, even a child's normal or resting blood pressure is high, creating a condition known as hypertension. Years of undetected, sustained hypertension can damage the fragile linings of the blood vessels in the heart, kidneys, and eyes.

There are varying degrees of hypertension, and varying degrees of risks. Blood pressure readings are given with two numbers: the "top" number, or systolic pressure, which is the pressure generated in the vessels when the heart contracts and pumps; and the "bottom" number, or diastolic pressure, which is the pressure in the vessels when the heart is between contractions.

Hypertension can be genetic but is usually related to diet and lifestyle. Being overweight is a major risk factor. Some secondary causes of hypertension are kidney disease, constriction of the aorta (the body's main artery), narrowing of the main arteries serving the kidneys, medication (hypertension can be a side effect), and malfunctioning adrenal and/or endocrine glands.

Symptoms associated with high blood pressure that require emergency attention include severe headache, confusion, numbness or weakness in an arm or a leg, shortness of breath, chest pain, and sudden decrease in urination.

Conventional treatment involves lifestyle changes (diet and exercise) and pharmaceutical medications.

■ BASIC PLAN

Diet

A high-fiber diet is recommended. You can get fiber from vegetables, whole grains, legumes, some fruits, nuts, and seeds. Onions, celery, and garlic are excellent foods to eat on a regular basis to help control high blood pressure. Saturated fats found in animal products should be reduced, while "good" fats found in cold-water fish such as salmon, mackerel, and herring should be consumed three times weekly.

Olive oil is the preferred cooking oil. Reduce the intake of salt while increasing potassium-rich foods (fruits and vegetables).

Regular water consumption is important. Not drinking enough fluids can cause an elevation in blood pressure.

Note: Some children may have what is called insulin sensitivity, where blood sugar tends to be elevated as well as blood pressure. These children do better on a diet that is low in simple sugars, and moderate in protein and complex carbohydrates. Work with a nutrition-oriented doctor.

Nutritional Supplements

Calcium and magnesium—Give 500 to 600 milligrams of calcium and 250 to 500 milligrams of magnesium daily. Relaxes blood vessels and may reduce blood pressure.

Herbal Remedies

Ginkgo biloba and **hawthorn berry** are two of the best herbs to use to reduce blood pressure. Use under the guidance of a doctor.

Homeopathy

A constitutional treatment from a homeopathic practitioner may be helpful.

■ ADVANCED PLAN

Nutritional Supplements

The following are all helpful for reducing blood pressure. Work with a nutrition-oriented doctor to find the safe and effective dosage for your child.

Vital Study

For a randomized, double-blind, placebo-controlled trial published in the *Journal of Pediatrics,* 101 fifth-grade students were studied to see what effect calcium supplementation had on their blood pressure. The children consumed 480 millileters of juice beverages, containing either no calcium or 600 milligrams of calcium (as calcium citrate malate) daily for 12 weeks. On school days, the beverages were consumed at school, and for the weekends, the beverages were taken home to drink. The calcium supplementation made the biggest difference in children whose diets were the lowest in calcium (on average, it reduced their blood pressures by 3.5 millimeters of mercury). Researchers concluded that calcium had a blood pressure lowering effect, especially in those who had a low dietary intake.

Coenzyme Q$_{10}$—Common dosages are 25 to 50 milligrams daily.

Vitamin C—A common daily dosage is the child's age in years times 50 milligrams.

Children's multivitamin—Provides a base of vitamins and minerals to help prevent deficiencies. Contains potassium, which is also known to help reduce blood pressure.

Flaxseed oil—The following are common daily dosages: children 2 and under, 1 teaspoon;

kids 3 to 6, 2 teaspoons; kids 7 and older, 2 to 3 teaspoons.

Herbal Remedy

Garlic extract—Give 200 milligrams daily for children 10 and under, or 400 milligrams daily for kids 11 and older.

Acupressure

Four Gates—This is a combination of Liver 3, located on top of the foot in the hollow between the big toe and second toe, and Large Intestine 4, located in the webbing between the thumb and index finger. Two people should push gently on all four points at the same time for 15 seconds. Repeat three times. Do this once daily.

Aromatherapy

Lavender—Add 1 or 2 drops to a vaporizer as the child sleeps. Or add 1 or 2 drops to a tissue and keep it under the child's pillow. If the child is taking a homeopathic remedy, use aromatherapy at a different time.

■ WHAT TO EXPECT

Lifestyle changes such as diet and exercise can make profound changes in a child's blood pressure, as can nutritional supplements. Improvements can be seen within 3 to 5 weeks. High blood pressure that is a result of a disease, such as kidney disease, may require pharmaceutical treatment, as can acute hypertension. Work with a doctor, particularly a naturopathic doctor, to incorporate the natural therapies listed in this chapter.

Hives

One in five children develops hives (also known medically as urticaria) sometime in his lifetime. The skin lesions are red, bumpy, itchy patches of skin that can spot the body anywhere. The rash can blanket the body or appear in just one area. It can appear and disappear, itch or not itch.

Children develop hives commonly in response to allergies or infections.

The comforting news is that most hives disappear on their own within a day or so, although some cases can become chronic. The unsettling news is that it can be a challenge to identify what's causing these irritating rash outbreaks.

Typical triggers for hives include food allergies (especially fish, eggs, nuts, and food additives), drug allergies (particularly penicillin and aspirin), sensitivity to plants (especially to pollen) or animals (pet dander or saliva), and insect bites.

Heat, cold, sunlight, or excessive sweat from exercise could spark hives. Also, hives can be symptoms of more serious conditions such as parasitic infections, hepatitis, cancer, hyperthyroidism, and rare blood disorders.

Hive reactions that occur in the throat area or that cause respiratory distress should be immediately evaluated at the nearest emergency room. Epinephrine and antihistamines are administered to reduce the allergic reaction and maintain an open airway. Oxygen may be administered and, in severe cases, a breathing tube is inserted into the throat to maintain the airway.

The conventional approach is to identify

the offending allergen by patient history or with the use of allergy testing (usually a skin scratch test or blood antibody testing). Your doctor may prescribe an epinephrine kit to have on hand if your child has experienced a severe hive reaction. Antihistamine medications such as Benadryl are also used to reduce hive symptoms. More serious cases of hives are treated with corticosteroids such as prednisone, which are used on a short-term basis.

■ BASIC PLAN

Diet

If your child breaks out in hives after eating food, write down what your child ate and review it with your doctor. It is important that the offending food be avoided in the future. Common hive-inducing foods include peanuts, nuts, and cow's milk.

Nutritional Supplement

Vitamin C—Supports the immune system and has mild anti-inflammatory effects. Dosage: the child's age in years times 50 milligrams, twice daily. Reduce the dosage if diarrhea occurs. Consider using a buffered vitamin C powder (nonacidic) or liquid vitamin C. Both work well for infants and children, and can be mixed in juice.

Herbal Remedy

Oatmeal bath—Add a cup of oatmeal powder such as Aveeno to a warm bath. The other alternative is to put regular oatmeal (such as Quaker Oats) into a cheesecloth bag, tie it with a string, and hang it under the faucet or float it in the tub. Have the child soak in the warm bath for 5 to 15 minutes. When done, pat the child dry so that a film of oatmeal is left on the skin. This film contains the anti-itch properties of the oatmeal.

Homeopathy

Pick the following remedy that best matches your child's symptoms. Unless otherwise indicated, give your child 2 pellets of a 30C potency every hour for up to three doses. (For infants, crush the pellets into powder and mix it with water.) If there is no improvement within 3 hours, try another remedy. After you first notice improvement, stop giving the remedy unless symptoms begin to return.

Note: Lower potencies (6X, 12X, 6C) may need to be given more often (every 2 hours).

Apis mellifica—The most common remedy for hives. The child experiences swelling and intolerable itching that is worse with warmth and better with cold applications. His face and eyelids become puffy.

Rhus toxicodendron—For hives that occur as the result of getting wet or chilled, or during a fever. The hives are very itchy and feel hot and burning. The child feels better with heat and warm applications. He is very restless.

Urtica urens—For hives from eating shellfish.

Acupressure

Large Intestine 4—Reduces inflammation in the body. Located in the webbing between the thumb and index finger. Gently press the acupressure point with a thumb for 10 to 15 seconds. Perform on both sides of the body and repeat three times each day.

■ ADVANCED PLAN

Nutritional Supplement

Quercitin—This flavonoid has anti-allergy properties to reduce swelling and itching. Dosage: 3 milligrams per pound of body weight, two or three times daily.

Homeopathy

Bach Flower Rescue Remedy cream applied topically helps to reduce itching. Apply it to the worst areas throughout the day. Discontinue use when the itching is gone. The liquid form of Rescue Remedy can also be taken internally to help with the restlessness that accompanies hives. Give 2 drops three times a day. (For infants, put the drops in ¼ cup of water, then give ¼ teaspoon of the water.)

■ WHAT TO EXPECT

Mild cases of hives should clear up within a couple of days. If your child is experiencing respiratory distress or severe symptoms, see a doctor immediately.

Hypoglycemia

Hypoglycemia means low blood glucose. This disorder has two types: fasting hypoglycemia, in which blood sugar levels get too low when a child goes too long without eating, and postprandial hypoglycemia, in which blood sugar levels rise and then quickly fall after the child eats a meal. Children with either type may experience racing pulses, headaches, uncontrolled sweating and hand trembling, tingling sensations, anxiety, hunger, mood and behavior changes, confusion, and even loss of consciousness.

Among low birth weight infants, hypoglycemia can be a serious, potentially life-threatening condition if left untreated. The infant can develop seizures and/or brain damage. Fortunately, pediatricians routinely check for signs of hypoglycemia within the first day or two following the birth of an infant.

The body needs normal levels of blood sugar to maintain its energy levels. Fasting hypoglycemia can develop for many reasons. Certain medical conditions can cause hypoglycemia, such as the excessive secretion of insulin, as can genetic diseases. Also, diet and exercise are important in maintaining stable blood sugar levels.

Severe acute cases are treated with intravenous solutions of dextrose (sugar). The conventional approach to chronic hypoglycemia is diet management and, in some cases, pharmaceutical medications.

■ BASIC PLAN

Diet

For more even blood sugar levels, have your child eat smaller, more frequent meals (four to six meals) throughout the day instead of three larger meals. If this is difficult, then have three main meals with snacks between each meal.

Focus on quality protein sources (nuts, fish, lean poultry, and legumes), complex carbohydrates (found in whole grains), and high-fiber foods (such as salads, steamed vegetables, and whole grains).

Do not eat fruit or drink fruit juice between meals. These items should be consumed with meals to avoid causing blood sugar fluctuation. Limit to no more than 6 to 8 ounces of fruit juice daily.

Avoid simple sugars such as soft drinks and candy, and avoid refined flour products such as white rice and baked goods made from white flour. If your child does have these foods, which she likely will on occasion, it is best for her to consume them during or around mealtime. Also, avoid the use of artificial sweeteners.

Nutritional Supplement

Chromium is involved with blood sugar metabolism. Use it under the supervision of a doctor. Common dosages are as follows: 1 to 3 years old, 20 to 80 micrograms; 4 to 6 years old, 30 to 120 micrograms; ages 7 and up, 50 to 200 micrograms.

■ ADVANCED PLAN

Nutritional Supplements

Children's multivitamin—Supplies many of the vitamins and minerals required for blood sugar control.

Vitamin C—Required for proper insulin action. Dosage: the child's age in years times 50 milligrams, daily. Reduce the dosage if diarrhea occurs. Consider using a buffered vitamin

Case History

Tierra, a 10-year-old girl, was brought by her parents to our clinic because she suffered from dizziness and mood swings throughout the day. She also had a ravenous appetite for a girl who was so thin. Her parents noticed that her symptoms would flare up if she went long periods of time without eating, or if she consumed sugar products. Some blood work confirmed what we had suspected: Tierra had hypoglycemia. We had Tierra avoid fruit juices on an empty stomach. (Before, she was drinking 4 to 5 glasses of apple or grape juice a day.) We also had her eat a mixture of quality protein (poultry, fish, or eggs) and complex carbohydrates (such as whole wheat pasta and brown rice), as well as a salad with lunch and dinner. For breakfast, Tierra had oatmeal or granola cereal with a boiled egg. In addition, we made sure that between meals, she ate nonsugar snacks, such as almonds or walnuts, or drank a soy protein shake. For supplements, we had her take a multivitamin and extra chromium and vanadium. The results were noticeable within 3 days. Her energy level increased, and her moods were much more stable. Afterward, dizziness was a problem only if Tierra waited too long to eat.

C powder (nonacidic) or liquid vitamin C. Both work well for infants and children, and can be mixed in juice.

Essential fatty acids—Help with insulin balance and can help prevent complications of high blood sugar levels. Give a children's complex containing omega-3 and omega-6 fatty acids; follow the directions on the container. Or give flaxseed oil at the following daily dosages: children 2 and under, 1 teaspoon; kids 3 to 6, 2 teaspoons; kids 7 and older, 2 to 3 teaspoons. Reduce the dosage if diarrhea occurs.

Zinc—Involved with proper insulin activity. The following daily dose of zinc should include the amount in any multivitamin that your child takes: children 2 and younger, 5 milligrams; 3 and older, 10 to 15 milligrams. Use long-term under the supervision of a doctor.

Homeopathy
See a practitioner for a constitutional remedy.

■ WHAT TO EXPECT
Children with chronic hypoglycemia that is unrelated to a genetic defect of sugar metabolism do very well with diet management and natural therapy. Improvement is usually seen within 2 weeks.

Hypothyroidism

Although hyperthyroidism, or an overactive thyroid gland, is not common in children, hypothyroidism (an underactive gland) can be. With hypothyroidism, the thyroid gland does not produce an adequate amount of thyroid hormone. This insufficient supply slows down all the chemical reactions in the body, resulting in mental and physical changes.

Although hypothyroidism is more common among middle-age people and senior citizens, children can develop it, especially if they have family histories of this condition.

Common symptoms associated with hypothyroidism include sleeplessness, fatigue, muscle weakness, constipation, weight gain, thick and dry skin, swollen eyelids, thick tongue, loss of hearing, numbness and tingling in the hands, and intolerance to cold.

Hypothyroidism can be caused by:

- Bacterial and viral infections that affect the thyroid
- Hashimoto's disease (thyroiditis), a condition that causes the thyroid gland to become inflamed. It is a disorder of the immune system.
- Radiation treatments for hyperthyroidism that result in destruction of the thyroid gland
- A malfunctioning pituitary gland. This gland is designed to stimulate the thyroid to produce an adequate supply of hormones.

The conventional therapy is thyroid hormone replacement.

■ BASIC PLAN

Diet
Have your child consume foods that contain naturally occurring iodine; they are healthy for

the thyroid. Sea vegetables such as dulse, kelp, hijiki, and kombu are good choices.

Certain vegetables known as goitrogens may suppress thyroid function. These include kale, broccoli, cauliflower, cabbage, soy, and Brussels sprouts. Cooking the vegetables inactivates the goitrogens so that they are safe for a person with low thyroid to eat.

Nutritional Supplements

Thyroid and pituitary glandulars—Discuss using these supplements with your health care practitioner. Useful in cases of mild hypothyroidism to stimulate the thyroid gland.

Homeopathy

Pick the following remedy that best matches your child's symptoms. Unless otherwise indicated, give your child 2 pellets of a 30C potency two times daily. Improvements should be seen within 3 to 4 weeks. If there is no improvement within 3 to 4 weeks, try another remedy. After you first notice improvement, stop giving the remedy unless symptoms begin to return.

Note: Lower potencies (6X, 12X, 6C) may need to be given more often (three times daily).

Calcarea carbonica—The child is large and flabby. He has trouble keeping his weight under control. His feet are cold.

Lycopodium—The child craves sweets and gets low blood sugar if he misses a meal. He is irritable.

Natrum muriaticum—For low thyroid that comes on after an emotional grief or trauma. The child craves salt.

Thyroid 1X, 2X, or 3X—Used to tonify

Vital Fact

Congenital hypothyroidism is a condition in which babies are born without thyroid glands, have thyroid enzyme defects, or have defective glands, and thus cannot produce thyroid hormones. This accounts for 1 in 4,000 live births.

---

a weak thyroid gland. Give 2 pellets twice daily for at least 8 weeks.

■ ADVANCED PLAN

Nutritional Supplements

Children's multivitamin—Supplies vitamins A and E and B vitamins, as well as zinc required for thyroid hormone production.

Children's whole food supplement—Give one that contains kelp, a natural source of iodine.

Essential fatty acid complex—Essential fatty acids are required for proper thyroid function. Choose a children's blend that contains omega-3's and omega-6's, and follow the directions on the container. Or give flaxseed oil at the following daily dosages: children 2 and younger, 1 teaspoon; kids 3 to 6, 2 teaspoons; kids 7 and older, 2 to 3 teaspoons. Reduce the dosage if diarrhea occurs.

Acupressure

Stomach 36—Located four finger-widths below the kneecap and one finger-width toward the outside of the leg (outside of the shinbone on the muscle). Gently press the acupressure point with a thumb for 10 to 15 seconds. Perform on both sides of the body and repeat three times each day.

■ WHAT TO EXPECT

Natural therapy is helpful for cases of mild hypothyroidism, where the thyroid gland is producing near normal levels of thyroid hormone. It is essential to work with a holistic doctor.

Immunity Problems

The immune system serves as the army within a child's body. Its mission is to protect the body against foreign invaders, especially bacterial and viral infections and cancers.

When foreign invaders try to infiltrate, a healthy immune system calls its team of white blood cells to serve as the body's frontline defense. Together, these white blood cells, known as leukocytes, ward off infection and repair damage caused by the invaders.

Certain diseases can weaken the immune system and make it vulnerable to bacterial and viral attackers. The biggest disease threat to the immune system is AIDS. AIDS is caused by the HIV virus, which disarms and destroys the body's white blood cells. Less deadly viruses and infectious agents such as the common cold can also weaken the body's immune system.

Common symptoms associated with a weakened immune system include physical exhaustion, colds, sore throats, swollen glands, susceptibility to repeated infections, muscle weakness, and unexplained weight loss.

Factors that may be involved in causing a weakened immune system include:

- Extreme and chronic physical and emotional stress
- Chronic depression
- Poor diets that are high in processed foods, sugar, and saturated and hydrogenated fat
- Obesity and lack of regular physical activity
- Certain medications, including antibiotics and cortisone
- Exposure to toxic substances such as heavy metals (including lead)
- Allergies (food and environmental)
- Nutritional deficiencies (such as of iron, vitamin C, or vitamin A)
- Not enough sleep

The conventional approach is to look for the metabolic cause of the weakened immune system. For example, blood work is done to look for infectious causes. Infections are most commonly treated with antibiotics.

Note that alternative treatment recommendations need to be based on the cause of the weakened immune system. A good history and lab work by your holistic doctor will be helpful in identifying the cause or causes.

■ BASIC PLAN

Diet

Follow a whole-foods diet. (See "Diet" on page 4 for more information.) Quality protein sources are important, such as fish, legumes, nuts, and lean poultry. Decrease the consumption of sugars and soft drinks, which leach minerals out of the body and have a suppressive effect on the immune system. Artificial sweeteners and preservatives should be avoided as well.

Foods that contain essential fatty acids are important for immune system health. Fish such as salmon, halibut, trout, and mackerel are good sources. Fresh fish two or three times weekly is recommended. Flaxseeds are an excellent source of the important alpha linolenic acid (ALA). They can be ground up and sprinkled on salads or added to healthy protein or fruit or vegetable shakes. Grind 1 teaspoon per 50 pounds of body weight (children weighing 30 to 50 pounds may also use 1 teaspoon) and give this amount daily, always with 8 ounces of water.

Breastfeeding is important for a healthy immune system, and in general, infants who are breastfed are more resistant to disease. What the mother eats is important. Food sensitivities passed on to the infant can lead to immune problems. For a bottlefed baby who has a weak immune system, switch to a nondairy formula or hypoallergenic formula. (See The Importance of Breastfeeding on page 123 for more on breast- and bottlefeeding.)

Food sensitivities can lead to a weakened immune system. (See "Food Allergies and Food Sensitivities" on page 298 for more information.)

Adequate fluid intake is important. Make sure that your child is consuming water throughout the day.

Nutritional Supplement

Children's multivitamin—Provides a base of the essential vitamins and minerals for a healthy immune system. Give as directed on the container.

Herbal Remedy

Either **echinacea** or **larix** is a good herb to use for immune system support. Give one of these herbs daily for 4 weeks, then take 2 weeks off, and repeat this cycle if necessary.

Note: Immune-enhancing herbs do not necessarily treat the cause of a child's weakened immune system, but they can be used while the underlying imbalance is being addressed.

■ ADVANCED PLAN

Nutritional Supplements

Vitamin C—Supports the immune system. Dosage: the child's age in years times 50 milligrams, once daily. Reduce the dosage if diarrhea occurs. Consider using a buffered vitamin C powder (nonacidic) or liquid vitamin C. Both work well for infants and children, and can be mixed in juice.

Children's whole food supplement—Choose one that contains a blend of vegetables and fruits. Available in capsule or powder form.

Probiotic—Choose a children's acidophilus with bifidus formula. Use it on a regular basis if your child has a history of antibiotic use, which can wipe out good bacteria and weaken the immune system. Give as directed on the container.

Aromatherapy

Lavender and Roman chamomile—Add 1 drop of each to a vaporizer, or add them to a tissue and keep it under the child's pillow.

Acupressure

Stomach 36—Located four finger-widths below the kneecap and one finger-width toward the outside of the leg (outside of the shinbone on the muscle). Gently press the acupressure point with a thumb for 10 to 15 seconds. Perform on both sides of the body and repeat three times each day.

■ WHAT TO EXPECT

Two to 4 weeks of natural therapy should improve a child's immune status and reduce the susceptibility to disease. Over the long term, natural therapies as outlined in this chapter are a superior way to optimize immune function.

Impetigo

This highly contagious skin infection can appear anywhere on the body, but it tends to show up on exposed areas, especially the face. The infected areas appear in patches ranging from dime to quarter size. They usually start as tiny blisters that erupt. Scratching spreads these eruptions and exposes moist, red skin. After a few days of infection, the affected skin areas are covered with a golden, grainy crust that spreads at the edges.

Impetigo easily spreads from child to child through skin-to-skin contact or shared objects such as desks, toys, and clothing. In severe cases, the infection penetrates a deeper layer of skin and develops into ecthyma, an ulcerated form of the disease. Ecthyma creates tiny, pus-filled ulcers with thick, dark crusts.

Impetigo is caused by either streptococcus or staphylococcus bacteria.

The disease occurs in two forms: bullous and nonbullous impetigo. Bullous impetigo—the less common type—typically affects infants and younger children and often begins on skin near the diaper area. A strain of staphylococcus, it causes transparent, fluid-filled blisters that break easily, releasing clear fluid and leaving shallow skin surrounded by a scaly rim.

Nonbullous impetigo, which accounts for about 70 percent of impetigo cases, generally affects children older than 2. The staphylococcus bacteria attacks the skin, forming tiny, red dots and leaving crusty, honey-hued patches of infected skin. This usually develops near a child's face, arms, and legs and commonly near skin that has been cut, burned, bitten by insects, or affected by chicken pox.

Conventional treatment involves antibiotics and or antibiotic topical cream. This condition should be monitored by a doctor no matter what course of treatment is chosen. If antibiotics are used, the natural recommendations can be used as well to speed up healing.

■ BASIC PLAN

Diet

Follow a whole-foods diet that is free of refined sugars (see "Diet" on page 4). Increase the intake of purified water to help skin healing. Soups, broths, and steamed vegetables are excellent.

Nutritional Supplements

Vitamin C—Supports the immune system. Dosage: the child's age in years times 50 milligrams, twice daily. Reduce the dosage if diarrhea occurs. Consider using a buffered vitamin C powder (nonacidic) or liquid vitamin C. Both work well for infants and children, and can be mixed in juice.

Zinc—Supports the immune system and enhances skin healing. Dosage: children 2 and younger, 5 milligrams; 2 and older, 10 to 15 milligrams. Use for 2 weeks and then stop.

Herbal Remedies

Echinacea and goldenseal combination—Taken internally, this combination has a strong antimicrobial effect by enhancing the immune system. Give until the infection has cleared up.

Propolis—This resinous substance from beeswax has potent antimicrobial effects when applied to the skin. Available as a tincture, a liquid spray, or a cream. Apply to the affected areas three times daily.

Homeopathy

Pick the following remedy that best matches your child's symptoms. Unless otherwise indicated, give your child 2 pellets of a 30C potency twice daily. (For infants, crush the pellets into powder and mix it with water.) Improvements should be seen within 48 hours. If there is no improvement within 48 hours, try another remedy. After you first notice improvement, stop giving the remedy unless symptoms begin to return.

Note: Lower potencies (6X, 12X, 6C) may need to be given more often (three times daily).

Antimonium crudum—For pustules and pimples that are itchy. Symptoms are worse after a bath or from the heat of bed. The child's tongue has a thick, white coating.

Arsenicum album—For a skin infection that burns and itches.

Graphites—For sticky, honey-colored fluid that oozes from the skin. Severe itching is made worse by heat and baths, and is better with cold.

Rhus toxicodendron—For moist eruptions that are itchy and that make the child very restless.

Sulphur—The child has a tendency to develop skin problems. She scratches her skin until it bleeds. She is very warm and has a high thirst for cold drinks.

■ ADVANCED PLAN

Nutritional Supplements

Vitamin A—Supports the immune system. Daily dosage: infants under 1 year, 1,875 international units (IU); children 1 to 3, 2,000 IU; kids 4 to 6, 2,500 IU; kids 7 to 10, 3,500 IU; males 11 and older, 5,000 IU; females 11 and older, 4,000 IU.

Note: These dosages are for short-term use (up to 10 days). Higher dosages may be used only under a doctor's supervision. Available in liquid drops.

Probiotic—If your child is given antibiotics, make sure to supplement with children's acidophilus and bifidus for 2 months to replace the good bacteria. Give as directed on the container.

Herbal Remedies

Tea tree oil—Best used as a cream with children, or dilute 5 drops in 2 cups of water and apply it to the skin with a cotton swab.

Calendula—Has disinfectant and antimicrobial properties. Apply topically as a tincture (diluted, 1 teaspoon of tincture in 4 teaspoons of water) or cream.

■ WHAT TO EXPECT

Improvements should be seen within 48 hours.

Insomnia

Forget that old saying "sleep like a baby." In reality, babies rarely sleep more than 6 hours at a stretch. More commonly, they awaken hungry and demand food by crying. Or they awaken due to teething pain or soiled diapers.

Regardless of a person's age, normal sleep patterns consist of alternating cycles of rapid eye movement (REM) sleep and non-REM sleep. REM, the lighter stage of sleep, is when we dream. The non-REM is the deeper, sound sleep. Babies and young children have shorter sleep cycles than adults.

Insomnia, or sleeplessness, can occur at any age. This condition is characterized by frequent difficulty falling and/or staying asleep. Insomnia can be a temporary or long-term problem.

Common symptoms beyond trouble falling asleep include waking up frequently in the night, a fatigued feeling the next morning, and a feeling of restlessness as bedtime approaches.

Nightmares, depression, anxiety, stress, or a chronic condition such as fever or an ear infection can cause insomnia. So can underlying medical problems such as hyperthyroidism, sleep apnea (a temporary cessation of breathing during sleep), or restless leg syndrome. And don't forget, a noisy environment, before-bedtime meals, and television before bed can disturb sleep.

Persistent sleeplessness can interfere with your child's (not to mention your own) ability to stay alert during the day.

■ BASIC PLAN

Diet

Sugar products should be avoided before bedtime, as they can cause nightmares. Foods that contain caffeine, such as soft drinks and chocolate, should be avoided in the evening, as they are too stimulating.

Avoid giving your child fluids for an hour or two before bedtime so that he does not wake to go to the bathroom.

Occasionally, food sensitivities can cause insomnia. (See "Food Allergies and Food Sensitivities" on page 298 for more information.)

Herbal Remedy

Passionflower—A gentle herb to relax the nervous system and promote sleep. Use for the relief of acute insomnia. Follow the herbal dosage information for acute conditions on page 139, up to a maximum of 30 drops. Give the remedy 30 minutes before bedtime.

Homeopathy

Pick the following remedy that best matches your child's symptoms. Unless otherwise indicated, give your child 2 pellets of a 30C potency 30 minutes before bedtime, and once more if he awakens. (For infants, crush the pellets into powder and mix it with water.) If there is no improvement with the second dose, try another remedy.

Aconitum napellus—For insomnia characterized by a child who is restless and fearful. Also for insomnia from fright or shock.

Arsenicum album—The child wakes up between midnight and 2:00 A.M. He is restless and anxious. He wakes up from a bad dream. The insomnia is due to anxiety and worry.

Chamomilla—For insomnia from ear infections or teething. The child is irritable, screaming, and wants to be carried or rocked (which helps only temporarily).

Coffea cruda—For a child who is overly excited from an event or from good or bad news that keeps him awake. He is hypersensitive to sound, and overstimulated and restless.

Ignatia—For insomnia from grief or disappointing news. The child cries uncontrollably. He twitches and jerks during sleep.

Kali phosphoricum—The child has anxiety and suffers from nightmares. If you are unsure which remedy to use, try this one or a combination insomnia remedy.

Nux vomica—The child wakes up between 3:00 and 4:00 A.M. He is worried or anxious about the next day's events at school or in sports. He is a competitive and irritable child. Also for insomnia from spicy or rich food.

Pulsatilla—The child has separation anxiety about sleeping by himself away from parents. He is a very emotionally sensitive child and is afraid of the dark.

Rhus toxicodendron—The child is very restless and has trouble falling asleep from stiff or aching muscles and joints.

Stramonium—For insomnia as the result of night terrors—visions of violence.

Staphysagria—For trouble sleeping as the result of suppressed emotions. This is a common remedy for abused children.

■ ADVANCED PLAN

Aromatherapy

Orange and lavender—Add 1 drop of each to a tissue and place it under the child's pillow. If the child is taking a homeopathic remedy, use aromatherapy at a different time.

Acupressure

Four Gates—This is a combination of Liver 3, located on top of the foot in the hollow between the big toe and second toe, and Large Intestine 4, located in the webbing between the thumb and index finger. Two people should push on all four points gently at the same time for 15 seconds. Repeat three times. Do this once daily.

■ WHAT TO EXPECT

If the child is having insomnia one night, then the correct treatment may help him fall asleep within an hour. For chronic insomnia, expect improved sleep within 5 to 7 days of natural therapy. Homeopathy is the best choice for infants.

Irritability

It is inevitable that at times your child is going to be irritable. This may be a normal part of her personality, or it can be a sign of imbalances in the body. The irritability may be the result of a condition such as the common cold or teething. Dietary or nutritional deficiencies can be a cause as well. If the irritability seems to be a chronic problem, have your pediatrician check to make sure there is no underlying illness. The following natural therapies can be helpful.

■ BASIC PLAN

Diet

Fluctuating blood sugar levels can cause or worsen irritability. Make sure that your child is eating regular meals. Sugar products can lead to blood sugar imbalances and irritability, as can food sensitivities, particularly to artificial preservatives and sweeteners. (See "Food Allergies and Food Sensitivities" on page 298.)

Foods may play a role in children who are breastfed, and a breastfeeding mother's diet should be analyzed for food sensitivities.

Herbal Remedy

Chamomile—Use for the temporary relief of irritability.

Homeopathy

Pick the following remedy that best matches your child's symptoms. Unless otherwise indicated, give your child 2 pellets of a 30C potency two times daily. (For infants, crush the pellets into powder and mix it with water.) Improvements should be seen within 5 days. If there is no improvement within 5 days, try another remedy. After you first notice improvement, stop giving the remedy unless symptoms begin to return.

Note: Lower potencies (6X, 12X, 6C) may need to be given more often (three times daily).

Calcarea phosphorica—The child is irritable and whiny and wants constant attention. She is dissatisfied and gets bored easily.

Chamomilla—The child gets angry and very irritable easily. She demands things, and when they are given to her, she throws them away. For irritability caused by colic, ear infections, or teething.

Lycopodium—The child wants to be the boss and is irritable when she does not get her way. Irritability is worse from missing a meal.

Pulsatilla—The child has a very changeable mood; she is sweet one moment and irritable the next.

Nux vomica—The child has a competitive and easily irritated personality type. She often suffers from digestive problems.

Kali phosphoricum 6X and Magnesia phosphorica 6X—This combination is useful to help relax a child when the irritability is caused by stress. Give 2 pellets of each remedy twice daily (alternating, with 2 to 3 hours between them).

■ ADVANCED PLAN

Homeopathy

Beech Bach Flower Remedy—The child is critical and intolerant. Give 2 drops twice daily. Stop when the child has improved. If there is no improvement within 2 weeks, try another Bach Flower Remedy or consult with a practitioner.

Aromatherapy

Lavender—Soothing. Add 1 drop to a vaporizer or add it to a carrier oil and massage the child with it. If the child is taking a homeopathic remedy, use aromatherapy at a different time.

Acupressure

Four Gates—helps to release tension. This is a combination of Liver 3, located on top of the foot in the hollow between the big toe and second toe, and Large Intestine 4, located in the webbing between the thumb and index finger. Two people should push on all four points gently at the same time for 15 seconds. Repeat two times. Do this once daily.

■ WHAT TO EXPECT

You should see a reduction in your child's tendency toward irritability over 1 to 2 weeks.

Irritable Bowel Syndrome

Irritable bowel syndrome (IBS), as its name implies, is not a disease but rather a functional disorder associated with spastic colon. IBS ranks as the number one gastrointestinal disorder, affecting women twice as often as men.

Although IBS can strike at any age, it usually first appears during the late teens and early twenties. The most common symptoms are severe stomach cramping, constipation and/or diarrhea, fatigue, and flatulence. Other symptoms may include bloating, a feeling of fullness in the rectum, heartburn, indigestion, and nausea. These symptoms can surface after eating a large meal or when under a lot of stress.

There are many causes of IBS. Stress, food sensitivities, and depression can trigger attacks. IBS is difficult to identify because there are no specific medical tests for it. It is diagnosed by ruling out other medical conditions such as ulcers, Crohn's disease, colitis, and colon cancer.

■ BASIC PLAN

Diet

It is very important that your child's food sensitivities be identified and dealt with. Common ones include cow's milk and dairy products, wheat, sugar, soy, citrus fruits, and sugar. (See "Food Allergies and Food Sensitivities" on page 298 for more information.)

Easy-to-digest foods are recommended, such as soups, broths, steamed and cooked vegetables (reduce the intake of raw vegetables), rice, and wheat alternative breads and pastas. Refined sugar products should be eliminated or reduced, as should artificial sweeteners and preservatives.

Fiber is important with this condition. You can add more fiber to your child's diet with steamed and cooked vegetables such as broccoli, cauliflower, and carrots. Oatmeal provides fiber as well. Ground flaxseeds help to provide additional fiber. Grind 1 teaspoon of flaxseeds per 50 pounds of body weight (children weighing 30 to 50 pounds may also use 1 teaspoon) and give this amount daily with 8 ounces of water.

Nutritional Supplement

Probiotic—A children's acidophilus supplement that contains bifidus can be helpful to improve digestion and elimination. It is especially important for infants who have been on antibiotics. Give as directed on the container.

Herbal Remedies

Use one of the following herbs with each meal or anytime to relieve digestive symptoms.

Ginger—Relieves nausea, cramps, and flatulence. Works best as a fresh tea but is helpful in the tincture or capsule form. If using fresh ginger root to make a tea, make a decoction. If using a tea bag, make an infusion. (See "Herbal Preparations" on page 30 for more on tea decoctions and infusions.)

Chamomile—Reduces intestinal cramping and bloating, and relaxes the nervous system. Use as a tea or in the tincture form.

Homeopathy

Pick the following remedy that best matches your child's symptoms. Unless otherwise indicated, give your child 2 pellets of a 30C potency two times daily. Improvements should be seen within 7 to 10 days. If there is no improvement within 10 days, try another remedy. After you first notice improvement, stop giving the remedy unless symptoms begin to return.

Note: Lower potencies (6X, 12X, 6C) may need to be given more often (three times daily).

Colocynthis—The child suffers from abdominal cramping and bends over to relieve pain. Discomfort is also relieved through pressure and hot applications (such as a hot water bottle on the abdomen).

Ignatia—For digestive problems from emotional stress. The child experiences cramping and changeable digestive symptoms.

Lycopodium—The child experiences a lot of gas and bloating. His abdomen feels better with warm applications. Symptoms are worse between 4:00 and 8:00 P.M.

Nux vomica—For problems with intestinal cramps and constipation. Symptoms are worse with anger. The child is chilly and irritable.

Phosphorus—For burning pains in the stomach. The child craves and feels better with cold drinks. He is anxious and gets easily excited. Symptoms are worse before bedtime and when he is hungry.

Pulsatilla—For digestive upset after eating greasy and rich foods, and also fruit. The stool is changeable. The child desires attention.

The following Bach Flower Remedies can help alleviate some of the stress associated with this condition. Give 2 drops twice daily. Stop when the child has improved. If there is no improvement within 2 weeks, try another Bach Flower Remedy or consult with a practitioner.

Aspen—For a child who has underlying issues with fear and anxiety.

White chestnut—For a child who has underlying issues with persistent worry.

■ ADVANCED PLAN

Nutritional Supplements

Plant-derived enzymes—Give 1 to 2 capsules of plant enzymes with meals to help break down food more efficiently. Especially helpful for hard-to-digest foods, such as fast foods.

L-glutamine—This amino acid helps in repairing the digestive tract. Give 3 milligrams per pound of body weight daily.

Colostrum—Helps to repair the digestive tract and improve digestion. Give as directed on the container.

Herbal Remedies

Peppermint—Reduces intestinal spasms and is soothing to the digestive tract.

Gentian—Stimulates the digestive organs to function more efficiently. Give 5 drops in ¼

Vital Study

A study done by the University of Missouri looked at 42 children, ages 8 to 17, with irritable bowel syndrome (IBS). Children took one or two capsules of enteric-coated peppermint oil or a placebo three times daily for 2 weeks. Each capsule contained 187 milligrams of peppermint oil. At the end of the 2-week study, 76 percent of the children receiving peppermint oil reported having less pain with IBS.

cup of water at the beginning of each meal. Avoid if heartburn is present.

Fennel—Reduces gas and spasms, and stimulates stomach function.

Note: Digestive formulas that contain a combination of digestive herbs (such as the ones listed) are also available.

Aromatherapy

German chamomile—Add it to a carrier oil and rub onto the child's abdomen. If the child is taking a homeopathic remedy, use aromatherapy at a different time.

Acupressure

Gently press each of the following acupressure points with a thumb for 10 to 15 seconds. Perform on both sides of the body and repeat two times each day.

Liver 3—Located on top of the foot in the hollow between the big toe and second toe.

Pericardium 6—Located 2½ finger-widths below the wrist crease, in the middle of the forearm (palm side).

■ WHAT TO EXPECT

Improvements should be noticed within 2 to 3 weeks of treatment.

Jet Lag

Jet lag, that fuzzy, out-of-sorts feeling that lingers after you deplane from a long flight, can affect anyone at any age. This woozy feeling especially impacts individuals who must pass through two or more time zones to arrive at their destinations.

Symptoms associated with jet lag vary among travelers, but they often include the following: fatigue, irritability, daytime drowsiness, difficulty concentrating, disorientation, sleeplessness, headaches, and leg swelling. These symptoms may be mild or severe.

Most commercial airlines reach cruising altitudes of 30,000 feet, but the aircraft is pressurized to about 8,000 feet. This altitude difference can cause some travelers to feel lethargic and develop swelling in their extremities. The stale air and lack of humidity inside the cabin can also aggravate jet lag symptoms.

It's important to realize how jet lag can occur. Crossing time zones plays havoc with your built-in body clock, known as the circadian rhythm. Your internal clock is regulated by the hypothalamus gland, located in the brain. This gland processes nerve signals.

Your body clock is designed to expect regular cycles of daylight and darkness. Crossing time zones can throw this cycle out of sync. Children traveling across the country (east to west or west to east) are more affected by jet lag than those traveling north to south or south to north within the same time zone. Low levels of dehydration can also contribute to symptoms.

■ BASIC PLAN

Diet

Adequate water intake is the most important dietary concern. Higher altitudes can lead to dehydration. Make sure that your child is drinking water before, during, and after the flight. Keep in mind that soft drinks cause dehydration.

Nutritional Supplement

Vitamin C—Supports the immune system while flying. The type with bioflavonoids is preferable. Dosage: the child's age in years times 50 milligrams, once daily while flying. Reduce the dosage if diarrhea occurs. Consider using a buffered vitamin C powder (nonacidic) or liquid vitamin C. Both work well for infants and children, and can be mixed in juice.

Herbal Remedy

Chamomile is great herb to help with all the postflight symptoms of jet lag, as well as with anxiety or digestive upset while flying.

Homeopathy

Gelsemium 30C—Helps relieve the symptoms of jet lag, including fatigue and dizziness. If needed, give your child 2 pellets right after landing and another 2 pellets 1 hour later.

Bach Flower Rescue Remedy—This is excellent to use the day of flying and while flying, to help prevent jet lag symptoms. Add 5 drops to a child's water bottle and have her sip on it before flying and during the trip.

■ ADVANCED PLAN

Herbal Remedy

Passionflower—Use if needed to help your child get to sleep. Give 20 minutes before bedtime.

Aromatherapy

Add 2 drops of linden blossom (10 percent strength) to a tissue and place it under the child's pillow. If the child is taking a homeopathic remedy, use aromatherapy at a different time.

Acupressure

Four Gates—This is a combination of Liver 3, located on top of the foot in the hollow between the big toe and second toe, and Large Intestine 4, located in the webbing between the thumb and index finger. Two people should push on all four points gently at the same time for 15 seconds. Repeat three times. Do once daily.

■ WHAT TO EXPECT

You should see a reduction in jet lag symptoms when the natural therapies in this chapter are followed. We do not recommend melatonin for children in the treatment of jet lag.

Jock Itch

A common fungal infection, jock itch causes itchiness, redness, and scaliness in the groin and upper thigh areas. Although it is medically known as tinea cruris, this condition got its nickname—jock itch—because it occurs more often among males than females.

Fungal growth develops when heat and moisture get trapped against the skin due to snug-fitting athletic supporters or tight underwear. Sharing or reusing damp towels can also cause the fungi to multiply quickly, especially during warm weather.

Jock itch creates semicircular, scaly rashes that itch and burn.

If the condition persists for more than 2 weeks or worsens despite self-treatment, check with your doctor. It is possible that you may have confused this rash for jock itch when the true diagnosis may be psoriasis or contact dermatitis. Your doctor can confirm the diagnosis by taking a skin scraping and examining it under a microscope.

Conventional treatment consists of topical antifungal creams.

■ BASIC PLAN

Diet

Avoid refined sugars; fungi thrive on them. Food sources to avoid include sugar, soft drinks, and highly processed foods. Include garlic and onions in your child's diet if he's not sensitive to them; they have antifungal properties. Yogurt with live cultures (no sugar added) helps to increase the good bacteria that fight off fungus. Choose plain yogurt, rather than flavored, and add your own fruit.

Nutritional Supplement

Probiotic—A children's acidophilus and bifidus formula supplies the good bacteria that keep yeast and other microbes in check in the body. Give as directed on the container.

Herbal Remedy

Tea tree oil—Apply a cream or salve to the area twice daily. Make sure that the concentration is not too strong by applying a small amount to the skin for a few hours first. If no reaction occurs, then use it for the next 2 to 3 weeks.

Homeopathy

Pick the following remedy that best matches your child's symptoms. Unless otherwise indicated, give your child 2 pellets of a 30C potency two times daily. Improvements should be seen within 7 to 10 days. If there is no improvement within 10 days, try another remedy. After you first notice improvement, stop giving the remedy unless symptoms begin to return.

Note: Lower potencies (6X, 12X, 6C) may need to be given more often (three times daily).

Psorinum—For long-standing cases of jock itch that do not respond to other remedies.

Sulphur—For skin that is red and very itchy.

You can also see a homeopathic practitioner for an individualized remedy.

■ ADVANCED PLAN

Herbal Remedy

Echinacea—Stimulates the immune system and has antifungal properties. Give twice daily for 2 weeks.

■ WHAT TO EXPECT

You should notice improvement within 10 days of treatment.

Lactose Intolerance

This condition occurs when a baby or child cannot digest lactose, the sugar found in milk. Lactose is a disaccharide, the main sugar found in the milk of most mammals.

In some children, a vital enzyme called lactase is missing from their digestive systems. This enzyme is necessary to break down these disaccharides into simple sugars for absorption. Most nonwhite North American children become lactase-deficient between the ages of 10 and 20.

When lactose is not digested properly, water is retained in the bowels. This can trigger bloating, watery diarrhea, abdominal cramping, flatulence, vomiting, irritability, and dehydration. These symptoms often emerge after cow's milk or lactose-containing formula is introduced into your baby's diet. In children, the symptoms usually appear within 6 hours after drinking one or two glasses of milk or consuming a large amount of dairy products, especially on an empty stomach.

Conventional treatment is similar to the natural approach—that is, to avoid foods containing lactose or to supplement with the enzyme lactase.

■ BASIC PLAN

Diet

Foods containing lactose should be avoided unless lactase enzymes are helpful. These foods include dairy products such as cow's milk, ice cream, and cottage cheese. Aged cheeses tend to have less lactose and may be tolerated, depending on the child. Yogurt with live cultures may be tolerated by some children, as the live cultures produce the lactose-digesting enzyme lactase.

Nutritional Supplement

Lactase enzymes—Work to break down the sugar lactose. They are available in grocery stores, pharmacies, and health food stores. Give as directed on the container.

■ WHAT TO EXPECT

You should see immediate improvement once lactose-containing foods are avoided or reduced. Lactase enzymes can also produce dramatic improvement.

Case History

Five-year-old Andrew had chronic digestive problems that mainly included bloating and diarrhea. His parents thought that he might have lactose intolerance, but they had never put him on a strict lactose-free diet. We told them that since Andrew was African-American, there was a good chance that he did have lactose intolerance. One week of a lactose-free diet confirmed the diagnosis, and Andrew's digestive problems disappeared. For times when the family eats out or when Andrew wants to eat dairy products, his parents give him an enzyme supplement containing lactase.

Laryngitis

Laryngitis robs babies and children of their ability to speak clearly and easily. The condition can lead to hoarseness and even to loss of voice.

For infants and young children, this condition can result in a narrowing of the airway, causing breathing problems. Parents often describe their babies as having a seal-sounding bark or croupy cough. Other symptoms may include hoarseness, difficulty breathing, and a noisy intake of breath.

In older children, the symptoms are typically a sore throat and a hoarse, whisperlike voice. A child will often complain that her throat hurts or tickles when she speaks. Her voice box becomes inflamed. There are usually no symptoms of fever, body aches, diarrhea, or vomiting.

Most cases of laryngitis are caused by a viral infection. Less frequently, laryngitis can develop from a simple irritation of the voice box or vocal cords. These throat irritations can be caused by a child who talks, shouts, or sings loudly or for a long time. Teenagers who smoke cigarettes or drink alcohol can also develop laryngitis. In rare cases, the hoarseness is due to a tumor or enlarged thyroid.

Seek medical attention if your child exhibits any of the following symptoms:

- Trouble swallowing or breathing
- Fever
- Chills
- Uncontrollable drooling (in older children)

Voice rest and steam inhalation are the conventional treatments. Since laryngitis is most often a viral infection, antibiotics are ineffective. Bacterial bronchitis that accompanies laryngitis is treated with antibiotics.

■ BASIC PLAN

Diet

Avoid refined sugars, which suppress the immune system. Food sources to avoid include sugar, soft drinks, and highly processed foods. Soups and broths containing garlic and onions are helpful for their antiviral effect.

Nutritional Supplement

Vitamin C—Supports the immune system and has mild anti-inflammatory effects. The type with bioflavonoids is preferable. Dosage: the child's age in years times 50 milligrams, twice daily. Reduce the dosage if diarrhea occurs. Consider using a buffered vitamin C powder (nonacidic) or liquid vitamin C. Both work well for infants and children, and can be mixed in juice.

Herbal Remedies

Slippery elm—Soothing to the throat. Give as a lozenge (for children old enough not to choke on it) or use the tincture, capsule, or powder form.

Echinacea—Supports the immune system and has antiviral effects.

Note: Avoid the use of the herb goldenseal, which can have a drying effect on the throat.

Homeopathy

Pick the following remedy that best matches your child's symptoms. Unless otherwise indicated, give your child 2 pellets of a 30C potency three times daily. (For infants, crush the pellets into powder and mix it with water.) Improvements should be seen within 2 days. If there is no improvement within 2 days, try another remedy. After you first notice improvement, stop giving the remedy unless symptoms begin to return.

Note: Lower potencies (6X, 12X, 6C) may need to be given more often (four times daily).

Aconitum napellus—For sudden onset of laryngitis, especially after the child is exposed to a cold, dry wind. There is fever, and the child is restless and anxious.

Arum triphyllum—For hoarseness from singing or too much talking.

Causticum—For a raw and burning throat. There is a tickling sensation and mucus formation. The child is constantly trying to clear her throat. Symptoms are worse with cold, dry weather and speaking. A good remedy for chronic laryngitis.

Phosphorus—The most common remedy for laryngitis. There is a raw, burning sensation in the throat and a tickling cough. The child's throat feels worse with talking and cold air, and better with ice-cold drinks or cold food.

Spongia tosta—For hoarseness and constriction in the throat. The child's throat feels worse when swallowing and better with warm food or drinks.

Hydrotherapy

Alternate a warm face cloth (3 minutes) and a cold face cloth (1 minute) over the throat area. Repeat three times, and end with the cold cloth.

■ ADVANCED PLAN

Nutritional Supplements

Zinc—Supports the immune system and enhances skin healing. Dosage: children 2 and younger, 5 milligrams; 2 and older, 10 to 15 milligrams. Use for 2 weeks and then stop. Available as a lozenge (zinc gluconate) for children old enough to suck it without choking (over age 5).

Vitamin A—Supports the immune system. Daily dosage: infants under 1 year, 1,875 international units (IU); children 1 to 3, 2,000 IU; kids 4 to 6, 2,500 IU; kids 7 to 10, 3,500 IU; males 11 and older, 5,000 IU; females 11 and older, 4,000 IU.

Note: These dosages are for short-term use (up to 10 days). Higher dosages may be used only under a doctor's supervision. Available in liquid drops.

Herbal Remedy

Licorice root—Very soothing to the throat. Also has antiviral, anticough properties.

Aromatherapy

Eucalyptus and lavender—Add 2 or 3 drops of each to a vaporizer in your child's room. This will help to clear and moisten her throat. If your child is taking a homeopathic remedy, use aromatherapy at a different time.

Acupressure

Triple Warmer 17—Located directly below the bottom of the earlobe, in the depression behind the jaw. Gently press the acupressure point with a thumb for 10 to 15 seconds. Perform on both sides of the body and repeat three times each day.

■ WHAT TO EXPECT

You should see improvement within 2 to 3 days of treatment and resolution within 7 days.

Lice

Lice are extremely small parasites that live and feed on skin. No bigger than the size of a sesame seed, these parasites bite into the skin and suck blood for food. Their saliva gets

Vital Fact

About 12 million cases of lice are discovered each year, mostly among preschool and elementary school age children. Children at these ages frequently share combs, brushes, hats, towels, school gym mats, sleeping bags, or bed linens.

trapped under the skin and causes it to redden and itch.

The six-legged adult lice lay grayish white, oval eggs called nits that cling to the base of hair shafts. The stage between nit and adult is called nymph. It takes a nymph about 7 days to evolve into adulthood. Unable to leap or fly, lice spread from one infested child to another by direct contact or when children share combs, hats, and clothing. A lice infestation is not a reflection of a child's hygiene. Lice live in warm and crowded environments, such as classrooms and day care centers.

Lice can easily be mistaken for dandruff, but unlike dandruff flakes, lice stick to the hair shaft, making the hair look matted. They can be tricky to detect because they move quickly and shy away from bright light. A flashlight can help to identify them more easily. Some children with lice may also develop swollen glands, especially at the back of the scalp or in the groin area.

Conventional treatment involves anti-lice shampoos and the quarantining of children infected with lice.

■ BASIC PLAN

Contact your child's day care or school if you discover lice. Other children who have been in contact with your child should be checked for lice. Your child should not be in contact with other children until the lice has cleared up, which usually takes a few days.

Diet

Soups and foods containing onions and garlic (if your child is not sensitive to these foods) are of some benefit for their antiparasitic effect.

Aromatherapy

Mix 2 drops each of tea tree oil and lavender oil into 4 ounces of olive oil or 4 ounces of your child's shampoo. Massage the mixture into your child's hair and scalp, and do not rinse. Cover your child's head with a shower cap until morning. In the morning, add 5 drops of tea tree oil to a nit or fine-tooth comb, and comb the hair to remove the eggs. Rinse your child's hair, then blow it dry for 5 to 10 minutes (this helps to destroy the eggs). Repeat this procedure for 7 days.

Note: This treatment requires more work than conventional anti-lice shampoos but is also far less toxic. Make sure to not get oils into your child's yes.

Homeopathy

Sulphur—Give your child 2 pellets of a 30C potency twice daily for 3 days. (For infants, crush the pellets into powder and mix it with water.) For a more aggressive treatment, give Sulphur once daily and the homeopathic Psorinum 30C once daily for 3 days.

Other Recommendations

Wash everything with which your child comes into contact, using hot water. This includes all clothes, towels, and bedding. Make sure that combs and similar items are not shared among family members.

■ WHAT TO EXPECT

Lice can be tricky to treat. Just when you think they have been cleared up, they show up again. Up to 2 weeks of treatment is often required.

Lyme Disease

This potentially serious, long-lasting infection is caused by a spirochete—a spiral-shaped bacterium—called *Borrelia burgdorferi*. Lyme disease is spread by infected deer ticks. These tiny ticks feed on deer and mice.

Lyme disease was first identified in Lyme, Connecticut, (hence its name) but cases have been documented in most of the United States and in other countries. It is most common in the Middle Atlantic and southern New England states, and in California—places abundant with wooded areas.

A child becomes infected when bitten by a tick that carries the bacteria. The bite is extremely hard to detect and usually painless.

Symptoms vary among children and can come and go. Lyme disease is dubbed the Great Imitator by medical experts because it often mimics other illnesses and can be easily missed in the early stages.

Here are the progressive stages of Lyme disease:

Early stage: Within a week of the tick bite, a bull's-eye, red, ring-shaped rash appears (50 percent of the time) at the site. Within a couple of weeks, the ring grows in size, up to 6 inches in diameter. During this stage, the child may suffer muscle soreness, headaches, fever, swollen glands, and red eyes. People who have experienced this condition describe the initial stage as flulike in its symptoms. Symptoms usually develop within 3 days to 3 weeks after the tick bites.

Middle stage: Left untreated, within weeks to months of the bite, the disease can evolve and cause meningitis (inflammation of the membranes covering the brain), carditis (swelling of the heart muscle, producing irregular rhythms), or facial nerve palsy.

Late stage: The child may develop arthritis, especially in his hips or knees. In rare instances, the central nervous system is impacted.

One of the reasons this condition can become chronic is that the infecting bacteria get into the immune cells (lymphocytes) and can trigger an autoimmune reaction, whereby the immune system attacks its own cells and tissues. This leads to the release of inflammatory chemicals by the immune system, which results in pain, fatigue, and swelling.

Vital Fact

The U.S. Environmental Protection Agency (EPA) is requiring changes to insect repellent labels to ensure that DEET (N,N-diethyl-meta-toluamide) is applied safely, particularly to children. Companies that make and distribute DEET products will no longer be able to claim that their products are child-safe, and new labels will direct parents not to allow children to handle these products. (Currently, "child safe" claims are allowed on products that contain 15 percent or less of the active ingredient DEET.) New directions for use will also include the following statements:

- Do not use on hands or near the eyes and mouths of young children.
- Do not use under clothing.
- Avoid overapplication of the product.
- After returning indoors, wash treated skin with soap and water, and wash treated clothing.

DEET is registered by the EPA for both human and veterinary uses to help prevent bites from mosquitoes, ticks, and other insects that may transmit diseases such as Lyme disease, malaria, and encephalitis.

Early diagnosis is key with Lyme disease. The conventional treatment is antibiotic therapy for 2 to 6 weeks (and sometimes longer), as well as pain relievers such as aspirin and acetaminophen. Most cases respond to early treatment with antibiotics, although every case is different. A vaccine is available but is not recommended for people under 15 years of age.

■ BASIC PLAN

Prevention

According to the U.S. Centers for Disease Control and Prevention, the following three recommendations are important in preventing Lyme disease:

1. Avoidance of tick habitat. Whenever possible, avoid entering areas that are likely to be infested with ticks—particularly in spring and summer, when nymph-stage ticks feed. Ticks favor a moist, shaded environment, especially that provided by leaf litter and low-lying vegetation in wooded, brushy, or overgrown grassy habitat.

2. Personal protection. Anyone who is exposed to tick-infested areas should wear light-colored clothing so that ticks can be spotted more easily and removed before becoming attached. Wearing long-sleeve shirts and tucking pants into socks or boot tops may help keep ticks from reaching the skin. Ticks are usually located close to the ground, so wearing high rubber boots may provide additional protection.

Applying insect repellents containing DEET (diethyl-meta-toluamide) or permethrin (which kills ticks on contact) to clothes should also help reduce the risk of tick attachment.

DEET can be used safely on both children and adults but should be applied according to Environmental Protection Agency guidelines to reduce the possibility of toxicity. (See "Vital Fact" on opposite page for more information.)

3. Tick check and removal. Since transmission of *B. burgdorferi* from an infected tick is unlikely to occur before 36 hours of tick attachment, daily checks for ticks and their prompt removal will help prevent infection. Embedded ticks should be removed using fine-tip tweezers. *Do not* use petroleum jelly, a hot match, nail polish, or other products. Grasp the tick firmly and as closely to the skin as possible. With a steady motion, pull the tick's body away from the skin. The tick's mouth parts may remain in the skin, but do not be alarmed. The bacteria that cause Lyme disease are contained in the tick's midgut. Cleanse the area with an antiseptic.

Diet

A whole-foods diet is recommended to optimize the immune system. (See "Diet" on page 4 for more information.) Avoid refined sugars, which suppress the immune system. Foods to avoid include sugar, soft drinks, and highly processed foods. In addition, limit dairy products and fast foods, both of which are potentially harmful to the immune system.

Nutritional Supplements

Children's multivitamin—Provides a base of the essential vitamins and minerals for a healthy immune system. In addition, B vitamins are depleted by antibiotics, which your child

> ## Vital Fact
> People of all ages and both sexes are equally susceptible to Lyme disease. But the highest occurrence rates are in children from birth to 14 years of age and in adults 30 years and older.

will most likely be given. A children's multivitamin helps to replenish these missing nutrients.

Probiotic—Give a children's acidophilus supplement that contains bifidus, to replenish good bacteria that antibiotics destroy. Give as directed on the container while your child is on the antibiotics, and for 2 months or longer after the antibiotics are done.

Herbal Remedy

Echinacea—Supports the immune system.

Homeopathy

Gelsemium 30C—For symptoms of muscle aches, fatigue, weakness, and dizziness. Give 2 pellets once daily as needed for relief of these symptoms.

You can also see a homeopathic practitioner for a specific constitutional remedy.

Constitutional Hydrotherapy

Use this for immune system support and to reduce pain in the muscles and joints. (See Hydrotherapy for Children on page 115 for details on this therapy.)

■ ADVANCED PLAN

Nutritional Supplements

Vitamin C—Supports the immune system and has mild anti-inflammatory effects. The type with bioflavonoids is preferable. Dosage: the child's age in years times 50 milligrams, twice daily. Reduce the dosage if diarrhea occurs. Consider using a buffered vitamin C powder (nonacidic) or liquid vitamin C. Both work well for infants and children, and can be mixed in juice.

Calcium and magnesium—These help to relax the nervous system and muscles, which may have a tendency to spasm. We recommend 500 milligrams of calcium and 250 to 500 milligrams of magnesium daily, given with meals.

Coenzyme Q$_{10}$—Necessary for energy production in cells. Also helps to combat fatigue. Depending on the age and weight of the child, 25 to 50 milligrams is recommended daily, given with a meal. Use under the direction of a doctor.

Thymus glandular extract—Works to balance and support the immune system. Give two 250-milligram tablets or capsules daily, or give as directed on the container.

■ WHAT TO EXPECT

We recommend antibiotic therapy as soon as the disease has been diagnosed. Natural therapy should be used as a complementary treatment to support the immune system. Early therapy improves the likelihood of recovery from the disease.

Measles

Also known as rubeola, measles is a highly contagious childhood viral infection distinguished by a red, bumpy rash.

Infected children (and sometimes adults) spread measles when they wipe their noses, sneeze, or cough, and their respiratory secretions and droplets come into contact with others.

The initial symptoms are usually a runny nose, a persistent cough, eyes that easily redden and tear, fatigue, and increasing fever. The next classic symptom is blue-white spots (called Koplik's spots) with a red background that occur on the inside of the mouth. Then, within 1 to 2 days after the Koplik's spots are visible, the characteristic measles rash appears. Next comes a red, slightly bumpy rash that first appears below the ears and neck and spreads all over the body within 24 hours. The fine, red spots on the body enlarge to splotches but are only mildly itchy or not itchy at all. The fever and rash resolve on their own within 4 to 5 days.

The measles takes about 9 to 10 days to complete its cycle; hence, it is also known as the 9-day measles. Serious complications of measles can occur. In young children, middle ear infections are the most common complication. Respiratory tract infections such as bronchitis, croup, or laryngitis occur in most cases of uncomplicated measles. Pneumonia is also a potential complication, especially in adults. Digestive-related conditions can occur as well. Finally, rare complications may include encephalitis (inflammation of the brain) and seizures.

Conventional treatment for measles involves the use of fever-reducing medications such as acetaminophen. It is important that aspirin not be given to a child with any viral infection, including measles, to prevent the possibility of a serious condition known as Reye's syndrome.

Children with secondary ear infections are given antibiotics. Fluids and bed rest are standard recommendations as well.

■ BASIC PLAN

Diet

Fluids are very important during a feverish illness such as measles. Water, herbal teas, diluted juices, soups, and broths are all excellent. Sugar products should be avoided, as they can suppress the immune system.

Nutritional Supplements

Vitamin A—Studies have found vitamin A to be very effective in reducing complications with children who have measles, but only in very high doses, which should be given only under the supervision of a physician. Certain conditions such as liver disease prevent the use of high dosages of vitamin A and other supplements.

Herbal Remedies

Echinacea and goldenseal combination—Echinacea strengthens the immune system, and goldenseal has a healing effect on the mucous membranes of the throat and lungs, helping to prevent a serious respiratory tract infection.

Homeopathy

Pick the following remedy that best matches your child's symptoms. Unless otherwise indicated, give your child 2 pellets of a 30C potency three or four times daily. Improvements should be seen within 24 hours. If there is no improvement within 24 hours, try another remedy. After you first notice improvement, stop giving the remedy unless symptoms begin to return.

Note: Lower potencies (6X, 12X, 6C) may need to be given more often (four times daily).

Aconitum napellus—For the first stage of measles, before a rash appears. There is a high fever, chills, and cough. The child is restless and anxious and has a dry, barking cough.

Belladonna—For the first stage of measles, where the child has a high fever, red face, and throbbing headache.

Bryonia alba—The child has a dry cough. He wants to remain still. The measles skin eruption is delayed.

Euphrasia—For burning tears and eyes that are very sensitive to light. The child has a runny nose with bland discharge and a dry cough. There is a measles rash.

Gelsemium—For the beginning stage of the measles. The child has alternating chills and fever. He sneezes and has a sore throat. His muscles ache and he has low thirst. There is a croup cough.

Pulsatilla—The child has dry cough at night and a mild to moderate fever. He has tearing eyes and loose stools. He wants to be held and wants windows to be open.

Sulphur—The child is very hot, with a high thirst for cold drinks. His skin itches. There is inflammation of the eyelids. There is an itchy measles rash.

Morbillinum—Give 2 pellets of a 30C potency twice daily for 2 days to reduce the symptoms and severity of measles. This homeopathic nosode can be used preventively when someone in the house or area has been exposed to measles.

■ ADVANCED PLAN

Nutritional Supplements

Vitamin C—Supports the immune system and has mild anti-inflammatory effects. The type with bioflavonoids is preferable. Dosage: the child's age in years times 50 milligrams, twice daily. Reduce the dosage if diarrhea occurs. Consider using a buffered vitamin C powder (nonacidic) or liquid vitamin C. Both work well for infants and children, and can be mixed in juice.

Zinc—Supports the immune system and enhances skin healing. Dosage: children 2 and younger, 5 milligrams; 2 and older, 10 to 15 milligrams. Use for 2 weeks and then stop.

Thymus glandular extract—For immune support. Give one to two 250-milligram tablets or capsules daily or as directed on the container.

Herbal Remedies

Licorice root—Antiviral and soothing to the respiratory tract.

Osha root (*Ligusticum porteri*)—Helps to relieve respiratory tract congestion and infection.

Yarrow—Helps to reduce high fever.

■ WHAT TO EXPECT

You should see gradual improvement over 3 to 5 days. Natural therapy helps to prevent ear and serious respiratory tract infections.

Memory Problems

There are three types of memory: short-term, long-term/recent, and long-term/remote.

Short-term memory deals with the ability to recall new information for a few seconds or minutes. For example, you are able to recite a telephone number you've just been given verbally.

Long-term/recent memory covers the ability to recall events and people you've experienced within the past few days. For instance, you're able to remember what you had for dinner 2 nights ago or the score of the baseball game you attended yesterday.

Long-term/remote memory is the ability to recall events and often certain specific details from your distant past. If you're a teenager, you may be able to remember, for instance, what you wore for your fourth-grade class photo.

Scientists still don't know precisely how memory is stored in the brain. Whether memories are stored at specific locations or widespread across various brain regions remains a mystery.

Many factors can contribute to loss of memory, including a poorly functioning thyroid gland, drug side effects, a head trauma, high fever, an epileptic attack, a poor diet and nutritional deficiencies, anxiety, stress, boredom, and lack of sleep.

■ BASIC PLAN

Diet

A whole-foods diet is important to supply the nutrients that are needed for proper brain function and memory. (See "Diet" on page 4 for more information.) Foods that contain essential fatty acids are very important for brain health. Fish such as salmon, halibut, trout, and mackerel are good sources. Fresh fish two or three times weekly is recommended. Flaxseeds are an excellent source of the important omega-3 fatty acid known as alpha linolenic acid, or ALA. They can be ground up and sprinkled on salads or added to shakes. Grind 1 teaspoon per 50 pounds of body weight (children weighing 30 to 50 pounds may also use 1 teaspoon) and give this amount daily, always with 8 ounces of water.

Nutritional Supplements

Essential fatty acid complex—Choose a children's formula that contains a blend of omega-3 fatty acids, including 100 to 200 milligrams daily of docosahexaenoic acid (DHA), as well omega-6's (especially gamma linolenic acid, or GLA). These essential fats are required by the brain for proper function. Alternatively, you can give flaxseed oil at the following daily dosages: children 2 and under, 1 teaspoon; kids 3 to 6, 2 teaspoons; kids 7 and older, 2 to 3 teaspoons. Reduce the dosage if diarrhea occurs.

Herbal Remedy

Ginkgo biloba—Improves circulation and nutrients to the brain. Use under the guidance of a natural health care practitioner.

Homeopathy

Pick the following remedy that best matches your child's symptoms. Unless otherwise indicated, give your child 2 pellets of a 30C potency two times daily. Improvements should be seen within 1 month. If there is no improvement within 1 month, try another remedy. After you first notice improvement, stop giving the remedy unless symptoms begin to return.

Note: Lower potencies (6X, 12X, 6C) may need to be given more often (three times daily).

Baryta carbonica—For a child who has delayed development and who is slow with thought. She forgets names, things learned, and other daily tasks easily.

Calcarea carbonica—The child learns slowly. She has the Calcarea carbonica constitution: large and flabby.

Kali phosphoricum 6X—Works to rejuvenate the nerves and memory. Give 2 pellets twice daily.

Lycopodium—The child has a loss of confidence. She forgets names and dates easily.

She has poor concentration. She may have dyslexia.

■ ADVANCED PLAN

Nutritional Supplements

Phosphatidylserine—A nutritional supplement specific for memory. Daily dosages: children 25 to 75 pounds, 100 milligrams; kids 75 to 100 pounds, 200 milligrams; kids 100 pounds or more, 300 milligrams. Nontoxic and safe to use.

Children's multivitamin—Provides a base of the essential vitamins and minerals.

Aromatherapy

Lavender may help improve memory. Use 1 or 2 drops in a vaporizer at home.

■ WHAT TO EXPECT

Improvements in memory should be noted within 1 to 2 months of natural therapy.

Mononucleosis

Infectious mononucleosis is an acute illness of the throat and lymph nodes. Often nicknamed "the kissing disease," mononucleosis is spread from one person to another, usually through infected saliva. Drinking out of a cup that has been used by someone with this virus, or even coughing and sneezing, can also spread this disease.

Mononucleosis can affect anyone at any age, but it most often occurs between the preteen years and the early twenties.

In most cases, the Epstein-Barr virus causes mononucleosis.

Once a person is exposed to the virus, it generally takes between 30 and 50 days to show any symptoms. Most infants and young children with mononucleosis show no outward signs. However, among teenagers and those in their twenties, initial symptoms include fatigue, fever, sore throat, swollen glands, headache, abdominal pain, nausea, muscle aches, abnormal liver function, and an enlarged spleen. The fever gradually intensifies. A small number develop rashes or swollen eyelids. In healthy teenagers and adults, symptoms usually lasts 2 to 3 weeks, although fatigue can linger on for months afterward.

People who have weakened immune systems are at the greatest risk for developing this infection, which can last for weeks. And it may recur later in life.

Conventional treatment involves rest and fluids. Fever medicines such as acetaminophen are given if a child is uncomfortable. Aspirin should be avoided with any viral illness, such as mononucleosis, due to the risk of developing Reye's syndrome. Antibiotics are given for secondary bacterial infections of the throat.

■ BASIC PLAN

Diet

Make sure that your child gets plenty of fluids. Older children should drink at least six glasses of water throughout the day. Fruit juices, if used, should be diluted with water by at least 50 percent, as simple sugars can weaken the immune system. Homemade warm broths and soups are best; they are easy to digest and moisten the respiratory tract. Good old chicken soup is soothing if there is a sore throat. Fresh garlic added to the soup is helpful as long as your child is not sensitive to it. Do not give fried foods, as they are hard to digest. Avoid giving your child dairy products as they can contribute to mucus formation and weaken the immune system.

Nutritional Supplement

Vitamin C—Supports the immune system. Dosage: the child's age in years times 50 milligrams, twice daily. Reduce the dosage if diarrhea occurs. Consider using a buffered vitamin C powder (nonacidic) or liquid vitamin C. Both work well for infants and children, and can be mixed in juice.

Herbal Remedies

There are several herbs that can be used to treat viral infections such as mononucleosis. Choose one of the following or a formula that contains a combination of them.

We frequently recommend a formula that we call the virus cocktail. It includes **echinacea**, **astragalus**, **lomatium**, **reishi**, and **licorice root**. It is safe to use with children. If a similar formula is not available, choose either echinacea or lomatium as the primary herbal treatment.

Echinacea—This herb has received the most study in regard to the common cold and upper respiratory tract infections. Look for a flavored children's glycerin-based formula.

Lomatium—A potent antiviral herb that helps fight the Epstein-Barr virus.

Homeopathy

Pick the following remedy that best matches your child's symptoms. Unless otherwise indicated, give your child 2 pellets of a 30C potency twice daily. Improvements should be seen within 48 hours. If there is no improvement within 48 hours, try another remedy. After you first notice improvement, stop giving the remedy unless symptoms begin to return.

Note: Lower potencies (6X, 12X, 6C) may need to be given more often (three times daily).

Arsenicum album—The child experiences fever that comes and goes; it increases between midnight and 2:00 A.M. He is restless and exhausted, and he may have liver and spleen enlargement.

Baptisia—For flulike symptoms with great muscle soreness, and a fever with chills. The child looks toxic: His eyes are bloodshot, with dark circles underneath, and his skin is pale.

Gelsemium—The child feels chilled. He has achy and sore muscles. He is dizzy, with severe fatigue. This is the most common remedy for mononucleosis.

■ ADVANCED PLAN

Nutritional Supplement

Zinc—Supports the immune system and enhances skin healing. Dosage: children 2 and younger, 5 milligrams; 2 and older, 10 to 15 milligrams. Use for 2 weeks and then stop.

Herbal Remedies

Larix—A good immune system enhancer. It is available in a powder form that blends into water and juice, and may have a mild, sweet taste.

Echinacea and goldenseal combination—For bacterial throat infections that may accompany mononucleosis.

New Jersey tea (*Ceanothus americanus*)—Specific for an enlarged spleen. If it is unavailable commercially, contact an herbalist.

Aromatherapy

Eucalyptus and Roman chamomile—Add 1 drop of each to a vaporizer, or add them to a tissue and place it under your child's pillow. If the child is taking a homeopathic remedy, use aromatherapy at a different time.

■ WHAT TO EXPECT

You should be able to see gradual improvement over 7 to 10 days. Natural therapy will make the child more comfortable and less likely to develop other infections. We have seen natural therapy speed up recovery time.

Mood Swings

One moment, your child is smiling and laughing. The next moment, he is pouting and crying or fussing and arguing. You're at a loss to explain the sudden shift in mood.

Attitudes, perceptions, habits, emotions, and behaviors shape a child's personality. So do events, nutrition, and chemical balances within the body.

Mood swings don't always signal the presence of a mental or physical problem. Sudden outbursts of anger or tears that last only a short duration should not be cause for concern. It's all part of learning how to grow up and develop an acceptable temperament.

Mood swings in children and teenagers may be connected to nutritional imbalances that lead to abrupt changes in blood sugar levels. Emotional stress, lack of adequate sleep, hypoglycemia, alcohol or drug abuse, and fluctuating hormones can also spur mood swings.

The conventional approach is to rule out a biochemical problem such as hypoglycemia or diabetes, or an underlying psychological problem, and then recommend treatment.

■ BASIC PLAN

Diet

Make sure that your child is not consuming too many simple sugars, such as are found in soft drinks and white bread. This can lead to imbalanced blood sugar levels that can cause mood swings. Complex carbohydrates, quality protein sources, and adequate amounts of fiber from vegetables are needed to regulate blood sugar levels. (See "Diet" on page 4 for more information.)

Food sensitivities can also be an underlying

cause of mood swings. (See "Food Allergies and Food Sensitivities" on page 298.) In addition, some children are very sensitive to artificial sweeteners and preservatives, which can lead to emotional changes.

Skipping breakfast often leads to blood sugar and biochemical changes. If your child is not hungry in the morning, offer her a protein powder shake.

Foods that contain essential fatty acids are very important for a balanced mood. Fish such as salmon, halibut, trout, and mackerel are good sources. Fresh fish two or three times weekly is recommended. Flaxseeds are an excellent source of the important omega-3 fatty acid known as alpha linolenic acid (ALA). They can be ground up and sprinkled on salads or added to shakes. Grind 1 teaspoon per 50 pounds of body weight (children weighing 30 to 50 pounds may also use 1 teaspoon) and give this amount daily, always with 8 ounces of water.

Nutritional Supplements

Children's multivitamin—Provides a base of the essential vitamins and minerals.

Essential fatty acid complex—Choose a children's formula that contains a blend of omega-3 fatty acids, 100 to 200 milligrams daily of docosahexaenoic acid (DHA), and omega-6's, (especially gamma linolenic acid, or GLA). These essential fats are required by the brain for proper function. Alternatively, you can give flaxseed oil at the following daily dosages: children 2 and under, 1 teaspoon; kids 3 to 6, 2 teaspoons; kids 7 and older, 2 to 3 teaspoons. Reduce the dosage if diarrhea occurs.

Herbal Remedy

Passionflower—Relaxing to the nervous system. Use as needed to help calm a child down.

Homeopathy

Pick the following remedy that best matches your child's symptoms. Unless otherwise indicated, give your child 2 pellets of a 30C potency two times daily. Improvements should be seen within 7 days. If there is no improvement within 7 days, try another remedy. After you first notice improvement, stop giving the remedy unless symptoms begin to return.

Note: Lower potencies (6X, 12X, 6C) may need to be given more often (three times daily).

Ignatia—The child is very high-strung. Mood swings may be related to emotional disturbances. The child wants to be by herself.

Lycopodium—The child is irritable, especially when going too long without eating. She is bossy, although underneath she has poor confidence.

Nux vomica—The child is demanding and irritable. She wants to be the boss. She is chilly and constipated.

Pulsatilla—The child has very changeable moods. She is clingy and wants to be comforted. She craves sweets.

Bach Flower Rescue Remedy— Helps calm down an emotional child. Give 2 drops twice daily until you notice improvement.

■ ADVANCED PLAN

Nutritional Supplements

B complex—Many of the B vitamins are involved with proper neurotransmitter function in the brain. Give a B complex at the following daily dosages: children under age 7, 25 milligrams; children 7 and older, 50 milligrams.

Phosphatidylserine—A brain nutrient that helps with concentration and cognitive function. Daily dosages: children 25 to 75 pounds, 100 milligrams; kids 75 to 100 pounds, 200 milligrams; children 100 pounds or more, 300 milligrams.

Aromatherapy

Lavender—Add 1 to 2 drops to a vaporizer, or add it to a tissue and place it under your child's pillow. If the child is taking a homeopathic remedy, use aromatherapy at a different time.

Acupressure

Four Gates—Helps to release tension. This is a combination of Liver 3, located on top of the foot in the hollow between the big toe and second toe, and Large Intestine 4, located in the webbing between the thumb and index finger. Two people should push on all four points gently at the same time, for 15 seconds. Repeat three times. Do this once daily.

■ WHAT TO EXPECT

Natural therapies can help reduce the frequency of mood swings. Improvements are usually noticed within 1 to 4 weeks.

Motion Sickness

Repeated acceleration and deceleration in stop-and-go traffic inside a car. Heavy waves slapping against the boat during a sail. The spinning, climbing, and diving of a roller-coaster ride: Whether they are traveling by car, boat, or airplane or participating in an amusement park ride, children seem to be affected more often than adults by motion sickness.

Motion sickness happens when the brain receives conflicting messages from the inner ears and the eyes. The inner ears are responsible for controlling the body's balance and equilibrium. The eyes are responsible for conveying what is being seen back to the brain. Abrupt, irregular body movements and postures inside moving objects can set off this conflict between the inner ears and the eyes.

This inner battle can cause a child to become pale, dizzy, nauseated, and clammy. He may complain of a headache or a feeling of uneasiness—or he may even vomit.

Why some children are prone to motion sickness while others aren't remains one of life's mysteries. Fortunately, motion sickness has no lasting effects.

The conventional treatment is to give medications that prevent motion sickness. But sometimes, simpler approaches may prevail. Open the car windows: Fresh air may be helpful. If your child is old enough, encourage him to look out the window at a fixed point, such as a distant hill or sign.

■ BASIC PLAN

Diet

Have your child avoid greasy and fried foods before traveling; these are more likely to upset his stomach. Some children get less motion sickness on an empty stomach, while others do better on a full stomach.

Herbal Remedy

Ginger—This can be an effective herb to prevent or relieve the symptoms of motion sickness, such as nausea. Give your child ¼ cup of fresh ginger tea (let it cool to room temperature first), or give ginger in the tincture or capsule form. If using fresh ginger root to make a tea, make a decoction. If using a tea bag, make an infusion. (See "Herbal Preparations" on page 30 for more on tea decoctions and infusions.)

Homeopathy

Use a combination homeopathic motion sickness formula (give as directed on the container). Or pick the one of the following remedies that best matches your child's symptoms. For the remedies that follow, unless otherwise indicated, give your child 2 pellets of a 30C potency every 15 minutes for up to three doses. If there is no improvement within 1 hour, try another remedy. After you first notice improvement, stop giving the remedy unless symptoms begin to return.

Note: Lower potencies (6X, 12X, 6C) can also be used (every 15 minutes).

Borax—Downward motions such as those from an airplane make the child sick.

Cocculus—For nausea and dizziness from moving objects such as a car or boat. The smell or thought of food makes nausea worse. Fresh air makes nausea worse. The child wants to lie down. This is the most common remedy for motion sickness. Try it if you don't know which one to use.

Petroleum—The child has nausea and dizziness from rising. There is nausea from the smell of food cooking. There is a sinking sensation in the child's stomach. He feels better from eating and worse from fresh air.

Sepia—For motion sickness from walking or reading in the car. The child has nausea from the smell of food.

Tabacum—For extreme nausea, dizziness, sweating, and faintness from the least motion. The child is cold, pale, and clammy. He feels much better in the cool air or from vomiting. He feels worse with heat.

Acupressure

Pericardium 6—Relieves nausea. Located 2½ finger-widths below the wrist crease, in the middle of the forearm (palm side). Gently press the acupressure point with a thumb for 10 to 15 seconds. Perform on both sides of the body and repeat as needed for relief .

Note: A special wristband can be used to prevent nausea (Sea-Bands are one brand). The wristband gently pushes on the acupressure point Pericardium 6. You can buy such a wristband at pharmacies, health food stores, or acupuncturists' offices.

■ WHAT TO EXPECT

The correct homeopathic remedy provides relief within minutes, as may acupressure.

Mumps

Mumps is a contagious viral infection that mainly affects children between the ages of 5 and 10. It occurs most commonly in the late winter and early spring. Mumps is spread by sneezing or coughing.

Mumps typically causes painful swelling on one side of the face and neck and then spreads to the other side. The saliva glands become swollen. These glands are located in front and below the ears. Pain intensifies when a child chews or swallows or yawns.

Symptoms can take up to a month to emerge once a child has become infected. Initially, mumps begins with chills, fatigue, mild fever, aching ears, sore throat, and headaches. These symptoms may not be present in milder cases. Then, the child's parotid glands (in the cheeks) start to swell and hurt. The earlobes are pushed upward and outward, peaking at day 3. Fever usually increases once the parotid glands begin to swell. Swelling of the glands usually resolves within 7 days. Swallowing, especially drinking acidic beverages such as lemonade or orange juice, aggravates the cheek pain.

Complications in boys can include swelling of the testicles (usually one side only), known as orchitis. Sterility and hormonal changes from orchitis are rare. In a small percentage of girls, mumps causes pelvic pain and tenderness.

Caution: If your child exhibits symptoms of a headache, stiff neck, and high fever, seek immediate medical attention to rule out a more serious complication of the mumps.

Conventional treatment of the mumps includes the use of pain- and fever-reducing medications. Aspirin should not be given due to the possibility of Reye's syndrome. A soft diet that reduces chewing is recommended as well as bed rest. Testicular swelling is treated with ice packs and (rarely) with corticosteroids. Antibiotics are ineffective against viral infections such as the mumps. Pediatricians recommend the mumps vaccine (part of the MMR series) for prevention.

■ BASIC PLAN

Diet

Soft foods are advised, since chewing and swallowing increases pain. Soups, broths, and stews are ideal, as are diluted vegetable juices. Vegetables should be steamed. Citrus fruits and acidic foods such as tomato sauce should be avoided, as they can increase throat pain. Purified water should be consumed throughout the day. Sugar and dairy products should be avoided, as they can suppress the immune system.

Nutritional Supplements

Vitamin A—Supports the immune system. Daily dosage: infants under 1 year, 1,875 international units (IU); children 1 to 3, 2,000

IU; kids 4 to 6, 2,500 IU; kids 7 to 10, 3,500 IU; males 11 and older, 5,000 IU; females 11 and older, 4,000 IU.

Note: These dosages are for short-term use (up to 10 days). Higher dosages may be used only under a doctor's supervision. Available in liquid drops.

Vitamin C—Supports the immune system. Dosage: the child's age in years times 50 milligrams, twice daily. Reduce the dosage if diarrhea occurs. Consider using a buffered vitamin C powder (nonacidic) or liquid vitamin C. Both work well for infants and children, and can be mixed in juice.

Herbal Remedy

Echinacea—Supports the immune system. Look for a flavored children's glycerin-based formula. If none is available, capsules or a regular tincture will work just as well.

Homeopathy

Pick the following remedy that best matches your child's symptoms. Unless otherwise indicated, give your child 2 pellets of a 30C potency three times daily. Improvements should be seen within 48 hours. If there is no improvement within 48 hours, try another remedy. After you first notice improvement, stop giving the remedy unless symptoms begin to return.

Note: Lower potencies (6X, 12X, 6C) may need to be given more often (four times daily).

Abrotanum—The testes begin to swell as the parotid glands become less swollen.

Belladonna—For inflammation of the right parotid gland. The child feels shooting pains, and his face is bright red.

Carbo vegetabilis—The mumps go to the testes or breasts after the child becomes chilled. The child is very chilly and is exhausted and wants to be fanned.

Mercurius solubilis or vivus—The glands on the right side of the throat are swollen. The child has a fever, increased salivation, and bad breath. He is sensitive to warm and cold.

Phytolacca—For hard glands on the right side of the throat. Swallowing radiates pain to the ear.

Pilocarpus jaborandi—For increased perspiration and salivation. Helps with complications of the mumps.

Pulsatilla—For mumps that spreads to the testicles in boys and the breasts in girls. The child wants to be held and comforted. She has low thirst and feels better in the fresh air and worse in a warm room.

Rhus toxicodendron—For inflammation of the left parotid gland. Symptoms are worse from the cold.

Parotidinum nosode—Used to shorten the course and severity of the disease. Give 2 pellets twice daily for 2 days. Also used preventively if a child is exposed to someone with the mumps.

■ ADVANCED PLAN

Nutritional Supplement

Zinc—Supports the immune system. Dosage: children 2 and younger, 5 milligrams;

2 and older, 10 to 15 milligrams. Use for 2 weeks and then stop.

Herbal Remedies

Larix—A good immune system enhancer. It is available in a powder form that blends into water and juice, and may have a mild, sweet taste.

Lomatium—A potent antiviral herb that helps fight the mumps virus.

Aromatherapy

Eucalyptus and German chamomile— Add equal parts to a carrier oil and massage into the back and sides of the child's neck. Or add these to a vaporizer, or add them to a tissue and place it under your child's pillow. If the child is taking a homeopathic remedy, use aromatherapy at a different time.

■ WHAT TO EXPECT

Natural approaches are particularly appropriate, as mumps is caused by a viral infection that is not responsive to antibiotics. You should see gradual improvement within 3 to 5 days of natural therapy. Natural treatments may also help prevent complications associated with the mumps.

Muscle Aches and Cramps

Your child may have general soreness after a long day of playing. Or maybe she has aching shoulders after overdoing it in the swimming pool, or painful calf pains during the night. The occasional muscle aches and cramps often just go along with growing up as an active child, and they are rarely a reason to worry.

Muscle aches can affect an active child as well as a sedentary child. The pain often occurs when muscles are overused and pulled or strained, particularly after a vigorous workout that didn't follow a warmup or stretching session. The pain can range from mild to severe and usually dissipates after a few restful days. Lingering or recurrent pain, especially when accompanied by a fever, decreased muscular strength, or joint swelling, could suggest a severe strain—possibly injury.

A feeling of a muscle turning into a knot indicates a muscle cramp. Muscle cramps can afflict any child, regardless of fitness or diet. Heat cramps, which are common to the calves, thighs, and abdomen, can strike a child who is exercising in hot weather or a hot gymnasium and who needs water. Night cramps, which often knot up the muscles of the calves, feet, and thighs, causing sharp pains and tightening muscles, commonly awaken a child from a sound sleep.

Deficiencies of nutrients such as calcium, magnesium, and B vitamins are often at the root of muscle aches and cramps. Lack of sleep can also contribute to the problem.

The conventional approach is to recommend rest and possibly an electrolyte solution to restore lost minerals. Massage of affected areas, and a regular program of stretching before doing any kind of physical activity, is also a good idea.

■ BASIC PLAN

Diet

If your child is having aches and cramps because of a deficiency of calcium, magnesium, or potassium, here are some food sources that can help remedy the problem.

- Calcium: Kelp, cheese, collards, kale, turnip greens, almonds, yogurt, milk, broccoli, and calcium-enriched rice and soy milk
- Magnesium: Whole grains, nuts, legumes, soy, and green leafy vegetables
- Potassium: Fruits and vegetables, especially apples, bananas, carrots, oranges, potatoes, tomatoes, cantaloupe, peaches, plums, and strawberries. Meat and fish are also sources of potassium.

Avoid products that lead to the loss of minerals, such as soft drinks, candy, coffee, and refined breads and pastas.

Electrolyte drinks such as Recharge or Gatorade, or Pedialyte for young children, can be helpful to quickly restore lost minerals. We recommend these drinks only on a short-term basis. Many contain artificial colorings and high amounts of sugar.

Consuming water during hot days or after physical activity is important.

Nutritional Supplements

Calcium and magnesium—Give 500 milligrams of calcium and 250 to 500 milligrams of magnesium daily. This is especially helpful for leg cramps that occur at night.

Homeopathy

Magnesia phosphorica 6X—Relaxes and prevents muscle spasms and cramps. Give 2 to 3 pellets every 5 minutes for the relief of acute spasms. For preventive purposes, a child should take 2 pellets twice daily.

■ ADVANCED PLAN

Nutritional Supplement

Children's multivitamin—Provides a base of the essential vitamins and minerals. Especially important for chronic muscle spasms and cramps.

Homeopathy

Pick the following remedy that best matches your child's symptoms. Unless otherwise indicated, give your child 2 pellets of a 30C potency every 15 minutes for up to three doses. If there is no improvement within 1 hour, try another remedy. After you first notice improvement, stop giving the remedy unless symptoms begin to return.

Note: Lower potencies (6X, 12X, 6C) can also be given (every 15 minutes).

Calcarea carbonica—For a child prone to cramps in the legs and feet, especially at night or after exertion. Symptoms are worse in cold, damp weather. The child craves milk. She tends to be large and flabby.

Calcarea phosphorica—For growing pains and cramps. The pain is worse in cold weather. Cramps are better when the area is rubbed. The child tends to be thin.

Cuprum metallicum—For spasms and twitching of different parts of the body, especially the legs and feet.

Aromatherapy

Lavender and peppermint—Add equal parts of these to a carrier oil and massage it onto the muscle. If the muscle aches or cramps are occurring at night, use black pepper instead of peppermint. If the child is taking a homeopathic remedy, use aromatherapy at a different time.

■ WHAT TO EXPECT

Acute cramps and spasms usually improve within 5 to 15 minutes.

Nail Biting

Nail biting is a nervous habit that is usually a sign of a child's anxiety or insecurity. Some psychologists say that biting nails can be a child's way of making himself comfortable during times of stress. Most children outgrow nail biting when they reach adolescence and learn how to take care of their nails.

If a child just bites off the tips of his nails, then nail biting is not a medical problem. But parents should be concerned if the nail biting is aggressive, such as when a child gnaws the nail deep below the top of the fingertip and so much that fingers bleed and swell.

With such aggressive nail biting, the child often chews, tears, and picks at the nail so much that the cuticle or nail root can be disturbed. The cuticle acts as barrier to keep bacteria and yeast from entering the body through the skin of the finger. Any damage to the cuticle could result in a low-grade infection and permanent nail deformity.

■ BASIC PLAN

Talk with your child about his nail biting. Try to find out if it is a habit or a symptom of stress or nervousness. Just talking with your child can help break the cycle of nail biting. When he starts to bite his nails, redirect his attention toward something else.

Diet

A whole-foods diet is important to make sure that enough B vitamins and other important nutrients are present to help your child deal with stress. (See "Diet" on page 4 for more information.)

Foods that contain essential fatty acids are very important for nail health. Fish such as salmon, halibut, trout, and mackerel are good sources. Fresh fish two or three times weekly is recommended. Flaxseeds are an excellent source of the important alpha linolenic acid. They can be ground up and sprinkled on salads or added to shakes. Grind 1 teaspoon per 50 pounds of body weight (children weighing 30 to 50 pounds may also use 1 teaspoon) and give this amount daily, always with 8 ounces of water.

Essential fatty acids can also be found in nuts and seeds.

Nutritional Supplement

Children's multivitamin—Provides a base of the essential vitamins and minerals.

Homeopathy

Kali phosphoricum 6X—To help reduce the effects of nervousness and stress. Give 2 pellets twice daily.

■ ADVANCED PLAN

Nutritional Supplements

Essential fatty acid complex—Choose a children's blend that contains omega-3 and omega-6 fatty acids. Or give flaxseed oil at the following daily dosages: children 2 and under, 1 teaspoon; kids 3 to 6, 2 teaspoons; kids 7 and older, 2 to 3 teaspoons. Reduce the dosage if diarrhea occurs.

Calcium and magnesium—These relax the nervous system. Give 500 milligrams of calcium and 250 to 500 milligrams of magnesium.

■ WHAT TO EXPECT

Natural therapy may help improve nail biting within 4 to 8 weeks. Or the child may simply outgrow it. We don't recommend finger lotions that are sold over the counter to deter nail biting. Kids just lick it off, and it rarely helps.

Nail Problems

The nails keep bacteria, yeast, and liquids from entering the body through the skin. Damage to the nails and surrounding tissues can leave the body vulnerable to infection. Injuries to the fingernails and toenails are common in childhood.

One typical nail problem is a hangnail, a flap of dried skin on the side of the nail that is formed from a child's biting or tearing her fingernails. Because it juts from the finger, a hangnail can easily be torn off, chewed on, or ripped from the finger, leaving a cut or a tear in the skin near the cuticle. Any opening in the skin is a hole in the body's defense against infection.

Crumbly, whitish nails that accumulate scales underneath them, and dry, peeling surrounding skin, can be symptoms of a fungal infection. If the skin adjacent to the nail is also tender and discolored and oozes pus when pressure is applied to it, a bacteria infection, or paronychia, has probably occurred. Severe finger pain, accumulation of pus, and swelling in the finger pad could indicate felon, an infection common after a minor finger injury or thorn prick.

Other nail problems include pitted nails, which are associated with psoriasis. Very pale-colored nail beds could indicate anemia. Horizontal ridges can indicate infection, low thyroid, or other illnesses. White spots suggest a zinc deficiency. Spoon-shaped nails point to an iron deficiency. Easily broken nails may signal a deficiency of protein, essential fatty acids, calcium, silica, and/or certain trace minerals. Abnormal nail shape and strength is often the result of poor digestion and absorption.

■ BASIC PLAN

First, rule out any health problems with your physician, such as a systemic illness or a localized nail infection (such as fungus or bacteria).

Diet

A whole-foods diet that includes adequate amounts of protein, minerals, and essential fatty acids is important for nail health. (See "Diet" on page 4 for more details.)

Nutritional Supplement

Children's multivitamin—Provides a base of the essential vitamins and minerals. Give as directed on the container.

Herbal Remedies

Fennel, gentian root, and ginger root—To improve digestion and absorption, have your child take one or a combination of these digestive herbs with each meal for 1 month.

Homeopathy

Silica 6X—Specific for brittle nails that may also have white spots. Give 2 pellets twice daily for at least 6 weeks.

■ ADVANCED PLAN

Nutritional Supplements

Essential fatty acid complex—Choose a children's blend that contains omega-3 fatty acids, including 50 to 200 milligrams of docosahexaenoic acid (DHA), as well as omega-6's (especially gamma linolenic acid, or GLA). Or give flaxseed oil at the following daily dosages: children 2 and under, 1 teaspoon; kids 3 to 6, 2 teaspoons; kids 7 and older, 2 to 3 tea-

spoons. Reduce the dosage if diarrhea occurs.

Calcium and magnesium—Give 500 to 1,000 milligrams of calcium and 250 to 500 milligrams of magnesium daily.

Silica or horsetail extract—Give 4 milligrams per pound of body weight daily.

■ WHAT TO EXPECT

You should see improvements in the health of your child's nails in 4 to 8 weeks.

Nausea and Vomiting

Nausea is the queasiness and general discomfort that comes with symptoms of stomach upset. It is often accompanied by vomiting. A child may first show a loss of appetite and complain of a full, cramping, or tender abdomen. Vomiting or diarrhea may follow, providing some temporary relief from the nausea.

The causes of a child's stomachaches range from physical to emotional. A single, short attack of nausea is likely to be a reaction to food or an emotional upset. When nausea is severe and continuing, the most likely cause is probably related to food poisoning, an infection, or a more serious underlying problem.

In older children, stomachache and vomiting are often linked to food poisoning, overeating, food allergies, or motion sickness.

Bacterial and viral infections are frequently at the root of the vomiting and diarrhea attacks associated with nausea. If you're able to eliminate infection, food reactions, and underlying physical problems from the list of reasons why your child continues to experience nausea, the cause is likely emotional.

Emotional disturbances can lead to stomach upset. Events that bring a child tension and anxiety—such as homesickness, a family's divorce, a new sibling, school phobia, and sorrow—can disrupt a child's normal eating and digestion tendencies, leading to nausea.

Make sure to rule out environmental causes of nausea, such as toxic chemicals and cleaning agents.

The conventional approach is to identify the cause of the nausea. If an infection is involved, antibiotics may be given. Antinausea and antivomiting drugs may be prescribed.

Caution: Contact your doctor right away if your child has projectile vomiting, vomits blood, or experiences severe abdominal pain with his nausea and vomiting. Also contact your doctor if your child has lost a lot of fluids from vomiting and/or diarrhea.

■ BASIC PLAN

Diet

Dehydration is the biggest concern. Make sure to replace lost fluids and electrolytes. Electrolyte drinks, such as Pedialyte for younger children or Gatorade, Powerade, or Recharge for older kids, are an easy way for your child to take in fluids and minerals. Do not force solid food on a child until he is fully recovered. Soups and broths are good, as they are easy to digest.

Nutritional Supplement

Probiotic—A children's acidophilus and bifidus supplement can be helpful to recover from food poisoning. Give as directed on the container.

Herbal Remedy

Ginger root—Helps to reduce nausea, vomiting, and diarrhea. Give as a fresh tea (cool to room temperature), or in the capsule or tincture form every 1 to 2 hours for relief of symptoms. If using fresh ginger root to make a tea, make a decoction. If using a tea bag, make an infusion. (See "Herbal Preparations" on page 30 for more on tea decoctions and infusions.)

Homeopathy

Use a combination digestive upset formula, or pick the one of the following remedies that best matches your symptoms. For the remedies below, unless otherwise indicated, give your child 2 pellets of a 30C potency every 2 hours. (For infants, crush the pellets into powder and mix it with water.) Improvements should be seen within 6 hours. If there is no improvement within 6 hours, try another remedy. After you first notice improvement, stop giving the remedy unless symptoms begin to return.

Note: Lower potencies (6X, 12X, 6C) may need to be given more often (every 1 hour).

Aethusa cynapium—For a baby who vomits milk (breast or cow's milk) due to intolerance.

Arsenicum album—For symptoms of nausea, vomiting, and diarrhea that all happen at once. There are burning pains. Symptoms are worse between midnight and 2:00 A.M. The child is thirsty but vomits up fluids. He is chilly.

Ipecacuanha—Specific for symptoms of constant nausea that are not relieved from vomiting.

Note: Do not confuse homeopathic Ipecacuanha with syrup of ipecac, which is completely different. (Syrup of ipecac makes one throw up.)

Nux vomica—For nausea, cramps, and painful vomiting. For bad reactions to medications or foods. The child is very irritable.

Phosphorus—For nausea and vomiting. There is burning in the stomach. The child craves ice-cold drinks but vomits the fluid back up. He may vomit blood.

Pulsatilla—For nausea and vomiting from eating rich and fatty foods.

Tabacum—For nausea and vomiting from motion sickness.

Veratrum album—For projectile vomiting that may be accompanied by diarrhea. The child is very cold but still sweaty.

Acupressure

Gently press each of the following acupressure points with a thumb for 10 to 15 seconds. Perform on both sides of the body and repeat as needed for relief of symptoms.

Stomach 36—Located four finger-widths below the kneecap and one finger-width toward the outside of the leg (outside of the shinbone on the muscle).

Pericardium 6—Located 2½ finger-widths below the wrist crease, in the middle of the forearm (palm side).

Aromatherapy

Peppermint—Add to a carrier oil and rub this onto the child's abdomen. If the child is taking a homeopathic remedy, use aromatherapy at a different time.

■ ADVANCED PLAN

Herbal Remedies

Soothing herbs include **peppermint**, **chamomile**, **licorice**, and **fennel**. These can be found in herbal formulas, or you can pick the one that is available to you.

Constitutional Hydrotherapy

This soothes the digestive tract. (See Hydrotherapy for Children on page 115 for details.)

■ WHAT TO EXPECT

Your child should experience relief of symptoms within 2 to 6 hours. If symptoms do not improve within 24 hours, see a doctor.

Night Terrors and Nightmares

A child may experience sudden, dramatic interruptions known as night terrors during sleep. He may thrash about violently, scream, and awaken frightened and confused with his pupils widened and his breath and heart racing. This episode may appear very frightening to parents and because of its violent nature can be confused with seizures or epileptic fits.

For reasons that doctors cannot explain, night terrors commonly occur between midnight and 2:00 A.M., often about 2 hours into normal sleep. Episodes of night terrors usually last about 5 to 10 minutes, after which the child may seem disoriented and even tearful before relaxing and falling asleep. Sometimes, a soothing parent is unable to stop a child in the middle of night terror.

Night terrors are experienced by about 1 to 5 percent of children, particularly boys between the ages of 5 and 7. The terrors usually stop by the time a child becomes a teenager. They can be triggered by a fever and/or emotional problem and influenced by heredity.

Nightmares can be symptoms of childhood anxiety in which negative or fearful thoughts interrupt or haunt the child during sleep. Nightmares can be triggered by upheaval in a child's life, such as a death, divorce, or family move. Rarely do nightmares bring a child to thrash violently as night terrors do, but they can be disruptive and awakening.

Diet can be a factor in night terrors and nightmares. Simple sugars, especially before bedtime, can cause a problem for some children.

Establish a calming routine before bed each night. A good example is a warm bath followed by a bedtime story that has a happy and positive theme. Also, relaxing and calming music for 15 minutes while the child prepares to go to sleep is helpful.

Night-lights work well for some children who experience nightmares. In addition, do not allow the child to watch television for at least ½ hour before bed. TV can be too stimulating.

■ BASIC PLAN

Diet

Foods that contain simple sugars (such as soft drinks and candy, and refined flours such as waffles) should not be consumed after 5:00 P.M. if your child is having problems with night terrors or nightmares. Simple sugars cause surges of adrenaline while the child is asleep, which can alter his normal sleep rhythms.

Food sensitivities may play a role in night terrors and nightmares for some children. (See "Food Allergies and Food Sensitivities" on page 298 for how to identify and treat them.)

Nutritional Supplements

Calcium and magnesium—Giving 500 milligrams of calcium and 250 to 500 milligrams of magnesium with the evening meal can be helpful to relax your child's nervous system and the effects of stress before sleep.

Homeopathy

Rock rose Bach Flower Remedy—Specific for nightmares and night terrors. Give your child 2 drops before bed, and stop when you notice improvement. Rescue Remedy would be a good second choice.

Or choose the one of the following remedies that best matches your child's symptoms. Give your child 2 pellets of a 30C potency before bedtime or if he cannot get back to sleep. For chronic nightmares, give the one of the following remedies that best matches your child's symptoms. Unless otherwise indicated, give your child 2 pellets of a 30C potency two times daily. Improvements should be seen within 5 days. If there is no improvement within 5 days, try another remedy. After you first notice improvement, stop giving the remedy unless symptoms begin to return.

Note: Lower potencies (6X, 12X, 6C) may need to be given more often (three times daily).

Aconitum napellus—The child wakes up in panic and fear. If he cannot get back to sleep due to a bad dream or night terror, use this remedy to help calm him.

Calcarea carbonica—The child gets nightmares after watching something scary or frightening on TV or from hearing a scary story.

Phosphorus—For nightmares about animals, ghosts, and monsters. Nightmares may start after watching a scary program on TV. The child has the Phosphorus constitution. (See "Phosphorus" on page 69 for a full description.)

Pulsatilla—The child has nightmares and sleep problems being alone in his bedroom. He has nightmares of abandonment. Stress felt from the family can bring on nightmares.

Stramonium—The child suffers from night terrors. He yells out in his sleep and dreams that someone is hurting him. He has violent dreams.

Aromatherapy

Lavender and myrtle—Add 1 drop of each to a tissue and place it under your child's pillow. If the child is taking a homeopathic remedy, use aromatherapy at a different time.

■ WHAT TO EXPECT

Your child should experience improvement within 1 to 2 weeks if the nightmares or terrors have been a chronic problem. Homeopathic remedies can work within a day or two for acute cases.

Nose, Runny

A child with a runny nose is as common as a child with sticky, candy-covered fingers. A runny nose can be a sign of the common cold. But it can also be caused by cold air and by allergens such as dust, animal dander, and pollen.

This isn't all bad. A sniffling child whose nose drips with mucus is a child with a working and maturing immune system. Mucus is one of the body's natural cleansing mechanisms, working to flush out bacteria, viruses, irritants, and debris particles that want to enter the body through the nose and cause inflammation and infection.

A child could get a runny nose from a cold virus. This might be accompanied by a fever, a decrease in appetite, and foul-smelling, yellowish mucus. If a runny nose lasts longer than 2 weeks, it's possibly caused by an allergic condition, which would be associated with intense sneezing and watery, itchy eyes.

Food sensitivities are a common cause of chronic runny noses in children. This is especially true if other symptoms such as watery eyes and sneezing are not present.

The conventional approach is to use over-the-counter cold medicines for viral infections such as the common cold, and antihistamine medications for allergy-related runny noses.

■ BASIC PLAN

It makes sense to let an occasional runny nose run its course unless the nose is becoming plugged up or the child is uncomfortable. A runny nose caused by allergies should be treated. (If caused by a cold, see "Colds" on page 233 for more information.)

Diet

Be suspicious of food sensitivities as the cause of a chronic runny nose. Common food triggers include dairy products, sugar, wheat, soy, and citrus fruits, but we have also seen that kids who drink apple juice all the time develop chronic runny noses, which improve when they drink it less often. (See "Food Allergies and Food Sensitivities" on page 298 for more on this subject.)

For runny noses attributed to viral infections, make sure that your child drinks water throughout the day.

Nutritional Supplement

Vitamin C—Supports the immune system and has an anti-allergy effect. Dosage: the child's age in years times 50 milligrams, twice daily. Reduce the dosage if diarrhea occurs. Consider using a buffered vitamin C powder (nonacidic) or liquid vitamin C. Both work well for infants and children, and can be mixed in juice.

Herbal Remedies

Nettle—Also known as stinging nettle. This herb is helpful for some children with environmental allergies. Freeze-dried nettle capsules are useful, as is the tincture form.

Echinacea and goldenseal—For virus-related runny noses. Echinacea supports the immune system, while goldenseal helps to dry up the mucus.

Homeopathy

Pollen desensitization formula—Contains common pollens in a homeopathic mixture. Taking these formulas can desensitize the immune system to the offending pollens. Give as directed on the container. Start using at the beginning of the pollen season. Homeopathic desensitization formulas for dust, mold, cat hair, and other allergens are also available.

Combination hay fever formula—If your child suffers from hay fever, a combination of the most common remedies for hay fever can be helpful. Give as directed on the container.

Or, pick the following remedy that best matches your child's symptoms. For the remedies below, unless otherwise indicated, give your child 2 pellets of a 30C potency two times daily. (For infants, crush the pellets into powder and mix it with water.) Improvements should be seen within 3 days. If there is no improvement within 3 days, try another remedy. After you first notice improvement, stop giving the remedy unless symptoms begin to return.

Note: Lower potencies (6X, 12X, 6C) may need to be given more often (three times daily).

Allium cepa—For watery eyes with burning nasal discharge. The child is sneezing. Symptoms are better in the open air.

Ambrosia—For children who react to ragweed pollen. The child's head and nose are stuffed up. Works well taken preventively for a month prior to and during hay fever season.

Arsenicum album—For burning eyes and a nonstop runny nose that causes the skin under it to become red and excoriated. The child is chilly and restless.

Euphrasia—For burning, tearing eyes that are bloodshot with a bland nasal discharge.

Sabadilla—For tremendous sneezing and runny nose. The child feels better in a warm room.

Wyethia—For intense itching on the roof of the mouth or behind the nose.

■ ADVANCED PLAN

Nutritional Supplements

The following supplements have anti-allergy effects:

Quercitin—Daily dosage: 3 milligrams per pound of body weight.

Grape seed extract or pycnogenol—Give 1 milligram per pound of body weight daily.

Flaxseed oil—Give at the following daily dosages: children 2 and under, 1 teaspoon; kids 3 to 6, 2 teaspoons; kids 7 and older, 2 to 3 teaspoons. Cut back the dosage if loose stools occur.

Herbal Remedies

Astragalus—This Chinese herb helps to balance the immune system to react less against allergies.

Licorice root—Has anti-allergy effects and reduces inflammation of the sinus and respiratory tract.

Acupressure

Gently press each of the following acupressure points with a thumb or thumbs for 10 to 15 seconds. Perform on both sides of the body and repeat three times each day.

Large Intestine 4—Relieves nasal congestion. Located in the webbing between the thumb and index finger.

Large Intestine 20—Reduces sneezing and nasal symptoms. Located on the lower, outer corner of each nostril.

Aromatherapy

Eucalyptus and frankincense—Add equal parts to a carrier substance such as aloe vera gel and rub underneath the child's nose once daily. If the child is taking a homeopathic remedy, use aromatherapy at a different time.

■ WHAT TO EXPECT

Homeopathic treatment usually provides some relief within 3 to 5 days. Chronic allergies can take longer to clear up. Runny nose as the result of food allergies usually clears within 1 week when the offending foods are avoided. Most children will notice improvement over the course of 2 to 4 weeks.

Obesity

Obesity refers to having too much body fat for a child's specific age, sex, and bone structure. An obese child often has a protruding abdomen, a large waist, sizeable thighs, fat deposits in the breast area, and skin streaked with crooked white or purple lines known as stretch marks.

It is important to note that obesity is not just a measure of weight but a proportion of body fat relative to the entire mass of a child's body. For instance, a child classified as overweight when compared with children of the same age, sex, height, and build may actually have extra pounds from dense, well-developed muscle, which is heavier than fat.

The American Academy of Pediatrics advises that doctors use the Body Mass Index (BMI) to determine childhood obesity. The BMI measurement is calculated by dividing the child's weight in kilograms by his height in meters squared. The number is then compared with a standard for children of a similar age, sex, and body build.

Obesity puts a child at a greater risk for developing high blood pressure, breathing problems, and many other health problems. An obese child may also have muscular and joint wearing associated with carrying the extra weight around. She may also be exposed to negative social teasing, which may lead to emotional and psychological problems.

A person may become obese at any age. Obesity, however, peaks during the first year of life, around age 5, and again during adolescence. A small percentage of childhood obesity is the result of a genetic or hormonal disorder. Many cases are due to lifestyle—the quality of a child's diet and the amount of exercise she gets.

Obesity affects 15 to 25 percent of all children in the United States, and this number continues to rise. It is common for children who are obese to come from families with parents and siblings who are also obese. Three of every 10 obese children grow up to become obese adults. The longer a child remains obese, the more likely she is to carry obesity into adulthood.

Emotional problems can be at the root of the cause for some children with obesity, and this should not be overlooked. Eating may be an emotional outlet for these children.

The American diet has a lot to do with the weight of our children today. Refined foods stripped of their nutrients (especially simple carbohydrates) are in essence empty calories that promote weight gain. Altered fats, such as hydrogenated fats, are also a problem and are found in most fast and packaged foods.

The conventional approach is to rule out any metabolic disorder (such as low thyroid) and recommend a reduced-calorie diet in combination with increased physical activity. Regular exercise is key in managing weight. Do not force a particular exercise program on your child. Instead, find one or two exercises or activities that she enjoys and help her with her commitment to them. Some fun examples might include soccer, biking, walking, and swimming. The duration of the exercise should be built up to 1 hour, done five times weekly. Exercise helps to stimulate thermogenesis, the body's internal fat-burning mechanism.

Counseling is recommended to help obese children with behavior modification and to help them cope with the emotional stresses that come with this condition.

Keep in mind that the best plan for weight loss is one that combines a balanced diet, exercise, and balancing of the hormonal systems (such as thyroid and insulin).

■ BASIC PLAN

Diet

The Standard American Diet promotes weight gain and obesity for many children. Junk foods, refined flour products, and a high-fat diet all promote fat storage. For long-term success in battling obesity, a child's family must focus on a whole-foods diet. (See "Diet" on page 4.) Whole grains, vegetables, legumes, fish, lean poultry, and lesser amounts of fruit are encouraged.

Skipping meals, especially breakfast, should be discouraged. This commonly used weight-loss technique actually causes the reverse reaction, whereby the body stores fat. Instead, smaller, more frequent meals are encouraged throughout the day. This promotes a feeling of satiety instead of binge eating, and it also encourages more level blood sugar levels. If a child is not hungry at breakfast, then a protein shake is recommended. Whey or soy protein powders are good options.

Foods that are high in saturated fat, such as red meat and dairy products, should be minimized. Products containing processed fats such as margarine and trans fatty acids or hydrogenated fats should be avoided. These are mainly found in fast foods and packaged foods. Fried foods should also be discouraged.

The ratio between carbohydrates, protein, and fats is important. As with adults, many children gain weight from a condition known as insulin resistance. In this condition, glucose is unable to enter cells effectively. As a result, there can be spikes of high blood sugar and hormonal reactions in the body that lead to fat storage and weight gain. A diet consisting of 40 percent carbohydrates, 30 percent protein, and 30 percent fat (good fats) is a ratio that will help many children lose weight. Fruit, fruit juices, and sugar products, if consumed, should be consumed with meals and not on an empty stomach, which further worsens insulin resistance.

To keep it simple, have quality complex

carbohydrates, proteins, and fats at each meal. A holistic doctor, nutritionist, or naturopathic physician can help you achieve this goal.

Adequate water is required to flush toxins out of the body and to prevent water retention. A child or adolescent should drink at least six 8-ounce glasses of water daily.

Food sensitivities can also cause water retention and thus weight gain. (See "Food Allergies and Food Sensitivities" on page 298 for more information.)

Nutritional Supplements

Children's multivitamin—Ensures a base of vitamins and minerals.

Chromium—Aids blood sugar metabolism. For children 7 years and older, a daily total of 100 micrograms (this includes the amount in any multivitamin they take) can be given. Use only under the guidance of a doctor.

Homeopathy

See a homeopathic practitioner for a constitutional remedy.

■ WHAT TO EXPECT

Work with a health care professional to follow a program as stated in this chapter. Long-term goals must be set. Weight loss may be slower than anticipated in the beginning as fat is replaced by muscle (muscle weighs more than fat). We recommend that you do not weigh your child more than once a month, as doing so puts too much stress on the child. Instead, rely on body fat measurements and the way the child's clothes fit. One pound of weight loss a week or every 2 weeks is very reasonable. We also encourage parents to exercise with their children and to follow the same dietary guidelines.

Osgood-Schlatter Disease

Osgood-Schlatter disease involves pain, tenderness, and often, swelling of the patellar tendon running from the kneecap to the leg when one frequently exerts the knees through heavy activity and exercise. The pain worsens with activity, particularly in the cases of competitive runners and jumpers.

The condition occurs in children and teenagers because repetitive running and jumping can stress and irritate a weakened developmental area where the patellar tendon meets the tibia (the shin) just below the kneecap. The open growth plate cannot handle the wear, thus allowing Osgood-Schlatter disease to occur. The result is that the skin above the injured area is red and inflamed, and persistent pain follows.

Children who participate in sports such as basketball, volleyball, and high-impact aerobics are especially prone to developing this overuse syndrome. It can affect one or both knees and can be detected by pinpointing the pain in a medical examination or through the use of diagnostic imaging.

Conventional treatment involves ice, rest, and in some cases, a supportive knee brace.

Vital Fact

Osgood-Schlatter disease is the most common cause of chronic knee pain in adolescents. It affects approximately 15 percent of boys and 10 percent of girls.

Physiotherapy and massage can also help to heal damaged tissue; see the Natural Health Care Modalities and Resource Guide on page 499 for more on these techniques.

■ BASIC PLAN

Diet

A whole-foods diet is recommended; fruits, vegetables, whole grains, and raw juices promote healing. Essential fatty acids are important, as is silica, found in rolled oats (as in porridge or Swiss muesli).

Nutritional Supplements

Vitamin E—Daily dosage: 100 international units per 50 pounds of body weight.

Selenium—Daily dosage: 1 microgram per pound of body weight.

Vitamin C—Dosage: the child's age in years times 50 milligrams, twice daily. Reduce the dosage if diarrhea occurs.

Herbal Remedy

Arnica oil—Apply this topically twice daily to reduce bruising or inflammation.

Homeopathy

Calcarea fluorica 6X—Strengthens and heals connective tissue. Give 2 pellets three times daily until the injury is healed and for an additional 2 months afterward.

Ruta graveolens 30C—For injuries to tendons. There is bruised pain and stiffness. Give 2 pellets twice daily for 2 weeks.

■ ADVANCED PLAN

Nutritional Supplements

Methylsulfonylmethane (MSM)—Acts as a natural anti-inflammatory and provides an organic form of sulfur that promotes tissue healing. Give 5 milligrams per pound of body weight per day internally, or apply as a cream to the site of the injury.

Children's multivitamin—Provides a base of vitamins and minerals for ligament and tendon health. Includes manganese, which is important for tendon healing.

Herbal Remedies

Bromelain—Has natural anti-inflammatory effects. Give 3 milligrams per pound of body weight two or three times daily, between meals.

Other herbs that have a natural anti-inflammatory effect include **turmeric**, **licorice**, **ginger root**, **devil's claw** (*Harpagophytum procumbens*), **white willow**, and **boswellia** (*Boswellia serrata*). They can be taken individually or as part of formulas.

Note: Do not give white willow during a fever or virus.

■ WHAT TO EXPECT

You should see more rapid healing when the listed natural therapies are used in addition to ice and rest. Healing time depends on the severity of the injury and how well the injury is rested. Most cases improve within 2 to 4 weeks. To prevent reinjury, the nutritional supplements recommended in this chapter should be used on a long-term basis at the dosages indicated. Many young athletes are concerned about taking time out from their high-impact sports. We recommend swimming laps or running in water to keep in shape as the body heals.

Parasites (Intestinal)

Microorganisms naturally inhabit and move through the body. Some are harmless, while others cause sickness. Infections can occur when parasites make their homes in your skin, gastrointestinal tract, lungs, liver, and other organs. Parasites require a host, such as human cells, to live and thrive.

Parasitic infections were once thought of as a problem mainly in underdeveloped countries. After all, diarrheal disease (from parasites and bacteria) is the greatest worldwide cause of death. Worldwide travel has been a major contributor to the spread of parasitic infections in North America. In addition, better diagnostic techniques have provided more accurate identification of parasites and have led researchers to conclude that parasitic infections are much more common than previously thought.

Diarrhea and abdominal pain are the most common symptoms of a parasitic infection. However, in many cases of parasite infection, these symptoms may not be present. A whole list of symptoms and conditions could be related to a parasitic infection. Examples include loss of appetite, fatigue, constipation, depressed immunity, food allergy, fever, chills, heartburn, stomach pain, inflammatory bowel disease, lower back pain, itchy anus, rash and skin itching, hives, weight loss, arthritis, bloody stools, mucus in the stool, colitis, Crohn's disease, flatulence, foul-smelling stools, malabsorption, rectal bleeding, mood changes such as depression and irritability, and vomiting.

Parasites interfere with the normal activities of the cells they infect, which may lead to symptoms and disease. The secretions released by a parasite can trigger an autoimmune reaction, in which the immune system attacks its own tissues. Examples include rheumatoid arthritis and Crohn's disease. Not all parasites are necessarily harmful. Some parasites live symbiotically in the digestive tract. It is thought that some parasites become a problem only when the environment of the body changes. For example, dysbiosis—the imbalance between friendly and potentially harmful bacteria in the digestive tract—can lead to certain parasites becoming pathogenic (disease-causing). The nutritional status of a person dictates whether a parasite can become a problem. A compromised immune system can also contribute to the outcome of a parasitic infestation.

Parasites are commonly transmitted through food that has been contaminated with fecal matter (this happens when food preparers do not wash their hands after going to the restroom) as well as through waste and the water supply.

There are many different types of parasites. Following are some of the more common ones in North America.

Blastocystis hominis: This parasite is detected in a high number of stool tests. Researchers are unclear about whether it is a pathogen, as many people carry it but do not have symptoms. However, it can cause many different digestive symptoms, including cramps, nausea, weight loss, and bloating. It is also associated with conditions such as irritable bowel syndrome, chronic fatigue, and arthritis.

Dientamoeba fragilis: Symptoms of this parasite, which resides in the large intestine, include diarrhea and abdominal pain.

Entamoeba histolytica: This amoeba is linked to diarrhea and a variety of other digestive symptoms.

Giardia: This is one of the most common parasites found in humans. It is transmitted through water and food, between children in day care centers, through fecal-oral contamination, or through sexual intercourse. Epidemics from contaminated streams and community water systems occur every year in the United States.

Cryptosporidium: Transmitted through contaminated food, water, and from person-to-person contact. Explosive diarrhea is a common symptom. This parasite is of particular concern for children who are HIV-positive. Their immune systems may not be able to fight off the parasite, making it a life-threatening condition.

Ascaris lumbricoides: This parasitic (worm) infection is the most common human worm infection in the world. Infection is common in the southeastern United States. Infection in children can cause abdominal cramps and malnutrition. Fecal-oral transmission often occurs from uncooked or unwashed vegetables.

Hookworm: Not as common in the United States as in other parts of the world, yet cases do occur. It usually causes no symptoms, although a skin itch may be present. Acute symptoms can include abdominal pain, diarrhea, weight loss, anemia, and many other symptoms. These worms can live up to 10 years. They are transmitted through direct contact with soil containing the eggs of hookworms.

Pinworms: Pinworms are scientifically known as *Enterobius vermicularis*. These are small, skinny, white worms no longer than ½ inch. Pinworms are one of the most common parasites to bring infection to people regardless of age or culture. They enter the body when their microscopic, infectious eggs, carried on a child's fingernails, clothing, bedding or even food, are ingested. The eggs are swallowed and then hatch in the warm haven that is the human body. Pinworms migrate to the large intestine, where they live and mature into adult form. Female pinworms travel at night or early morning through the anus to deposit their eggs. The deposit of the eggs is irritating and itchy, leading to scratching around the anus. One way to test whether your child has pinworms is to swab a small piece of transparent tape across the child's anus at night. Take the tape to your doctor to be examined microscopically. This may need to be done several times to rule out pinworms. You may be able to see the pinworms with a flashlight. If you can, collect some with tweezers to take to your doctor.

Strongyloides: The eggs of these worms can penetrate the skin and migrate to the lungs and intestines. Most infections occur via the fecal-oral route. Infected people may be asymptomatic, or they may have various digestive problems. Liver and nervous system infection can also be a serious complication.

Trichinosis: Infection occurs from eating undercooked or processed meat. There may be no symptoms, or there may be nausea, abdominal cramps, fever, and muscle pain (larvae can invade muscle tissue).

Conventional treatment of parasitic infections focuses on antiparasitic medications to eradicate the parasite. Toxicity and side effects vary for each medication.

■ BASIC PLAN

The first step in treating a parasitic infection is to get a proper diagnosis. This is mainly dependent on a stool analysis. We highly recommend using a laboratory that specializes in comprehensive parasitology testing. Many of the stool tests done by clinics are not sensitive enough to pick up many different forms of parasites. We recommend labs such as Great Smokies that specialize in this area. (See "Parasitology Testing" on page 506 for contact information.) Your child's doctor can order specialized parasite stool kits from them.

Certain blood tests by your doctor can also be helpful in pinpointing a diagnosis.

Note: Natural treatment of parasitic infections should be done under the guidance of a knowledgeable health care practitioner or doctor.

Diet

Sugar products should be reduced or avoided to optimize immune system health. Fresh garlic, ginger, and onions are excellent as prepared foods, as they have been shown to have antiparasitic effects. If your child is old enough to chew them, raw pumpkin seeds kill worms and parasites. They can be ground as well: Grind up $1/8$ to $1/4$ cup of pumpkin seeds daily, and give them with 8 ounces of water. Papaya juice also has antiworm effects.

Make sure that all fruits and vegetables are washed and cleaned properly. Meat and seafood products need to be cooked thoroughly. Avoid giving raw seafood to children.

Vital Fact

It is estimated that more than 1 billion people are infected with the worm infection ascariasis worldwide, of whom 20,000 die each year.

Nutritional Supplement

Probiotic—A children's acidophilus supplement that contains bifidus as well can be helpful to improve the amounts of these good bacteria, which help to fight and prevent the overgrowth of harmful parasites. It is especially important for infants who have been on antibiotics or antiparasitic medication. Give as directed on the container.

Herbal Remedy

Black walnut—Has antiworm and antiparasitic properties. Give 5 drops two or three times daily. Do not use for longer than 4 weeks.

Homeopathy

See a practitioner for an individualized remedy. Or pick the one of the following remedies that best matches your child's symptoms. For the remedies below, unless otherwise indicated, give your child 2 pellets of a 30C potency two times daily. (For infants, crush the pellets into powder and mix it with water.) Improvements should be seen within 14 days. If there is no improvement within 14

days, try another remedy. After you first notice improvement, stop giving the remedy unless symptoms begin to return.

Note: Lower potencies (6X, 12X, 6C) may need to be given more often (three times daily).

Cina—The child is very irritable and does not want to be touched. He picks at his nose and rectum. His appetite is very high. There may be pale, dark circles under the eyes. The child grinds his teeth at night.

Filix mas—A specific remedy for tapeworms.

Natrum phosphoricum—This remedy can be used for all types of worms. The tongue has a yellow, creamy coating.

Sabadilla—The child has itching of the rectum that alternates with itching of the nose or ears.

Spigelia—A homeopathic remedy for worms. The child has an itchy rectum and pain around the navel. He has bad breath.

Teucrium marum—For pinworms, threadworms, and roundworms. The child has itching in his nose and rectum. He is very irritable and nervous.

■ ADVANCED PLAN

Nutritional Supplement

Grapefruit seed extract—An effective antiparasitic supplement. Use under the guidance of a practitioner.

Herbal Remedies

More antiparasitic herbs include **wormwood, elecampane, ginger, goldenseal, Oregon**

grape root, and **coptis** *(Coptis chinensis)*. Look for formulas that contain combinations of these herbs, and use them under the guidance of a doctor.

Chinese herbal therapy also works very well for parasitic infections. See a qualified practitioner.

Oregano oil kills yeast and parasites. This is one of the few essential oils that can be ingested. Two drops diluted in ½ cup of water twice daily can be helpful. Use under the supervision of a doctor.

■ WHAT TO EXPECT

Work with a holistic doctor to eradicate harmful parasitic infections. A comprehensive stool analysis can help your doctor to identify the parasites, and then your child can be retested after treatment to make sure that the infection has cleared. Improvements are usually seen within 2 to 4 weeks.

Phobias

Monsters hiding in the closets or beneath a bed. Strangers lurking in the dark. Falling from a high place: These are just some of the fears and phobias that haunt children at different developmental stages.

At one time or another, most children carry with them a fear that makes them uneasy, nervous, and just plain scared. But a phobia is a continuous, excessive, or sometimes unaccountable fear triggered by the presence or occurrence of a person, object, or situation. It can be based upon something real or imaginary.

Most phobias eventually go away. In fact, most phobias don't pose significant restrictions on a child's life. If a phobia does interfere with the normal functioning of a child's life, it can become a serious anxiety disorder. But before a child comes to terms with her fears, she may show the typical signs of anxiety, which include the loss of appetite, crying, interrupted sleep, and irritability, as well as feelings of panic and avoidance.

For young children, the subjects of their phobias are often imaginary, such as the bogeyman. Older children are often troubled by what they hear about on television—crime, AIDS, and shootings—or by more realistic social fears—a school dance, report cards, and first dates.

The key to how a child survives her fear is the way in which the parents react to the phobia to make it less scary for the child.

■ BASIC PLAN

Talking with your child about what she is experiencing is the first step to take. Reassuring her that she is safe and secure will help reduce the anxiety associated with phobias. A children's counselor should treat phobias that seem to get worse or that restrict a child's daily activities and happiness.

Homeopathy

Pick one of the following Bach Flower Remedies and give 2 drops twice daily. Or make a formula containing a mixture of them, and have the child take it two or three times daily. (For a formula, add 2 drops of each to ¼ cup water.) Discontinue use if the problem disappears or if there is no improvement within 10 days.

Aspen—For fear and anxiety.

Holly—For loneliness.

Mimulus—For fear.

Rock rose—For states of terror such as nightmares.

■ WHAT TO EXPECT

The correct Bach Flower Remedy or other homeopathic remedy can help lessen a child's phobias. Counseling is indicated for phobias that interfere with a child's daily activities.

Pneumonia

Pneumonia is an acute inflammation and infection of the lung tissue, filling the tiny air sacs that line the lungs with fluid, mucus, and pus. It can take several weeks to recover from pneumonia.

A child suffering from pneumonia is likely to have a persistent, possibly severe cough; a fever; difficulty breathing; and lethargy. Telltale signs are rapid breathing, straining of the chest muscles to breathe, and a high fever.

Pneumonia often occurs as a complication of an illness such as a cold, the flu, or bronchitis. Pneumonia is usually viral or bacterial, with bacterial pneumonia being the most dangerous form. The symptoms of bacterial pneu-

monia include high fever, lethargy, chest pain, sweating, and paleness—all of which come on suddenly and frequently as a complication of other illnesses. A child looks and seems very sick.

If you suspect that your child has pneumonia, you should see a doctor right away. The conventional approach is to order an x-ray and blood work to confirm the suspicion of pneumonia.

Bacterial pneumonia is treated with antibiotics, and any fever is treated with acetaminophen, such as Tylenol. Cough medications are usually prescribed as well. Natural therapies can play a complementary role in treating bacterial pneumonia.

Viral pneumonia is treated with bed rest, physiotherapy (to reduce lung congestion; see "Physiotherapy" on page 506), and sometimes antibiotics to prevent a secondary bacterial infection. For viral infections, natural therapy may play a main role.

■ BASIC PLAN

Diet

Have your child go on a low-mucus diet by avoiding foods such as dairy products and bananas. Eliminate sugar products, as they can lower immune function. Warm soups, stews, and steamed vegetables are preferred, as they are easy to ingest and help to prevent dehydration. Simple sugars should be avoided. Make sure that your child consumes plenty of fluids. Water, warm herbal teas such as peppermint and licorice, and diluted fruit juices are good.

Nutritional Supplements

Vitamin A—Supports the immune system. Daily dosage: infants under 1 year, 1,875 international units (IU); children 1 to 3, 2,000 IU; kids 4 to 6, 2,500 IU; kids 7 to 10, 3,500 IU; males 11 and older, 5,000 IU; females 11 and older, 4,000 IU.

Note: These dosages are for short-term use (up to 10 days). Higher dosages may be used only under a doctor's supervision. Available in liquid drops.

Vitamin C—Supports the immune system. Dosage: the child's age in years times 50 milligrams, twice daily. Reduce the dosage if diarrhea occurs. Consider using a buffered vitamin C powder (nonacidic) or liquid vitamin C. Both work well for infants and children, and can be mixed in juice.

Herbal Remedies

Echinacea and goldenseal combination—Echinacea supports the immune system, and goldenseal helps with the excess mucus production.

Osha—An excellent herb to support the immune system and to help rid the lungs of mucus.

Homeopathy

Use a combination respiratory tract formula or pick the one of the following remedies that best matches your child's symptoms. For the remedies that follow, unless otherwise indicated, give your child 2 pellets of a 30C potency three times daily. Improvements should be seen within 2 days. If there is no improvement within 2 days, try another remedy. After you first notice improvement, stop giving the remedy unless symptoms begin to return.

Note: Lower potencies (6X, 12X, 6C) may need to be given more often (four times daily).

Case History

Four-year-old Launa had been suffering from viral pneumonia for 9 days. Her parents were concerned that she had not improved and were told that she may need to be hospitalized. That's when they brought her to see us at our clinic for the first time. Launa had shortness of breath, and she said that it felt like a weight had been placed on her chest. She had a fever that would come and go during the day. She was chilly and wanted to stay in bed and keep the covers on at all times. Her throat and chest felt better after drinking ice water. In addition to the antibiotics her family doctor had prescribed, we recommended echinacea and goldenseal, the homeopathic remedy Phosphorus, and constitutional hydrotherapy. Once she started the hydrotherapy, she was able to expectorate mucus that she previously had not been able to bring up. Within 2 days, she felt about 50 percent better. Her energy was improved and she was able to walk around her house. She made a complete recovery over the next 5 days.

Arsenicum album—The child is restless and chilly. He may feel a burning sensation in his lungs. A good remedy for right-sided pneumonia.

Antimonium tartaricum—For mucus production in the lungs that does not come out. There is a rattling sound in the child's chest.

Bryonia alba—The child is feverish with a high thirst, and he feels better in a cool room. There is a lot of rib pain with each cough. The child is irritable and feels worse with any movement.

Kali carbonicum—The child's symptoms are worse from 2:00 to 4:00 A.M. He feels better sitting upright or bent forward. His eyelids may be swollen. He is chilly.

Lycopodium—For right-sided pneumonia. Symptoms are worse from 4:00 to 8:00 P.M. The child feels better with warm drinks. His nostrils flare open to help breathing.

Phosphorus—The child's chest feels heavy, as if a weight were on it. He has a great thirst for cold drinks and feels worse lying on his left side.

Pulsatilla—The child is warm but has no thirst. He wants to be held and is weepy. He desires open air.

Sulphur—For burning in the lungs. The child is very hot and sweats easily. He has a high thirst for cold drinks.

Acupressure

Lung 1—Located on the outer portion of the chest, right below the collarbone. Gently press the acupressure point with a thumb for 10 to 15 seconds. Perform on both sides of the body and repeat three times each day.

Hydrotherapy

Constitutional hydrotherapy is highly recommended for all types of pneumonia. It stimulates the immune system, brings immune cells to the lungs, and reduces congestion in the respiratory tract. (See Hydrotherapy for Children on page 111 for directions.) Also, light patting on the back is helpful after a hydrotherapy treatment to help break up mucus.

■ ADVANCED PLAN

Nutritional Supplements

Zinc—Supports the immune system. Dosage: children 2 and younger, 5 milligrams; 2 and older, 10 to 15 milligrams. Use for 2 weeks and then stop.

Thymus glandular extract—Give one to two 250-milligram tablets or capsules daily for immune support.

N-acetylcysteine—Helps to thin mucus secretions. Give 2 milligrams per pound of body weight daily.

Herbal Remedies

There are many herbs that are helpful for lung infections. Look for formulas that contain herbs such as **astragalus**, **yerba santa**, **licorice root**, **usnea** (*Usnea* species), *lungwort* (*Pulmonaria officinalis*), **ginger**, and **marshmallow root**, in addition to the herbs listed in the Basic Plan section.

Aromatherapy

Add 1 drop of **eucalyptus**, 2 drops of **tea tree oil**, and 1 drop of **frankincense** to a vaporizer in the child's room. If the child is taking a homeopathic remedy, use aromatherapy at a different time.

■ WHAT TO EXPECT

You should notice improvement within 5 days. Bacterial pneumonia is treated with antibiotics. It is a good idea to also use the listed natural therapies for bacterial pneumonia to quicken recovery and make the child more comfortable.

Poison Ivy, Poison Oak, and Poison Sumac Rashes

The world's most common allergy is an allergic reaction to the plants poison ivy, poison oak, and poison sumac. These plants trigger allergic reactions when they touch a person's skin, leaving an intensely itchy, red rash with tiny blisters across the contact area.

The itch results from urushiol oil, a potential toxin that can transfer from clothes to skin and from touch to touch, spreading the irritant around a child's body and potentially from person to person. Get as little as one-billionth of a gram on your skin and you could soon start scratching.

Poison ivy, oak, or sumac starts a reaction that is a form of allergic contact dermatitis. The reaction will show its symptoms within 4 hours to a couple of days after contact. In addition to the pesky rash, this skin disease causes fluid-filled blisters that can break, forming scaly crusts atop the infected areas. Symptoms can last up to 10 days or longer if left untreated. Not everyone reacts adversely to contacting poison ivy, oak, or sumac.

See your doctor under any of the following circumstances:

- The rash is painful or swollen.
- The rash is located on the face or genitals.
- Your child shows signs of infection (such as a fever).
- Your child cannot get any relief from treatment.
- The rash is accompanied by severe itching and oozing of fluid to the extent that the clothes stick to the skin.

Caution: If your child has difficulty breathing, go to the closest emergency room.

Conventional treatment focuses on soothing lotions such as calamine and others. Antihistamine medications such as Benadryl may be prescribed. Topical hydrocortisone cream may be prescribed to reduce the inflammation and itching. For severe cases, steroids such as prednisone may be given for short-term use.

■ BASIC PLAN

If possible, wash the child with soap and warm water immediately after exposure. Do not use a washcloth, so that the allergic oil is not spread around. Washing with soap and water within the first 10 minutes of contact works most effectively.

Make sure to wash all of your child's clothes (including shoes) that may have some of the poisonous oil on them. While wearing a pair of gloves, hose the items down, then rinse out any washable items in the washer before you add detergent.

Diet

A whole-foods diet is recommended. (See "Diet" on page 4 for more information). Avoid simple sugars, which can hinder the immune system. Detoxifying juices such as carrot juice diluted with water is good.

Nutritional Supplement

Vitamin C—Supports the immune system and has mild anti-inflammatory effects. The type with bioflavonoids is preferable. Dosage: the child's age in years times 50 milligrams, twice daily. Reduce the dosage if diarrhea occurs. Consider using a buffered vitamin C powder (nonacidic) or liquid vitamin C. Both work well for infants and children, and can be mixed in juice.

Herbal Remedy

Calendula—Helps to relieve itching, prevents secondary infections, and promotes skin healing. Apply the liquid form (succus is preferable) three or four times daily to the affected area(s). You can apply a nonsuccus tincture as 1 teaspoon diluted in 4 teaspoons of water.

Homeopathy

Pick the following remedy that best matches your child's symptoms. Unless otherwise indicated, give your child 2 pellets of a 30C po-

tency every hour for up to three doses. If there is no improvement within 3 hours, try another remedy. After you first notice improvement, stop giving the remedy unless symptoms begin to return.

Note: Lower potencies (6X, 12X, 6C) can be used also (give them every hour).

Anacardium orientale—For serious itching and burning, which gets worse after the child scratches. Rubbing and eating bring temporary relief. Skin feels better in hot water.

Croton tiglium—Poison ivy rash and diarrhea occur at the same time. The rash mainly affects the face and/or genitals. Scratching the skin is painful.

Graphites—The skin oozes a thick, honey-colored fluid.

Rhus toxicodendron—For blistering, itchy and burning lesions that are better from a hot bath. The child is very restless. Start with this remedy if you do not know which one to use.

Sulphur—For an itchy and burning rash that is worse with warm applications. The child scratches the skin until it bleeds.

■ ADVANCED PLAN

Nutritional Supplement

Zinc—Supports the immune system and enhances skin healing. Dosage: children 2 and younger, 5 milligrams; 2 and older, 10 to 15 milligrams. Use for 2 weeks and then stop.

■ WHAT TO EXPECT

There should be a reduction in itching and skin symptoms within 24 hours with the correct natural therapy.

Psoriasis

Psoriasis is one of the world's most common chronic skin disorders. The condition causes inflammation and silvery scaling. Raised skin patches appear typically on the scalp, the backsides of the wrists, and on the elbows, navel, lower back, knees, buttocks, and ankles. These patches can range in size from less than ¼ inch to several inches in diameter.

Although it is common, psoriasis is not contagious. Psoriasis can develop at any age, but it usually first appears during adolescence and surfaces most among teenagers and young adults. Symptoms including itching, burning, or stinging lesions and can wax and wane over many years. In many cases, there is a family history of psoriasis.

Based on the appearance and location of the scaly patches, psoriasis can be identified as one of four specific types:

- Plaque psoriasis—Red, rounded or oval patches are covered with a silvery scale.
- Inverse psoriasis—The patchy surface is usually moist and found in skin creases, especially in the underarm, navel, or under the breast.
- Pustular psoriasis—Skin patches are studded with pimples.
- Guttate psoriasis—Red, scaly, dime-size or smaller patches surface suddenly and simultaneously, often following a bout with strep throat or a viral upper respiratory infection.

In some instances, psoriasis can be associated with arthritis or nail thickening.

The underlying cause of psoriasis remains unclear, but it is known that in this condition, the skin cells replicate too rapidly. As a result, the skin thickens and becomes scaly. Infections, stress, climate changes, and lack of sunlight can trigger flare-ups.

The conventional approach is to use either topical steroids, coal tar products combined with ultraviolet treatment, synthetic vitamin D₃ (calcipotriene), or other topical treatments.

■ BASIC PLAN

Various factors may need to be addressed from a holistic viewpoint. These include digestive and elimination function, liver and kidney detoxification ability, food sensitivities, nutritional deficiencies and imbalances, and stress.

Diet

A whole-foods diet high in fiber is recommended. Fiber found in vegetables, some fruits, whole grains, and legumes helps in the elimination of toxins through the colon. (For more information, see "Diet" on page 4.)

Fresh fish such as salmon is recommended, as the omega-3 fatty acids promote skin health and reduce inflammation. A minimum of three servings a week is recommended. Dairy products and red meat should be limited as they contain arachadonic acid, which flares up inflammatory conditions such as psoriasis. Flaxseeds are an excellent source of the important omega-3 fatty acids. They can be ground up and sprinkled on salads or added to healthy protein, fruit, or vegetable shakes. Grind 1 teaspoon per 50 pounds of body weight (children weighing 30 to 50 pounds may also use 1 tea-

Vital Fact

An estimated 6.4 million Americans have been diagnosed with psoriasis. Children who have one or both parents with psoriasis have a 10 to 25 percent chance of developing this skin condition.

spoon) and give this amount daily, always with 8 ounces of water.

If tolerated, yogurt with live cultures is good, as it helps to increase the good bacteria needed for intestinal and thus skin health.

Food sensitivities play a major role in the flare-up of psoriasis in some individuals. Food sensitivities should be identified and treated. (See "Food Allergies and Food Sensitivities" on page 298 for more information.)

Nutritional Supplements

Essential fatty acids—Essential fatty acids are very important in the treatment of psoriasis. An essential fatty acid formulation containing omega-3 fatty acids (from fish or flaxseed oil) and gamma linolenic acid (GLA) is good. Otherwise, use a fish oil (such as salmon oil), as most of the research has been done on high doses of fish oil. The fish oil daily dosage is 1 gram per 50 pounds of body weight.

Herbal Remedy

Sarsaparilla (*Smilax* species) and burdock root—The combination of these two herbs works well to help improve underlying toxicity associated with psoriasis. They can be taken on a long-term basis.

Homeopathy

Pick the following remedy that best matches your child's symptoms. Unless otherwise indicated, give your child 2 pellets of a 30C potency two times daily. Improvements should be seen within 2 days. If there is no improvement within 2 weeks, try another remedy. After you first notice improvement, stop giving the remedy unless symptoms begin to return.

Note: Lower potencies (6X, 12X, 6C) may need to be given more often (three times daily).

Arsenicum album—For red, dry, scaly patches that burn or itch very intensely. Lesions feel better with warm water and are worse from the cold.

Graphites—For oozing lesions that scar easily. For thick, hard scales that are itchy.

Petroleum—For dry, leathery skin. For deep, raw cracks in skin that do not heal easily.

■ ADVANCED PLAN

Nutritional Supplements

Microbial-derived enzymes—Taken with each meal, these improve digestion and absorption problems that can be related to psoriasis. Sold as a digestive enzyme complex.

Probiotic—Give a children's supplement that contains bifidus and acidophilus, which help to balance gut bacteria. Give as directed on the container.

Children's multivitamin—Provides a base of the essential vitamins and minerals.

Vitamin C—Supports the immune system and has mild anti-inflammatory effects. The type with bioflavonoids is preferable. Dosage: the child's age in years times 50 milligrams, twice daily. Reduce the dosage if diarrhea occurs. Consider using a buffered vitamin C powder (nonacidic) or liquid vitamin C. Both work well for infants and children, and can be mixed in juice.

Herbal Remedy

Milk thistle—Supports liver detoxification, which is necessary for healthy skin.

Aromatherapy

Add equal parts **lavender**, **Roman** or **German chamomile**, and **geranium** to a carrier oil and apply it to the affected area. If the child is taking a homeopathic remedy, use aromatherapy at a different time.

■ WHAT TO EXPECT

About 50 percent of psoriasis cases improve with nutritional therapy. Improvements can be seen within 1 to 2 months.

Ringworm

Despite its name, ringworm is a contagious infection caused by fungi, not worms. The "worm" part of its name comes from the wavy, ring-shaped, scaly, red blotches that sur-

face on a child's skin, including the scalp area as well as the nails.

Early signs include flakes or little bumps on the skin. As the infection progresses, circles or ovals with flat centers and raised, red borders appear. These patches can be itchy and tend to spread from one area of the body to another. The patch's center may clear as it spreads. On the scalp, ringworm can cause bald patches or patches of short, broken hairs. Fortunately, hair loss is temporary.

Although it is not serious, ringworm is persistent and easily spreads from one child to the next through sharing of contaminated hats or combs or contact with infected surfaces such as shower stalls or gymnasium floors. Less commonly, a child may contract ringworm by playing with a dog, cat, or other animal that is infected.

Conventional treatment focuses on the use of antifungal creams and on antifungal medicines such as griseofulvin that are taken internally. In addition, shampoos that contain selenium sulfide 2.5 percent are used daily. Treatment can take up to 6 weeks or longer.

■ BASIC PLAN

Diet

Avoid giving your child sugar products, as sugar feeds the fungus. This includes soft drinks, candy, and processed foods such as sugar-sweetened cereal. Fruit juices should be diluted and kept to a minimum. Follow a whole-foods diet. (See "Diet" on page 4 for more information.)

Garlic, oregano, and onions have anti-fungal effects and can be included in prepared meals. Be careful with younger children, as they may have difficulty with spices.

Nutritional Supplements

Probiotic—A children's acidophilus with bifidus formula builds up good bacteria, which help to fight a fungal infection and keep it from overgrowing. Give as directed on the container.

Zinc—Supports the immune system and enhances skin healing. Dosage: children 2 and younger, 5 milligrams; 2 and older, 10 to 15 milligrams. Use for 2 weeks and then stop.

Herbal Remedy

Tea tree oil—The herb of choice for fungal infections. Use a tea tree oil shampoo daily for 1 month.

Homeopathy

Pick the following remedy that best matches your child's symptoms. Unless otherwise indicated, give your child 2 pellets of a 30C potency two times daily. Improvements should be seen within 2 weeks. If there is no improvement within 2 weeks, try another rem-edy. After you first notice improvement, stop giving the remedy unless symptoms begin to return.

Note: Lower potencies (6X, 12X, 6C) may need to be given more often (three times daily).

Calcarea carbonica—The child has ringworm on her scalp. For a large, flabby child who sweats easily on the back of her head.

Sulphur—The area of infection is red, irritated, and burning. The child may have other skin rashes as well.

Thuja occidentalis—For long-standing cases of ringworm that do not respond to treatment.

■ ADVANCED PLAN

Herbal Remedies

Echinacea—Taken internally to support the immune system's response to the fungal infection.

Calendula—Soothing and healing to dry and cracked skin. Apply topically twice daily to the affected area.

■ WHAT TO EXPECT

Improvement is usually noticed within 4 to 6 weeks of treatment.

Roseola

Roseola is a contagious, viral disease that generally affects children under age 2. It is characterized by a fever of 103° to 105°F that begins suddenly and lasts for 3 to 5 days. Usually by the fourth day, the fever comes down and is followed quickly by an itchy pink rash that appears on the chest and abdomen (and to a lesser extent on the face and extremities). The rash usually lasts for a few hours to 2 days. Roseola may also result in swollen lymph glands, an enlarged spleen, a runny nose, a sore throat, irritability, fussiness, and loss of appetite.

This disease is caused by a member of the herpes family (different from the herpes viruses that cause cold sores or genital herpes). Roseola tends to be most prevalent during the spring and summer months in northern climates. It can quickly spread in places frequented by babies and toddlers, especially day care centers and shopping malls. A child with roseola can be infectious for up to 5 days after the fever subsides.

Usually, roseola goes away without any treatment. A child with a fever and a rash should be excluded from day care until seen by a physician. Complications are rare, though febrile seizures can occur due to the prolonged high fever. Seek immediate medical attention if your child has any of the following symptoms:

- Acts confused, lethargic, or delirious
- Experiences a seizure
- Vomits or has diarrhea
- Complains of a stiff neck or has dilated pupils
- Has had the fever for more than 72 hours
- Cries continuously
- Is difficult to awaken

- Has a significant decrease in urine output
- Has trouble breathing

The conventional approach is to use fever-reducing medications such as acetaminophen to control the fever and make the child more comfortable.

Caution: Never give aspirin to a child who has a fever. This can cause an immune reaction leading to the development of Reye's syndrome, a potentially fatal illness where liver and brain damage can occur. The herb white willow, which contains active ingredients similar to aspirin, may pose the same risk, so avoid using it as well.

■ BASIC PLAN

Diet
Dehydration is the biggest concern. Regular water intake is important to prevent dehydration. Herbal teas and highly diluted fruit juices can also be given. Frozen fruit juice pops are popular with kids but should be used sparingly due to their sugar content, which can hinder immune function.

Do not force your child to eat if he is not hungry. Instead, offer light, easy-to-digest soups and broths.

Do not give your child sugar products, which can lower immune function.

Breastfeeding should be maintained for nursing infants.

Nutritional Supplement
Vitamin C—Supports the immune system and has mild anti-inflammatory effects. The

type with bioflavonoids is preferable. Dosage: the child's age in years times 50 milligrams, twice daily. Reduce the dosage if diarrhea occurs. Consider using a buffered vitamin C powder (nonacidic) or liquid vitamin C. Both work well for infants and children, and can be mixed in juice.

Herbal Remedies

Echinacea—Has fever-reducing properties and helps stimulate immune cells to fight an infection. Alcohol-free, flavored products are available for children.

Yarrow, chamomile, and elder flower—One or a combination of these herbs in tea or tincture form helps to reduce a fever and make a child more comfortable. **Peppermint** is also cooling and adds a pleasant taste.

Homeopathy

Combination fever remedies are available. Or pick the one of the following remedies that matches best to your child's symptoms. For the remedies below, give 2 pellets of a 30C potency every hour for up to 3 doses. (For infants, crush the pellets into powder and mix it with water.) If there is no improvement, switch to another remedy. For very high fevers (104°F), give the indicated remedy every 15 minutes and seek medical attention.

Note: Lower potencies (6X, 12X, 6C) can be used with the same frequency.

Aconitum napellus—Useful at the very beginning of a fever when there is a sudden onset. Often occurs after the child has been exposed to the cold or wind. The child is restless and fearful, and he may be crying. This remedy is most useful in the first few hours of a sudden fever. One cheek may be red and the other pale during a fever.

Arsenicum album—For a fever that occurs or increases between midnight and 2:00 A.M. The child is chilly along with the fever. Anxiety and restlessness are usually present. The child feels better with sips of warm water.

Belladonna—For a sudden, intense fever. The child's body feels very hot, but his feet are cold. The child does not usually get any chills. His pupils may be dilated, and his cheeks and face are often bright red. He may be sensitive to light and have a throbbing headache.

Bryonia alba—The child has a fever with a tremendous thirst. His face is flushed. He is very irritable and does not want to move.

Chamomilla—For fever that accompanies teething. One cheek is red while the other is pale. The child is very irritable and feels better temporarily being carried or rocked.

Ferrum phosphoricum—The child has a fever but does not act sick. Use this remedy if you do not know which remedy to use.

Pulsatilla—The child has a fever with low thirst. He wants to be held and is very clingy. He feels better with an open window or in the open air. Symptoms change a lot during the fever.

Pyrogen or pyrogenium—The child has a high fever and appears very sick. His body feels bruised and aching. His pulse does not match up to his fever (for instance, he has a high fever but a slow pulse). This is not a common remedy in stores, so you may need to see a homeopathic practitioner.

Sulphur—For acute or long-lasting fevers where the whole body is warm. The child has a high thirst for cold drinks. His feet get really hot and he wants them and the rest of his body uncovered. The top of his head gets very hot.

Hydrotherapy

Constitutional hydrotherapy works very well in helping to control fevers and fight infections. The next best choice is foot hydrotherapy. (See Hydrotherapy for Children on page 115 for directions.) Perform either therapy one or two times daily.

■ WHAT TO EXPECT

The child should feel better within 48 hours of natural treatment.

Scabies

Appropriately, *scabies* is derived from the Latin word for "to scratch." Microscopic, crablike creatures called mites (*Sarcoptes scabiei*) cause this highly contagious skin rash infection. They are passed on from other people or from infested items such as clothing or bedding. Animals such as sheep can also harbor scabies.

Classic signs that a child has scabies include prolonged and intense itching or scratching of bumps the size of flea bites, about 7 to 10 days after the mites lay eggs just under the top surface of the skin. These pests leave their calling cards: linear, bumpy, pinkish or light gray trails that indicate that the mites are burrowing under the skin and creating an allergic reaction. The itching seems to accelerate at night (the mites travel then, while the child is sleeping). The rash may progress to scaly and crusty lesions.

Prime places for scabies are between the toes and the fingers, in the armpits, and on the wrists, genitals, breasts, and buttocks.

Scabies can quickly spread from one child to the next through skin-to-skin contact or by the sharing of infected clothing, towels, or bed linens. Everyone in the household is at risk, including family pets. Children with scabies are also vulnerable to a secondary bacterial infection due to cuts in the skin created by scratching with dirty fingernails.

The conventional treatment is the use of permethrin cream (sold under the brand names Nix and Elimite). Topical cortisone cream may be prescribed to reduce itching, or in more severe cases, prednisone may be prescribed for internal use. Antibiotics are given only if there is a secondary bacterial skin infection. Wash everything that the child contacts, using hot water. This includes all clothes, towels, and bedding. These items should not be allowed to come into contact with other children and adults.

■ BASIC PLAN

Diet

Follow a whole-foods diet. (See "Diet" on page 4 for more information.) Garlic and onions are good foods to add to meals for their immune-protective effects.

Herbal Remedy

Tea tree oil cream—After washing the skin, apply the cream or gel form of tea tree oil to the affected areas two or three times daily. Also, add 5 drops of tea tree oil to the child's bathwater when filling the bathtub, swish it around, and then place the child in the water.

Homeopathy

Pick the following remedy that best matches your child's symptoms. Unless otherwise indicated, give your child 2 pellets of a 30C potency twice daily. Improvements should be seen within 48 hours. If there is no improvement within 48 hours, try another remedy. After you first notice improvement, stop giving the remedy unless symptoms begin to return.

Note: Lower potencies (6X, 12X, 6C) may need to be given more often (three times daily).

Psorinum—For children who repeatedly contract scabies.

Sulphur—Helps with the itching and scratching associated with scabies.

■ WHAT TO EXPECT

The infection should resolve within 10 to 14 days. Proper natural therapies help to reduce the itching quickly, often in 24 to 48 hours.

Scarlet Fever

Years ago, before antibiotics, scarlet fever was a serious condition that could do irreversible harm to a child's heart and kidneys. It got its name from the bright red rash that accompanies an infection of group A streptococcal bacteria.

Today, scarlet fever is less prevalent, but it still merits serious attention. Beyond the spotty, spreading rash, other common symptoms include a severe sore throat, painful swallowing, high fever, chills, headache, swollen lymph glands in the neck, nausea, and a loss of appetite. In some cases, yellowish gray patches appear at the back of the throat, and the tongue may be coated white with dots of red. If you notice symptoms of scarlet fever, see a doctor.

The rash first appears on the neck, upper chest, and back areas, and within a day or two, it will spread to the lower trunk, legs, and arms. The tongue has a strawberry color. After 5 days or so, the rash will turn a spotty brown as it fades and begins to peel. Peeling and flaking may last between 2 and 6 weeks.

Children with scarlet fever are at greater risk of developing other medical problems, including strep throat, sinusitis, middle ear infection, rheumatic fever, and kidney tissue damage. In the body's zeal to dispatch immune defenders to attack the bacteria, kidney or heart tissues may get accidentally caught in the crossfire and become damaged. Conventional treatment is to administer antibiotics.

■ BASIC PLAN

Diet

Eliminate sugar products, as they can lower immune function. Warm soups, stews, and steamed vegetables are preferred foods, as they are easy to eat without irritating the throat. Make sure that your child consumes plenty of fluids. Water, warm herbal teas (especially ginger tea), and diluted fruit juices are good.

Nutritional Supplements

Vitamin C—Supports the immune system and has mild anti-inflammatory effects. The type with bioflavonoids is preferable. Dosage: the child's age in years times 50 milligrams, twice daily. Reduce the dosage if diarrhea occurs. Consider using a buffered vitamin C powder (nonacidic) or liquid vitamin C. Both work well for infants and children, and can be mixed in juice.

Probiotic—Choose a children's acidophilus supplement that also contains the good bacteria bifidus. It is especially important for infants who have been on antibiotics. Give as directed on the container.

Herbal Remedies

Echinacea and goldenseal—This combination stimulates the immune system and fights bacterial infection of the throat.

Homeopathy

Pick the following remedy that best matches your child's symptoms. Unless otherwise indicated, give your child 2 pellets of a 30C potency three times daily. Improvements should be seen within 48 hours. If there is no improvement within 48 hours, try another remedy. After you first notice improvement,

stop giving the remedy unless symptoms begin to return.

Note: Lower potencies (6X, 12X, 6C) may need to be given more often (four times daily).

Arsenicum album—The child has burning pains and is very restless and anxious.

Belladonna—The main remedy for this condition. The child has a high fever and a flushed face, and her pupils may be dilated. She has low thirst.

Streptococcinum—Used to prevent a strep bacterial infection or to help the immune system eradicate the infection more efficiently.

Hydrotherapy

Alternate a wrung-out, warm face cloth (2 minutes) with a cold face cloth (5 minutes) and apply to the throat three times. Repeat this twice daily. This alternation of temperatures brings immune cells into the throat area and helps to reduce throat pain.

■ ADVANCED PLAN

Nutritional Supplements

Vitamin A—Supports the immune system. Daily dosage: infants under 1 year, 1,875 international units (IU); children 1 to 3, 2,000 IU; kids 4 to 6, 2,500 IU; kids 7 to 10, 3,500 IU; males 11 and older, 5,000 IU; females 11 and older, 4,000 IU.

Note: These dosages are for short-term use (up to 10 days). Higher dosages may be used only under a doctor's supervision. Available in liquid drops.

Zinc—Supports the immune system and

enhances skin healing. Dosage: children 2 and younger, 5 milligrams; 2 and older, 10 to 15 milligrams. Use for 2 weeks and then stop.

Herbal Remedies

Licorice root—Supports the immune system and soothes a sore throat.

Propolis—Taken as a tincture or as a spray, it has direct antibacterial effects when it contacts the throat.

■ WHAT TO EXPECT

Use the natural therapies in this chapter under the supervision of a doctor. You should notice improvement within 5 days.

Sciatica

Nerve pain and muscle spasm characterize sciatica. In this condition, there is an irritation or compression of the nerves that exit the lower back and the sacral areas of the spine. This can occur from lifting an object improperly, or from a herniated disc, a muscle spasm, or misalignment or subluxations of the lower spine. Pain radiates down the front, side, or back of the leg depending on which area of the spine is affected. Also, leg weakness and abnormal sensations such as numbness can occur. Sciatica is more common in adults but can happen in children.

The conventional approach is to rule out a serious condition of the spine, such as a herniated disc. Treatment involves bed rest, painkillers and anti-inflammatories, and physiotherapy. Chiropractic adjustment or osteopathic manipulation can be quite effective. (See the Natural Health Care Modalities and Resource Guide on page 499 for more on these therapies.)

■ BASIC PLAN

Diet

Avoid foods that can further worsen inflammation, including products that contain caffeine (such as soft drinks and chocolate), saturated fat (such as red meat and dairy products), and sugar. Have your child consume foods rich in calcium and magnesium, and make sure that he drinks plenty of fluids. Also, feed him cold-water fish such as salmon for the omega-3 fatty acids, which have anti-inflammatory properties.

Nutritional Supplements

Calcium—Relaxes muscle spasms. Give 500 milligrams daily.

Magnesium—Relaxes the nerves and muscles. Give along with calcium at 250 to 500 milligrams daily.

Herbal Remedy

Bromelain—Acts as a natural anti-inflammatory. Give 3 milligrams per pound of body weight two or three times daily, between meals.

Homeopathy

Pick the following remedy that best matches your child's symptoms. Unless otherwise indi-

cated, give your child 2 pellets of a 30C potency three times daily. Improvements should be seen within 24 hours. If there is no improvement within 24 hours, try another remedy. After you first notice improvement, stop giving the remedy unless symptoms begin to return.

Note: Lower potencies (6X, 12X, 6C) may need to be given more often (four times daily).

Arsenicum album—For right-sided sciatica with burning nerve pain. The child is restless. Sciatica feels better with warm applications. Symptoms are worse between midnight and 2:00 A.M.

Bryonia alba—For severe lower back pain and sciatica where the child must lie flat. He feels better lying on the painful side.

Colocynthis—For sciatica accompanied by spasms and cramps. The pain tends to be more right-sided. Symptoms feel better with heat and pressure, and lying on the side that hurts. Worse from movement and cold. The child is irritable from the pain.

Gnaphalium polycephalum—For alternating leg numbness and pain. Symptoms are worse lying down. Right-sided sciatica.

Hypericum perforatum—For sciatica resulting from direct injury of the sciatica nerve or the spine. There are cutting, shooting pains along the nerve.

Lachesis—For left- or right-sided sciatica with severe pain and sensitivity. There is burning pain. The skin of the legs is very sensitive. Symptoms are worse at night or upon waking from sleep.

Rhus toxicodendron—For lower back pain and stiffness. There is burning sciatica pain. For sciatica brought on from overexertion. Symptoms are worse in the morning and from being still, from cold, and from lifting. The child feels better with heat and gentle motion.

Note: If you don't know what remedy to give, you can alternate 2 pellets of **Kali phosphoricum 6X** and 2 pellets of **Magnesia phosphorica 6X** to reduce nerve pain and muscle spasm. Give one remedy one hour, and the other an hour later.

■ ADVANCED PLAN

Nutritional Supplement

Methylsulfonylmethane (MSM)—Give 5 milligrams per pound of body weight internally each day, or apply topically as a cream. Use until the problem is resolved. No toxicity.

Acupressure or Acupuncture

Both of these techniques are helpful to relieve sciatica. See a practitioner of oriental medicine.

■ WHAT TO EXPECT

Pick a practitioner that specializes in musculoskeletal problems, such as a chiropractor, for specific treatment. Also, incorporate the natural therapies listed in this chapter. Acute cases can be improved in 24 to 48 hours.

Seizures

In general terms, a seizure is an abrupt, uncontrollable contraction of muscles that may be

Vital Fact

More than 2 million Americans have epilepsy, and 30 percent of them are children under age 18. About 180,000 new cases of epilepsy are diagnosed each year.

mild or severe. During a seizure, the normal electrical activity of the brain is altered, resulting in a sudden change in movement, behavior, sensation, or consciousness triggered by an abnormal electrical discharge to the brain. Epilepsy is a neurological condition that covers a variety of seizure disorders. Children who have reoccurring seizures are diagnosed to have epilepsy.

During a seizure, brain cells fire uncontrollably at rates up to four times normal, temporarily impacting the way a child moves, thinks, feels, or behaves.

When this abnormal electrical activity affects the entire cerebral cortex of the brain, it is called a primary generalized seizure. When it is restricted to one brain area, it is called a partial seizure. Here is some specific information on the two types.

Primary generalized seizure: Of this type, there are two main subtypes: grand mal and petit mal. Grand mal seizures are characterized by the loss of consciousness, falling to the ground, and the temporary cessation of breathing. A child's body muscles contract simultaneously, and the seizure lasts less than 2 minutes. Petit mal seizures usually involve rapid blinking, blank stares, stationary positioning, and chewing movements of the mouth.

Partial seizure: The primary types of partial seizures are called simple partial and complex partial. Simple partial is a very localized seizure that a person may feel without it affecting her level of awareness. One arm or leg may jerk, or a person may feel nausea or unexplained rage, or notice abnormal smells. Complex partial is more common. In this type, a person loses her awareness of her surroundings, displays a blank stare, makes chewing movements with her mouth, and cannot recall the episode once the seizure is over. Some people may repeat a string of inappropriate words or phrases during this type of seizure.

Seizures are caused by a host of conditions, including brain injuries suffered before or after birth, infections (especially encephalitis and meningitis), genetic disorders (such as tuberous sclerosis), a high fever (this type of seizure is called a febrile seizure), poisoning, epilepsy, shock, an allergic reaction, and brain tumors. In many cases, there is no identifiable cause for the seizures.

■ IMMEDIATE TREATMENT

If your child is having her first seizure, call for emergency medical help.

Talk to your child with reassuring and calming words.

Watch to make sure that your child is breathing and has an open airway. Do not try to hold down her tongue or insert anything in her mouth, as it may cause choking or you may be bitten.

Do not touch your child during a seizure or try to hold her down. Instead, clear the surrounding area of anything that could cause injury. Try to place a pillow or blankets underneath your child's head. Loosen her clothes if possible.

Call for emergency help if your child is turning pale or blue or has difficulty breathing, or if the seizure is lasting longer than 10 minutes.

■ BASIC PLAN

Note: It is important that you do not take your child off any anticonvulsant medications and start the following natural protocol. This all needs to be done with medical supervision. Work with your doctor to implement some of these natural therapies while your child's seizures are under control on pharmaceutical medication. After 4 to 6 months of natural treatment, work with your doctor to see whether your child's medication can be reduced. For some children with severe epilepsy, this may not be possible.

Diet

First used as a treatment in 1921, the ketogenic diet has shown to be helpful for myoclonic, focal, and temporal lobe epilepsy. The exact mode of action is still unknown. The classical 4-to-1 ketogenic diet contains four times as much fat as carbohydrates plus protein. The diet be-

Vital Study

A study published in *Pediatrics* evaluated the effectiveness and tolerability of the ketogenic diet in children who were unresponsive to seizure medications. This diet contains four times as much fat as carbohydrates plus protein, and begins with a 24-hour fast (allowing fluids). One hundred fifty children ages 1 to 16 years, virtually all of whom continued to have more than two seizures per week despite therapy with at least two anticonvulsant medications, were prospectively enrolled in this study, treated with the ketogenic diet, and followed for a minimum of 1 year. Researchers found that 3 months after the children began the diet, 83 percent of those starting remained on the diet, and 34 percent had a greater than 90 percent decrease in seizures. At 6 months, 71 percent still remained on the diet, and 32 percent had a greater than 90 percent decrease in seizures. At 1 year, 55 percent remained on the diet, and 27 percent had a greater than 90 percent decrease in seizure frequency. The authors of the study concluded that the ketogenic diet should be considered as an alternative therapy for children with difficult-to-control seizures. It is more effective than many of the new anticonvulsant medications and is well-tolerated by children and families when it is effective.

Vital Study

For a double-blind study published in *Epilepsia,* 24 children who did not respond to anticonvulsant medications were given either vitamin E (400 international units per day) or a placebo in addition to their medication. Researchers found that after 3 months, there was a significant improvement in those given the vitamin E (10 of 12 improved), while no improvement was noted in the control group (zero of 12 improved). No adverse effects were noted in the group of children given vitamin E.

gins with a typical 24-hour fast (allowing fluids such as water). This diet needs to be done under medical supervision with a doctor who has experience with the ketogenic diet.

Food sensitivities can be involved. Keep a diet diary and see if you notice any correlation between seizures and what your child has eaten. Dairy products and gluten products should be taken out of the diet to see if there is improvement. Food sensitivity testing is advised. (See "Food Allergies and Food Sensitivities" on page 298 for more information.)

Regular meals can be important to maintain adequate blood sugar levels.

Caffeine-containing products should be avoided, as caffeine is a stimulant.

Avoid all artificial sweeteners, and minimize artificial dyes and colorings as much as possible.

Nutritional Supplements

Calcium and magnesium—Help to relax the nervous system. Have your child take 500 milligrams twice daily of calcium and 500 milligrams of magnesium daily as part of a preventive supplement program. This combination is available in liquid form.

Vitamin B$_6$—Some studies have shown vitamin B$_6$ to be of value in the treatment of epilepsy. Anticonvulsants may lower the levels of this vitamin. A supplemental B$_6$ dosage of 25 to 50 milligrams daily is recommended in addition to any multivitamin the child might be taking. It should be used under the guidance of a doctor. Higher dosages may interfere with anticonvulsant medications.

Vitamin E—Up to 400 international units per day may be helpful with epileptic children.

Homeopathy

Kali phosphoricum 6X and **Magnesia phosphorica 6X** are good nerve tonics and can be used long-term even if the child is on medication. Give 2 pellets of both remedies together, twice daily.

There are many different remedies that can be used to treat a child to prevent epilepsy. This is best done with a homeopathic practitioner and the collaboration of the child's neurologist.

■ ADVANCED PLAN

Nutritional Supplements

The following supplements may also be helpful for children with epilepsy. Typical daily dosages are listed, but these supplements are best used under the guidance of a nutri-tion-oriented doctor.

Zinc—Dosage: children 2 and younger, 5 milligrams; 2 and older, 10 to 15 milligrams. Use with 1 milligram of copper long term.

Selenium—Dosage: 1 microgram per pound of body weight.

Manganese—Dosage: 1 to 3 milligrams.

Choline—Dosage: 10 to 30 milligrams.

GABA—Gamma-aminobutyric acid has an inhibitory action on the nervous system. Use it under the guidance of a knowledgeable practitioner.

■ WHAT TO EXPECT

Work with a nutrition-oriented or holistic doctor, as this can be a complex condition to treat. It needs to be approached very carefully with the help of a specialist when a child is on anticonvulsant medication.

Separation Anxiety

Signs of separation anxiety may start surfacing around 6 months of age, tied in to the crawling phase for infants. This emotional feeling of un-easiness and desire to be within eyesight of a parent, usually the mother, intensifies when a baby begins walking and developing coordina-tion skills.

It can be very upsetting for parents to hear their baby begin a loud crying outburst each time they leave the room. Separation anxiety is quite common among infants between the ages of 12 months and 18 months. Some re-search suggests that this time period is when the baby's body has the physical skills to walk and move away from the parents but does not have the mental maturity yet to cope with this temporary separation.

■ BASIC PLAN

First, prepare your child by letting him know that you will be coming back to get him.

Second, do not have a long goodbye, which heightens the child's anxiety. Give him a kiss, and tell him that you love him and will be back soon to pick him up.

Homeopathy

Bach Flower Rescue Remedy—Helps to calm the child down and lessen anxiety. Give the child 2 drops as needed, just before drop-ping him off or leaving.

Pulsatilla 30C—For a child who gets weepy and does not want his parents to leave him with someone else. A very clingy and shy child. Give 2 pellets (crushed up and mixed into water for infants) as needed.

Aromatherapy

Lavender and orange—Add 1 drop of each to a vaporizer. Leave it on in the room with the babysitter while you are gone. If the child is taking a homeopathic remedy, use aro-matherapy at a different time.

■ WHAT TO EXPECT

With time, your child should become more comfortable with you leaving. Homeopathic remedies can help a child with this transition period.

Shinsplints

Do you have a child who loves to run? Or one who is addicted to playing tennis? She may be prone to a condition called shinsplints. Shinsplints are muscle pain in the lower legs usually caused by exercise or other kinds of repetitive physical activity.

Certain repetitive movements common in jogging, power walking, and playing tennis can irritate the tendons and connective tissue that connect the leg muscles to the lower leg bones. Running on hard surfaces such as pavement increases the risk of shinsplints. This constant taxing of the muscle can evoke excessive stress on the muscle found on the front of the shinbone. There may also be swelling in addition to the constant leg pain. If the leg pain continues or worsens while the child rests, check with your doctor. That's a signal of a potential stress fracture.

The conventional approach is rest and pain-relieving medications such as acetaminophen. Physiotherapy may be recommended in more severe cases. (See "Physiotherapy" on page 506 for more information.)

■ BASIC PLAN

Rest is important so that more damage is not done and to give the tissues time to heal.

Apply an ice pack for 20 minutes at a time, three times daily, during the first 24 to 48 hours. Then, alternate hot and cold applications after the first 24 to 48 hours until the shinsplints are healed. Massaging the muscles around the injured site helps to bring circulation to the area and speed healing.

As a preventive measure, make sure that your child has shoes that fit properly and that have adequate cushioning for shock absorption. If your child likes to run or jog, have her do so on grass instead of concrete whenever possible in order to lessen the trauma to her legs.

Diet

Foods rich in vitamin C, such as fruits and vegetables, are needed to help repair the damaged connective tissue on the shin area. Good choices include citrus fruits, tomatoes, green peppers, dark green leafy vegetables, broccoli, cantaloupe, strawberries, Brussels sprouts, potatoes, and asparagus.

Nutritional Supplement

Vitamin C—Required to repair damaged connective tissue and has mild anti-inflammatory effects. The type with bioflavonoids is preferable. Dosage: the child's age in years times 50 milligrams, twice daily. Reduce the dosage if diarrhea occurs. Consider using a buffered vitamin C powder (nonacidic) or liquid vitamin C. Both can be mixed in juice.

Herbal Remedy

Arnica—Applied topically twice a day as an oil, cream, or gel to reduce pain and inflammation. Do not apply if the skin is broken.

Homeopathy

Pick the following remedy that best matches your child's symptoms. Unless otherwise indicated, give your child 2 pellets of a 30C potency twice daily. Improvements should be seen within 2 to 3 days. If there is no improvement within 3 days, try another remedy. After you first notice improvement, stop giving the remedy unless symptoms begin to return.

Note: Lower potencies (6X, 12X, 6C) may need to be given more often (three times daily).

Calcarea fluorica 6X—Use on a long-term basis to strengthen the patellar ligament and connective tissue that has become damaged with shinsplints.

Ruta graveolens—Heals sprained tendons and connective tissue that results in stiffness.

Rhus toxicodendron—Can be alternated with Ruta graveolens to help reduce stiffness and soreness.

■ ADVANCED PLAN

Nutritional Supplements

Methylsulfonylmethane (MSM)—Apply topically as a cream to reduce pain and inflammation, or give 5 milligrams per pound of body weight internally each day in supplement form. Use until the pain is gone.

Children's multivitamin—Provides a base of vitamins and minerals for tissue healing.

Manganese—Important for shinsplint healing. Give 3 milligrams daily for 2 weeks.

■ WHAT TO EXPECT

You may see rapid improvement within 7 days if the child does not stress the injury. Severe cases may take weeks to heal.

Side Stitches

Side stitches are those unexpected—and unwelcome—muscular pains that tug at a child's abdomen. They usually strike when a child is sprinting after a soccer ball, running for first base, or challenging a buddy to a friendly speed sprint. The next thing you see is your child stopping abruptly, leaning forward, and holding his side.

What causes a side stitch remains a mystery. However, experts theorize that short, spasmodic bursts of pain occur when the diaphragm (the muscle we use to breathe) fails to get an adequate supply of oxygen. As a consequence, the diaphragm starts to tighten and release a series of muscle spasms.

Although even champion runners can get them, people are more apt to suffer side stitches when they are out of shape or are exerting themselves too hard. Also, physical activity after a meal can lead to side stitches.

Fortunately, side stitches usually subside quickly. However, check with your doctor if your child experiences any of these symptoms:

- A mild fever
- Pain that persists beyond 3 hours
- Severe pain
- Pain that continues after a bowel movement

- Pain that remains even after several weeks of training

These symptoms could indicate a more serious condition such as appendicitis.

■ BASIC PLAN

Have your child build up his exercise activity gradually over time. Deep breathing exercises can also be helpful in preventing side stitches. Teach your child to breath more effectively through abdominal breathing exercises. Also, it is helpful if your child warms up before strenuous exercise.

Diet

Make sure that your child does not participate in strenuous activity right after eating, especially if he is prone to side stitches. Have him wait 30 minutes after eating. Large meals should be avoided before bouts of exercise. Food sensitivities may aggravate this condition. (See "Food Allergies and Food Sensitivities" on page 298.)

Nutritional Supplements

Calcium and magnesium—Give 500 milligrams of calcium and 250 of magnesium daily to prevent muscle tightening.

Homeopathy

Bryonia alba 30C—For sharp, stitching pain that is worse with movement. Give 2 pellets every 5 minutes for relief of side stitches.

Magnesia phosphorica 6X—Reduces muscle spasms and cramping. Give 2 pellets every 5 minutes for relief of side stitches.

■ WHAT TO EXPECT

If they are regularly active, most children will avoid side stitches. However, homeopathic remedies can provide relief within minutes.

Sinusitis

Sinusitis is an infection of the sinuses—the four sets of moist air cavities located in the forehead above the eyes, just below each eye, behind the cheeks, and surrounding the bridge of the nose. Actually, there are two types of sinusitis: acute sinusitis, which lasts for less than 1 month; and chronic sinusitis, which persists beyond 1 month.

In a healthy child, mucous membranes line the sinuses and effectively warm, moisten, and filter incoming air that is heading toward the trachea and lungs. Problems develop when nasal passageway membranes swell and obstruct the ducts that lead to the sinuses. This makes the sinuses irritated, inflamed, blocked, and prone to bacterial or viral infections.

In preteen children, sinusitis tends to hover around the nose and cheek regions. A child may complain of a runny or stuffy nose. Then, a fever emerges, followed by a thick white or green-yellow nasal discharge, swelling around the eyes, bad breath, and cheek pain or tenderness.

In teens, sinusitis is often characterized by pain or heaviness in the forehead as well as a headache and fever.

Sinusitis often happens after the onset of a

cold (with a secondary bacterial infection of the sinus). Also, pollen allergies such as hay fever can be at the root of sinusitis. An underestimated cause of chronic sinusitis is food sensitivities.

The conventional treatment for an infection-related sinusitis is antibiotics and pain- and fever-reducing medications such as acetaminophen. Antihistamines may be prescribed for pollen-related sinusitis.

■ BASIC PLAN

Diet

Food sensitivities are often involved with cases of chronic sinusitis. Dairy products are the most common offender. (See "Food Allergies and Food Sensitivities" on page 298 to identify and treat possible food sensitivities in your child.)

Nutritional Supplement

Vitamin C—Supports the immune system and has mild anti-inflammatory effects. The type with bioflavonoids is preferable. Dosage: the child's age in years times 50 milligrams, twice daily. Reduce the dosage if diarrhea occurs. Consider using a buffered vitamin C powder (nonacidic) or liquid vitamin C. Both work well for infants and children, and can be mixed in juice.

Herbal Remedies

Echinacea and goldenseal—This combination works well to treat virus- or bacteria-related sinusitis.

Homeopathy

Use a combination sinusitis formula, or pick the one of the following remedies that best matches your child's symptoms. For the remedies below, unless otherwise indicated, give your child 2 pellets of a 30C potency three times daily. Improvements should be seen within 24 hours. If there is no improvement within 24 hours, try another remedy. After you first notice improvement, stop giving the remedy unless symptoms begin to return.

Note: Lower potencies (6X, 12X, 6C) may need to be given more often (four times daily).

Belladonna—For the first stage of a sinus infection. There is fever and throbbing pain, especially on the right side of the sinus. The pain is worse when the child bends her head forward.

Bryonia alba—Movement of the child's head, especially bending the head downward, causes sinus pain.

Hepar sulphuris—For a painful, stuffy nose. The child is irritable. Her nose runs when exposed to cold air.

Kali bichromicum—For thick, stringy, yellow and/or green mucus that causes pain at the root of the nose.

Mercurius solubilis or vivus—The child is feverish and has pain around her nose and cheekbones. She salivates excessively and has a coated tongue. The nasal discharge is foul-smelling, and so is the breath.

Nux vomica—For a head cold where the child's nose is stuffed up at night and runs when she wakes up in the morning. The child is irritable, chilly, and impatient.

Pulsatilla—For thick, yellow-green mucus discharge. The child feels better in the open air or with a window open. She feels worse in a warm room. She has low thirst.

Silica—A good remedy for chronic sinusitis where the nasal cavities will not drain. The child feels worse in cold air, but her sinuses feel better with cold applications.

Hydrotherapy

Alternate hot cloths (2 minutes) and cold cloths (3 minutes) over the nose and across the cheeks. Repeat this twice, and do twice daily. This helps to reduce congestion and inflammation.

Acupressure

Gently press each of the following acupressure points with a thumb for 10 to 15 seconds. Perform on both sides of the body and repeat three times each day.

Large Intestine 20—Located on the lower, outer corner of each nostril.

Large Intestine 4—Located in the webbing between the thumb and index finger.

■ ADVANCED PLAN

Nutritional Supplements

N-acetylcysteine—Thins mucus secretions. Give 2 milligrams per pound of body weight, twice daily.

Vitamin A—Supports the immune system. Daily dosage: infants under 1 year, 1,875 international units (IU); children 1 to 3, 2,000 IU; kids 4 to 6, 2,500 IU; kids 7 to 10, 3,500 IU; males 11 and older, 5,000 IU; females 11 and older, 4,000 IU.

Note: These dosages are for short-term use (up to 10 days). Higher dosages may be used only under a doctor's supervision. Available in liquid drops.

Vitamin C—Supports the immune system. Dosage: the child's age in years times 50 milligrams, twice daily. Reduce the dosage if diarrhea occurs. Consider using a buffered vitamin C powder (nonacidic) or liquid vitamin C. Both work well for infants and children, and can be mixed in juice.

Zinc—Supports the immune system and enhances skin healing. Dosage: children 2 and younger, 5 milligrams; 2 and older, 10 to 15 milligrams. Use for 2 weeks and then stop.

Quercitin and bromelain combination—Acts as a natural anti-inflammatory. Especially useful for pollen-related sinusitis. Give 3 milligrams of each per pound of body weight, twice daily.

Pycnogenol or grape seed extract—Has a natural antihistamine effect and is especially useful for pollen-related sinusitis. Daily dosage: 1 milligram per pound of body weight.

Aromatherapy

German chamomile and lavender—Add 1 drop of each to a vaporizer. Or add equal parts of these oils to a carrier oil and rub it into skin below and around the sinuses. Be careful to avoid getting any in your child's eyes. If the child is taking a homeopathic remedy, use aromatherapy at a different time.

■ WHAT TO EXPECT

If your child has acute sinusitis, she should feel relief within 24 to 48 hours. Chronic sinusitis should respond within 7 days.

Snoring

Snoring sounds are produced when the fleshy parts of a child's mouth and airway vibrate in the gusts of air he exhales while sleeping. These vibrating parts include the tonsils, the adenoids, the palate, and the back of the tongue.

During sleep, throat and mouth muscles relax, allowing these other parts to droop a bit and narrow the airway. The narrower this airway, the faster the rush of air that goes through it, making these fleshy parts flap and produce snoring sounds.

Although snoring is much more common among people over age 50, it can occur in children. Sleep position can cause snoring, especially if a child likes to sleep on his back. In this position, the tongue falls back and partially obstructs the airway. An arid climate can also dry out and irritate the linings of the airway, causing snoring.

Children may temporarily snore when they have colds, allergies, or tonsillitis. In all these cases, the throat tissues swell and the tonsils, palate, and adenoids vibrate and partially block the airway. Snoring should stop when these conditions clear up.

Snoring also can be a symptom of a serious condition such as obstructive sleep apnea. This disorder is characterized by brief interruptions of breathing during sleep for 5 and even up to 30 seconds. These breathing pauses may total up to 30 per hour and are almost always accompanied by snoring. A child with this condition will snore loudly and irregularly and experience restless sleep. The louder the snoring, the greater the obstruction to the airway. Besides pauses of silence while your child sleeps, other symptoms that should make one suspicious of sleep apnea include:

• Reduced rate of growth
• Poor speech habits
• Poor school performance
• Hyperactivity

Tape recording your child's breathing sounds while he sleeps can help the doctor identify sleep apnea. If you suspect sleep apnea, have your child evaluated by a doctor who specializes in sleep disorders.

The conventional approach for snoring if it is caused by mucus irritation is a nasal decongestant. Have your child sleep on his side, not his back. Different sleeping positions can be helpful. Saltwater nasal drops are helpful for pollen allergies that clog the sinuses and lead to snoring.

Structural problems in the nasal cavity and/or throat may require surgery.

■ BASIC PLAN

Diet

Food sensitivities can lead to a mucus buildup that can be related to snoring. Dairy and wheat products are the most common offender, but many other foods can be allergens as well. (See "Food Allergies and Food Sensitivities" on page 298 to learn how to identify and treat food sensitivities.)

Nutritional Supplements

Bromelain and quercitin combination— Has a natural anti-inflammatory effect on the mucous membranes. Give 3 milligrams of each per pound of body weight, twice daily.

Herbal Remedies

If the snoring is related to pollen allergies, try freeze-dried **stinging nettle** (150 milligrams daily for children under 10; 300 milligrams daily for kids 10 and older). Or consult with an herbal practitioner for an individualized formulation.

Homeopathy

See a homeopathic practitioner for an individualized remedy.

Other Recommendations

Chiropractic, osteopathic, and craniosacral therapies may be helpful, since they improve drainage of the sinuses. (See the Natural Health Care Modalities and Resource Guide on page 499 for more on these therapies.)

■ WHAT TO EXPECT

Snoring can be a challenge to treat. Look for improvements within 2 weeks of using natural therapies. Otherwise, consult with a doctor or natural health care practitioner.

Sore Throat

The throat, also called the pharynx, is the tubelike funnel that divides into separate tracts for digestion and breathing. Mucous membranes coat the smooth throat muscles. In addition to serving as the passageway for air and food, the mucous membranes of the throat take on the role of protector against invading viruses and bacteria.

You may notice your child grimacing when swallowing or tenderly fingering her throat. Her voice may become hoarse. A sore throat typically features a persistent burning or scratchy throat, often accompanied by difficulty swallowing, a fever, fatigue, headaches, a runny nose, swollen neck glands, and an ear infection.

Almost like clockwork, many children develop sore throats during the early spring and late winter. Viruses are responsible for most sore throats—about two-thirds of all cases. The throat pain tends to go away within a few days. However, some sore throats can be bacterial infections that can persist for a week or longer.

As a safety precaution, have your child examined by a doctor if the sore throat tends to linger or worsen. Symptoms of a sore throat are very similar to a more serious condition called strep throat, which is caused by a bacterial infection.

Also, see a doctor if your child refuses to drink, has a high fever, has difficulty swallowing or excessive drooling, has white patches visible on the back of her throat, or has a history of rheumatic fever.

The conventional approach is to use pain relievers such as acetaminophen, cool drinks, and rest. If a bacterial infection is found with a throat culture, antibiotics are prescribed.

Caution: Do not give your child aspirin if she has a sore throat, as it can lead to a serious condition known as Reye's syndrome. The combination of a viral infection and aspirin use can lead to this problem in rare cases. Most sore throats are caused by viral infections.

■ BASIC PLAN

Diet

Avoid refined sugars, which suppress the immune system. Foods to avoid include sugar, soft drinks, and highly processed foods. In addition, limit dairy products and fast foods, both of which are potentially harmful to the immune system.

Frozen fruit juice pops can help give temporary relief of sore throats but should be used sparingly, as their sugar content can suppress immune function.

Encourage lots of liquids to moisten the throat. Soups, broths, and herbal teas are excellent.

Nutritional Supplements

Vitamin C—Supports the immune system and has mild anti-inflammatory effects. The type with bioflavonoids is preferable. Dosage: the child's age in years times 50 milligrams, twice daily. Reduce the dosage if diarrhea occurs. Consider using a buffered vitamin C powder (nonacidic) or liquid vitamin C. Both

work well for infants and children, and can be mixed in juice.

Herbal Remedies

Echinacea—Stimulates the immune system and fights infections. The liquid form is preferred for sore throats, as direct contact stimulates the lymphatic part of the immune system in the throat. Nonalcoholic, glycerin-based formulations are available, and they also come in different flavors.

Note: Because of its drying effect, do not use the herb goldenseal if the child's throat is very dry.

Homeopathy

Pick the following remedy that best matches your child's symptoms. Unless otherwise indicated, give your child 2 pellets of a 30C potency three times daily. Improvements should be seen within 24 hours. If there is no improvement within 24 hours, try another remedy. After you first notice improvement, stop giving the remedy unless symptoms begin to return.

Note: Lower potencies (6X, 12X, 6C) may need to be given more often (four times daily).

Aconitum napellus—For a sudden onset of a sore throat after the child is exposed to cold air. The throat is dry, red, and hot. The child is restless and anxious. Useful in the first hours of a sore throat.

Apis mellifica—For a red, inflamed throat that comes on quickly. Symptoms feel better with cold drinks (although thirst is low) and worse with warm drinks. The child may describe the pain as stinging or burning. The tonsils and uvula (the tissue in the middle of the throat that hangs down) are swollen and bright red. The soreness tends to be right-sided.

Arsenicum album—For burning pain in the throat that is relieved by warm drinks or warm food and worse with cold drinks or cold food. Pain is often worse on the right side, and the child sips on water frequently throughout the day.

Belladonna—For the first stage of a sore throat where there is high fever (this comes on quickly) and burning pain. The tonsils and throat are a bright or scarlet red color. The child has difficulty swallowing even water. The soreness tends to be right-sided.

Ferrum phosphoricum—The child has a sore throat and fever but does not act or feel really sick.

Hepar sulphuris—The child feels like there is a stick in her throat. The tonsils are often enlarged. The pain is better with hot drinks. The child is very irritable.

Lachesis—For a left-sided sore throat, or one that starts on the left side and moves to the right side. For tickling pain that is better when swallowing food and worse with empty swallowing. The child does not want anything to touch her throat.

Lycopodium—For a right-sided sore throat, or one that starts on the right side and moves to the left. The soreness feels better with warm drinks and worse with cold drinks.

Mercurius solubilis or vivus—The throat looks red and raw, with a lot of burning. The child salivates a lot (even though her throat is dry) and has bad breath and body odor. She is feverish. Glands are often swollen around the neck. There is a metallic taste in the mouth. Symptoms are worse at night.

Phytolacca—Pain radiates from the throat to the ears (particularly the right ear) when swallowing. The child may have pain at the root of her tongue. The throat feels better with cold drinks and worse with warm. The neck glands are enlarged.

Sulphur—The child is warm and sweaty. Her throat burns and is better with ice-cold drinks.

Hydrotherapy

Alternating hot cloths (2 minutes) and cold cloths (3 minutes) over the throat helps to reduce congestion and inflammation. Repeat this twice daily.

■ ADVANCED PLAN

Nutritional Supplements

Vitamin A—Supports the immune system. Daily dosage: infants under 1 year, 1,875 international units (IU); children 1 to 3, 2,000 IU; kids 4 to 6, 2,500 IU; kids 7 to 10, 3,500 IU; males 11 and older, 5,000 IU; females 11 and older, 4,000 IU.

Note: These dosages are for short-term use, up to 10 days. Higher dosages may be used only under a doctor's supervision. Available in liquid drops.

Zinc—Supports the immune system. Dosage: children 2 and younger, 5 milligrams; 2 and older, 10 to 15 milligrams. Use for 2 weeks and then stop.

Herbal Remedies

Propolis—Destroys bacteria and viruses on contact. Best used as a spray or tincture.

Licorice root—Stimulates the immune system and reduces inflammation of the throat.

Slippery elm lozenges—These are very soothing to the throat. If the child is 5 or older (to avoid choking), she can suck the lozenges throughout the day.

Lomatium root—A strong antiviral herb that supports the immune system.

Garlic as a food or supplement is effective to treat viral or bacterial sore throats.

■ WHAT TO EXPECT

You should see improvements within 48 hours of starting natural therapies. If the symptoms get worse, see a doctor.

Sprains and Strains

One misstep or lunge can easily lead to a muscle sprain or strain. Ankles, knees, and wrists are particularly vulnerable to these painful muscle problems, especially among active children.

Although both are usually treated the same way, a sprain differs from a strain. A sprain occurs when ligaments or other nonmuscle tissues surrounding a joint are torn. A strain is the result of overstretching or overtaxing muscle fibers. Both are characterized by swelling, painful movement, and bruising. If the sprain or strain is on a weight-bearing joint such as an ankle, a child may have to walk gingerly or use crutches.

The conventional approach to sprains and strains is to use pain relievers such as acetaminophen, as well as ice and rest. In more severe cases, the site of injury is wrapped or put in a brace or cast. Massage relaxes the muscles, reduces swelling, and increases mobility. Physiotherapy may also be recommended to speed healing. (See the Natural Health Care Modalities and Resource Guide on page 499 for more on these therapies.)

■ BASIC PLAN

Diet

A whole-foods diet is recommended for healing. (See "Diet" on page 4 for more information.)

Nutritional Supplements

Vitamin C—Has mild anti-inflammatory effects and is required for ligament and tendon healing. The type with bioflavonoids is preferable. Dosage: the child's age in years times 50 milligrams, twice daily. Reduce the dosage if diarrhea occurs. Consider using a buffered vitamin C powder (nonacidic) or liquid vitamin C. Both can be mixed in juice.

Bromelain—Has a natural anti-inflammatory effect. Best taken between meals. A common children's dosage is 3 milligrams per pound of body weight, taken twice daily.

Homeopathy

A combination trauma or injury formula contains common homeopathic remedies for an injury. Or you can pick the one of the following remedies that best matches your child's symptoms. Unless otherwise indicated, give your child 2 pellets of a 30C potency twice daily. Improvements should be seen within 48 hours. If there is no improvement within 48 hours, try another remedy. After you first notice improvement, stop giving the remedy unless symptoms begin to return.

Note: Lower potencies (6X, 12X, 6C) may need to be given more often (three times daily).

Arnica montana—Given immediately after a sprain or strain to reduce swelling and pain.

Bryonia alba—Useful for sprains where the least movement causes pain. Use when Rhus toxicodendron is not helping.

Calcarea fluorica 6X—Use long-term to heal and strengthen ligaments and tendons that sprain easily.

Ledum—For ankle sprains that feel cold to the touch and feel better in cold water.

Rhus toxicodendron—A good remedy to use for strains and sprains causing stiffness and immobility. The injury feels better with warm applications, stretching, and movement, and worse from cold.

Ruta graveolens—For sprained ligaments that involve the wrist, spine, knee, and ankle. Follows Arnica montana well.

Hydrotherapy
Alternating hot (3 minutes) and cold (3 minutes) cloths on the affected area helps to improve circulation and relieve swelling and inflammation. Repeat three times.

■ ADVANCED PLAN

Nutritional Supplements
Methylsulfonylmethane (MSM)—Taken internally (5 milligrams per pound of body weight daily) or applied as a cream, this has muscle-relaxing and pain-relieving effects. Use until the injury is healed.

Children's multivitamin—Provides a base of essential vitamins and minerals such as manganese, silica, zinc, copper, and many others that are involved with ligament and tendon healing.

Herbal Remedy
Arnica oil—Apply this twice daily over the sprain to reduce swelling and pain.

Aromatherapy
German chamomile—Apply 2 drops to a warm compress and apply it to the injured area once daily. If the child is taking a homeopathic remedy, use aromatherapy at a different time.

■ WHAT TO EXPECT
Your child should experience improvement within 5 to 7 days. A child's susceptibility to sprains and strains can be reduced with proper nutrition and stretching.

Stomachache

In the middle of the night, the silence is disrupted by a tender voice saying, "Mommy, I got a tummyache."

You enter your child's bedroom and witness him gingerly holding his stomach and wincing in pain. These pains can be sharp, burning, or muscle-cramping. Other symptoms present may include belching, nausea, a loss of appetite, bloating, gas pains, or diarrhea. Children with stomachaches often have bad breath due to the regurgitation of stomach acid up the esophagus.

Stomachaches in children are associated with a variety of physical and emotional causes. Topping the list are hunger, constipation, indigestion, nervous upset, anxiety, stress, the onset of the flu, irritation, food poisoning or sensitivity, and ulcers. A stomachache can also be a symptom related to motion sickness (from riding in a car or boat), hepatitis, overeating, or muscle strain.

The biggest fear among parents is that the stomachache is actually an appendicitis attack. Look for these key clues: writhing in pain, fever with nausea, and vomiting that is not associated with meals. If your child displays these symptoms, contact your doctor immediately. Also contact your doctor if the stomachache does not get better or gets worse as the day goes on.

Among infants, stomachaches can be linked to serious medical conditions, including feeding difficulties, anatomical defects, meningitis, and urinary tract infection.

See a doctor immediately if your child is in severe pain or cannot move because of the abdominal pain.

The conventional approach is to identify the cause of the stomachache and to make sure that nothing serious is occurring. Pain relievers such as acetaminophen may be recommended. A hot water bottle on the stomach helps to relieve abdominal discomfort. Make sure that the bottle is not too hot or left on the skin too long.

If stomachaches are a chronic problem and your doctor cannot find any physical cause, then make sure to talk to your child about stress in his life. Inquire about school, friends, and other factors that may be causing ill health and showing up as stomach problems. Anxiety and stress are common causes of digestive upset.

■ BASIC PLAN

Diet
If your child experiences chronic stomachaches, food sensitivities may be involved. (See "Food Allergies and Food Sensitivities" on page 298 for more information.)

If your child is hungry, feed him soups, stews, or steamed vegetables during bouts of stomachaches. These foods are easier to digest. Avoid giving fried foods.

If your child's stomachaches are due to constipation, then he is likely not getting enough fluids or fiber in his diet. (See "Constipation" on page 245 for more information.)

Nutritional Supplement
Probiotic—Choose a children's acidophilus supplement that also contains the good bacteria bifidus. It is especially important for infants who have been on antibiotics and then suffer from frequent stomachaches and digestive upset. Give as directed on the container.

Herbal Remedy

Chamomile is an excellent herb to relieve acute stomachaches. Make a fresh cup of tea and let it sit until it cools to room temperature. Other good choices include peppermint, ginger, and fennel.

Homeopathy

Pick the following remedy that best matches your child's symptoms. Unless otherwise indicated, give your child 2 pellets of a 30C potency every 30 minutes for up to three doses. (For infants, crush the pellets into powder and mix it with water.) If there is no improvement within 2 hours, try another remedy. After you first notice improvement, stop giving the remedy unless symptoms begin to return.

Note: Lower potencies (6X, 12X, 6C) can be given at the same frequency.

Chamomilla—The child screams and kicks from stomachache. Carrying the infant or child provides temporary relief.

Colocynthis—The child pulls his legs up to his abdomen and feels better with pressure against his abdomen or when bending over.

Ignatia—For stomachaches from emotional stress.

Lycopodium—For stomach pain where the child has a lot of gas and bloating. He feels better with warm drinks or warm applications to the tummy.

Magnesia phosphorica—The child lies down with his knees up to his abdomen. He feels better with a warm water bottle on his abdomen, with warm drinks, or when his abdomen is rubbed.

Nux vomica—For stomachache that results from constipation. Also for stomach pain from eating spicy foods or from adverse reactions to other foods. The child may also have heartburn.

Pulsatilla—For stomachache from eating pastries, ice cream, pork, or other rich and fatty foods. The child wants to be held.

Constitutional Hydrotherapy

This improves circulation to the digestive organs and relieves abdominal pain. (See Hydrotherapy for Children on page 115 for details.)

■ ADVANCED PLAN

Acupressure

Gently press the following acupressure points with a thumb for 10 to 15 seconds. Perform on both sides of the body and repeat three times each day.

Pericardium 6—Located 2½ finger-widths below the wrist crease, in the middle of the forearm (palm side).

Stomach 36—Located four finger-widths below the kneecap and one finger-width toward the outside of the leg (outside of the shinbone on the muscle).

Aromatherapy

Lavender and ginger—Add equal parts to a carrier oil and massage it onto the child's abdomen in a clockwise direction. If the child is taking a homeopathic remedy, use aromatherapy at a different time.

■ WHAT TO EXPECT

Your child should feel a reduction of stomach pain within 15 to 30 minutes of using natural therapies. If the stomachache persists, see a doctor.

Strep Throat

Strep throat is the most virulent version of a sore throat. The key difference is that strep throat is caused by the group A streptococcus bacteria, but sore throats can be caused by other bacteria and viruses, as well as by irritating smoke or chemicals.

With strep throat, the mucous membranes that line the throat become inflamed and the tonsils turn bright red. There may also be white craters or specks of pus on the tonsils. In addition, a child may suffer headaches, a high fever (104°F), abdominal pain, queasiness, and vomiting. Difficulty swallowing occurs because the glands on the front and sides of the neck become painfully swollen.

To definitively identify the condition as strep throat, it is necessary to perform a throat culture test at a doctor's office.

Children between the ages of 5 and 15 are the most susceptible to this contagious illness. Infants can also develop strep throat, but the symptoms are usually milder. Prime targets include children with weakened immune systems due to battling colds and sore throats during the midwinter to early spring. One child can spread the infection to another susceptible person by coughing or sneezing.

Strep throats rarely progress to the more serious conditions known as scarlet fever (marked by a high fever and a florid red rash) and rheumatic fever (which can potentially damage heart tissue).

The conventional therapy is antibiotic treatment and fever- and pain-relieving medicines such as acetaminophen.

■ BASIC PLAN

Diet

Avoid refined sugars, which suppress the immune system. Foods to avoid include sugar, soft drinks, and highly processed foods. In addition, limit dairy products and fast foods, both of which are potentially harmful to the immune system.

Frozen fruit juice pops can help give temporary relief of sore throats but should be used sparingly, as their sugar content can suppress immune function.

Encourage lots of liquids to moisten your child's throat. Soups, broths, and herbal teas are excellent.

Nutritional Supplements

Vitamin C—Supports the immune system and has mild anti-inflammatory effects. The type with bioflavonoids is preferable. Dosage: the child's age in years times 50 milligrams, twice daily. Reduce the dosage if diarrhea occurs. Consider using a buffered vitamin C powder (nonacidic) or liquid vitamin C. Both work well for infants and children, and can be mixed in juice.

Vital Fact

Studies show that up to 20 percent of individuals in certain populations have positive throat cultures for group A streptococci, the bacteria that cause strep throat. These same people have no symptoms and do not require treatment.

Herbal Remedies

Echinacea and goldenseal combination—Stimulates the immune system and fights infections. Goldenseal is specific for infections of mucous membranes such as the throat. The liquid form is preferred for sore throats, as direct contact stimulates the lymphatic part of the immune system in the throat. If your child's throat is very dry, use echinacea by itself or in combination with licorice root. Goldenseal can dry the throat.

Licorice root—Soothing to the throat and has immune-enhancing properties.

Homeopathy

Pick the following remedy that best matches your child's symptoms. Unless otherwise indicated, give your child 2 pellets of a 30C potency three times daily. Improvements should be seen within 24 hours. If there is no improvement within 24 hours, try another remedy. After you first notice improvement, stop giving the remedy unless symptoms begin to return.

Note: Lower potencies (6X, 12X, 6C) may need to be given more often (four times daily).

Aconitum napellus—For sudden onset of a sore throat after the child is exposed to cold air. The throat is dry, red, and hot. The child is restless and anxious. Useful in the first hours of a sore throat.

Apis mellifica—For a red, inflamed throat that comes on quickly. The throat feels better with cold drinks (although thirst is low) and worse with warm drinks. The child may describe the pain as stinging or burning. The tonsils and uvula (the tissue in the middle of the throat that hangs down) are swollen and bright red. The soreness tends to be right-sided.

Arsenicum album—For burning pain in the throat that is relieved by warm drinks or warm food and worsened with cold drinks or cold food. Pain is often worse on the right side, and the child sips on water frequently throughout the day.

Belladonna—For the first stage of a sore throat where there is high fever (this comes on quickly) and burning pain. The tonsils and throat are a bright or scarlet red color. The tongue is often a strawberry color. The child has difficulty swallowing even water. The soreness tends to be right-sided.

Ferrum phosphoricum—The child has a sore throat and fever but does not act or feel really sick.

Hepar sulphuris—The child feels like there is a stick in her throat. The tonsils are often enlarged. The pain is better with hot drinks. The child is very irritable.

Lachesis—For a left-sided sore throat, or one that starts on the left side and moves to the right side. There is tickling pain that is better swallowing food and worse with empty swallowing. The child does not want anything to touch her throat.

Lycopodium—For a right-sided sore throat, or one that starts on the right side and moves to the left. The pain feels better with warm drinks and worse with cold drinks.

Mercurius solubilis or vivus—The throat looks red and raw with a lot of burning. The child salivates a lot (even though her throat is dry) and has bad breath and body odor. She is feverish. Glands are often swollen around the neck. She has a metallic taste in her mouth. Symptoms are worse at night.

Phytolacca—The pain radiates from the throat to the ears (particularly the right ear) when swallowing. The child may have pain at the root of her tongue. Her throat feels better with cold drinks and worse with warm. Neck glands are enlarged.

Streptococcinum—Helps the immune system fight the strep infection more effectively. Can also be given preventively when a child is exposed to someone with strep throat.

Sulphur—The child is warm and sweaty. Her throat burns and is better with ice-cold drinks.

Hydrotherapy

Alternating hot (2 minutes) and cold (3 minutes) cloths over the throat helps to reduce congestion and inflammation. Repeat this twice daily.

■ ADVANCED PLAN

Nutritional Supplements

Vitamin A—Supports the immune system. Daily dosage: infants under 1 year, 1,875 international units (IU); children 1 to 3, 2,000 IU; kids 4 to 6, 2,500 IU; kids 7 to 10, 3,500 IU; males 11 and older, 5,000 IU; females 11 and older, 4,000 IU. *Note:* These dosages are for short-term use (up to 10 days). Higher dosages may be used only under a doctor's supervision. Available in liquid drops.

Zinc—Supports the immune system and enhances skin healing. Dosage: children 2 and younger, 5 milligrams; 2 and older, 10 to 15 milligrams. Use for 2 weeks and then stop.

Probiotic—Choose a children's acidophilus supplement with bifidus. Use for 2 months after your child has been on antibiotics. Give as directed on the container.

Herbal Remedies

Propolis—Destroys bacteria on contact. Best used as a spray or tincture.

Lomatium root—A strong antiviral and antibacterial herb that supports the immune system.

Slippery elm lozenges are very soothing to the throat. Most children over age 5 are able to suck on them without choking.

Garlic as a food or supplement is effective to help treat bacterial sore throats.

■ WHAT TO EXPECT

Your child's doctor will likely prescribe antibiotics for this condition. The natural therapies in this chapter can be used in conjunction with antibiotics to help relieve throat pain and fight the infection. Improvement should be seen within 3 days.

Stress

Stress knows no age limits. Like adults, children can experience the physical and emotional drawbacks associated with stressful situations. As parents, it is important not to lightly dismiss any comments from our children about what makes them feel worried, angry, or sad.

Just like adults, children seek loving, supportive environments in which they feel safe and secure.

Each day, children face new stressful challenges: learning to use manners, the first day of school, trying out for the school band, or taking a math test.

Here is a list of the top 12 stressful things that affect children:

- Moving to a new neighborhood
- Coping with a best friend moving away
- Changing schools, especially in the middle of the semester
- Death of a beloved relative such as a grandparent
- Death of a family pet
- Addition of a new baby brother or sister
- Parents who constantly fight
- Divorce of parents
- Remarriage of a parent to someone with children

- Attending summer camp for the first time
- Being picked on or ridiculed by a bully
- Getting into a tiff with a close friend

Faced with stress, a child may exhibit physical and/or emotional symptoms. He may complain of headaches, stomachaches, malaise, fatigue, or trouble sleeping. Or, he may display temper tantrums, tears, or withdrawal. Or he may feel anxious, worried or depressed. He may begin nervous habits such as fingernail biting or frequent swallowing.

Stress becomes unhealthy when it starts to take a toll on a child's physical and emotional well-being. A child's hormone and immune systems can become worn and weakened, making him more prone to infections and injuries.

Take time to talk to your child about how he feels. Talking about their problems allows children to let out suppressed feelings. Let kids be themselves. While it is important to emphasize discipline, don't be overdemanding with your children. Regular physical activity is a great way to help relieve the effects of stress. Counseling is important if your child cannot cope with or adapt to the stress he is dealing with. Also, if the stress is related to members of the family, then a third party such as a children's counselor is advised.

■ BASIC PLAN

Diet

A whole-foods diet is important; it provides the nutrients your child needs to combat stress. (See "Diet" on page 4 for more information.) Limit the consumption of sugar products, as they deplete minerals and weaken the immune system.

Nutritional Supplement

Children's multivitamin—Provides a base of the essential vitamins and minerals required to combat stress.

Herbal Remedy

Passionflower—Stress that is causing anxiety, tight muscles, and insomnia can be helped with passionflower. Give twice daily for relief of symptoms while the cause is being addressed.

Homeopathy

Bach Flower Remedies—You can give a Bach Flower Rescue Remedy, which helps to ease the effects of stress. Or pick one or a combination of the Bach Flower Remedies that best fits your child's picture of stress. **Aspen**, for instance, is a good remedy for fear and anxiety. **Walnut** is good for a child going through emotional adjustments that cause stress. **White chestnut** is used to combat persistent worry. Give 2 drops one or two times daily. (To combine remedies, see "How to Use Bach Flower Remedies" on page 76.) If there is no improvement within 2 weeks, try another Bach Flower Remedy or consult with a practitioner.

Ignatia 30C—The child is uptight and has mood swings as the result of stress. He cries but wants to be left alone. Give 2 pellets two times daily for 1 week, and then as needed.

Kali phosphoricum 6X and Magnesia phosphorica 6X—If you do not know what to give, this combination is helpful for the effects of stress. Give 2 pellets of each remedy twice daily, alternating remedies for a total of 4 doses.

■ ADVANCED PLAN

Nutritional Supplement

Vitamin C—Supports the immune system and is easily depleted under times of stress. The type with bioflavonoids is preferable. Dosage: the child's age in years times 50 milligrams, once daily. Reduce the dosage if diarrhea occurs. Consider using a buffered vitamin C powder (nonacidic) or liquid vitamin C. Both can be mixed in juice.

Acupressure

Four Gates—Helps to release tension. This is a combination of Liver 3, located on top of the foot in the hollow between the big toe and second toe, and Large Intestine 4, located in the webbing between the thumb and index finger. Two people should push on all four points gently at the same time for 15 seconds. Repeat three times. Do this once daily.

■ WHAT TO EXPECT

By talking with your child and using nutritional and natural therapy support, you can help your child become more resistant to the effects of stress.

Sty

A sty, also known medically as hordeolum, is a common infection that causes lumps to form on the inside or outside of eyelids, usually near the root of an eyelash. Sties develop more often on the edge of the upper eyelid than on the lower eyelid. A chalazion is very similar to a sty and is an enlargement of one of the glands near the eyelid. A chalazion can last for months, while a sty usually starts to clear up in a few days.

Beyond the visible lump, other sty symptoms including swelling in the eyelid, sensitivity to light, excessive tearing, and a yellow, pus-filled blister. Some sties are painful; others are pain-free. They are rarely regarded as a serious eye problem.

Sties develop when the eyelid glands and their ducts become clogged or infected. When this happens, secretions accumulate and harden to form a bump. Large sties can press on the cornea and cause blurred vision.

Most sties are caused by bacterial infection, particularly the staphylococcus bacteria. Acute swelling and inflammation of a gland leads to the production of pus and a hardened blister. Dust, smoke, and pollution can aggravate this condition.

See your doctor if your child's sty is not improving after 3 days or if it is causing too much discomfort. The conventional approach is to apply a warm compress to the sty. Most rupture on their own. Antibiotics are rarely prescribed.

■ BASIC PLAN

The best treatment is to apply a warm compress to the sty for 5 to 10 minutes, four times daily. The sty should rupture on its own, and when it does, your child will feel more relief than pain.

Homeopathy

Homeopathic remedies work well to alleviate the pain of a sty and to accelerate it coming to a head. They also can be helpful in reducing your child's susceptibility to sties. Pick the following remedy that best matches your child's symptoms. Unless otherwise indicated, give your child 2 pellets of a 30C potency three times daily. Improvements should be seen within 24 hours. If there is no improvement within 24 hours, try another remedy. After you first notice improvement, stop giving the remedy unless symptoms begin to return.

Note: Lower potencies (6X, 12X, 6C) may need to be given more often (four times daily).

Apis mellifica—For burning pain from the sty. The eyelid is very puffy and swollen. It feels better with cold applications.

Belladonna—For sties that come on quickly. The eye is red and dry. The skin is very red and swollen.

Hepar sulphuris—For a red eyelid that is filled with pus and very painful. It is sensitive to cold air and better with warm applications.

Pulsatilla—For a sty with a thick, yellow discharge. The eye is watery and itchy and feels worse with warm applications and better with cold and fresh air.

Silica—For a sty that has built up pus but does not erupt. Silica helps with rupture and drainage of the sty.

Staphysagria—The most common remedy for chronic sties. These often occur in children with a history of abuse or suppressed anger.

Sulphur—For hot, burning pain from sties that is worse with warm applications.

■ WHAT TO EXPECT

You should see quick improvement within 48 hours using a hot compress and homeopathy.

Sunburn

Parents encourage their children to go outside and play, but too much sun can be a bad thing. Sunburn is a skin injury caused by overexposure to sunlight. Melanin, the dark pigment found in the top layers of skin, is no longer able to protect the skin from the effects of too much sunlight. Too much of this sort of exposure can cause premature aging of the skin and can increase a child's risk for skin cancer later in life.

Ultraviolet rays create most of sunlight's damage by penetrating radiation through layers of skin and harming deep skin cells. There are two kinds of UV radiation: ultraviolet A (UVA) and ultraviolet B (UVB). UVA exists year-round, and UVB becomes more prevalent during warm months. The sun's rays are the most powerful between 10:00 A.M. and 2:00 P.M. on sunny days, but children can also develop sunburns during cloudy days.

As a result of this radiation exposure, the outer layer of skin (the epidermis) turns red, swells, becomes painful, and may blister. A child may complain of a headache. Symptoms usually surface within 6 to 12 hours after sun exposure and peak at 24 hours. Within a couple of days, the sunburned skin may tan or peel. Sunburn can be categorized as a first-degree burn or a second-degree burn (characterized by blisters).

Severe cases of sunburn can cause restlessness at night.

Children who are fair-skinned with light-colored eyes and blond or red hair are at the greatest risk for sunburn. In addition, children taking certain antibiotics (such as tetracycline) are more prone to sunburn than other children.

Generally, sunburn can be effectively treated at home. However, consult your doctor if your child has any of these accompanying symptoms that may indicate sun poisoning or heatstroke:

- Severe blisters (risk of infection)
- Fever
- Nausea
- Chills

The conventional treatment for sunburns is water compresses and pain-relieving medications such as aspirin or acetaminophen. Although it is controversial, prednisone use for a few days may be prescribed in severe cases.

As a practical preventative, apply sunscreen with an SPF (sun protection factor) of at least 15—and higher for children with sensitive skin (30 SPF)—at least 30 minutes before your child goes outdoors. Cover the entire body. Have your child wear a hat and sunglasses to protect against the ultraviolet rays of the sun. Be aware that UV exposure continues on cloudy days and through the glass of windows in the home and car. Be particularly careful with infants, and make sure that they are covered well when in the sun.

■ BASIC PLAN

If your child appears to be getting sunburn, get her indoors and into a cool bath.

An oatmeal bath is also very soothing. Add a cup of oatmeal powder such as Aveeno to a warm bath. The other alternative is to put regular oatmeal (such as Quaker Oats) into a cheesecloth bag, tie it with a string, and hang it under the faucet or float it in the tub. Have the child soak in the warm bath for 5 to 15 minutes. When done, pat the child dry so that a film of oatmeal is left on the skin. This film contains the anti-itch and soothing properties of the oatmeal.

Diet

Fluid intake is very important. Make sure that your child drinks lots of water the day she gets the sunburn, and for the following 3 days as the tissues heal.

Nutritional Supplement

Vitamin C—Enhances tissue healing and has mild anti-inflammatory effects. The type with bioflavonoids is preferable. Dosage: the child's age in years times 50 milligrams, twice daily. Reduce the dosage if diarrhea occurs. Consider using a buffered vitamin C powder (nonacidic) or liquid vitamin C. Both work well for infants and children, and can be mixed in juice.

Herbal Remedy

Aloe vera—After a cool bath, pat the child dry and apply aloe vera gel to the sunburned skin.

Homeopathy

Cantharis 30C—Give this remedy when it becomes clear that your child has a sunburn. Helps to prevent blistering and reduces pain. Give 2 pellets two times daily on the first day, to stimulate healing.

■ ADVANCED PLAN

Nutritional Supplements

Zinc—Enhances skin healing. Dosage: children 2 and younger, 5 milligrams; 2 and older, 10 to 15 milligrams. Use for 2 weeks and then stop.

Carotenoid complex—Best taken preventively. Many of the carotenoids help to absorb the sun's ultraviolet rays and prevent sun damage. Give as part of a multivitamin.

■ WHAT TO EXPECT

In many cases, prompt natural treatment will prevent blisters from developing. Pain relief is usually noticed the same day using homeopathy or aloe vera.

Surgery, Preparation for and Recovery from

When your child requires surgery, even a minor procedure, it can be a time of stress, anxiety, and worry for the whole family.

Children who eat well-balanced diets, exercise regularly, and are informed about the surgery and the reasons behind it tend to be the best surgical candidates.

You can also do your part to ensure that your child has a speedy and complete recovery and reduce the risk of complications. Natural therapies speed up the healing process.

The conventional approach is pain-relieving medications, rest, and/or physiotherapy. (See "Physiotherapy" on page 506 for more information.)

■ BASIC PLAN

Diet

Depending on the surgery and how your child feels, he may need to consume liquefied foods. Soups, broths, stews, and fresh juices are good. Regular water intake is important to keep the body hydrated. Check with your child's surgeon for the type of diet that is indicated. Once a whole-foods diet can be eaten, follow the guidelines under "Diet" on page 4.

Also, vitamin C–rich foods are important for tissue healing. Good examples include citrus fruits, tomatoes, green bell peppers, dark green leafy vegetables, broccoli, cantaloupe, strawberries, Brussels sprouts, potatoes, and asparagus.

Foods that contain essential fatty acids are very important for hair health. And essential fatty acids are helpful for tissue repair. Fish such as salmon, halibut, trout, and mackerel are good sources and are recommended two or three times weekly. Flaxseeds are an excellent source of the important alpha linolenic acid (ALA). They can be ground up and sprinkled on salads or added to shakes. Grind 1 teaspoon per 50 pounds of body weight (children weighing 30 to 50 pounds may also use 1 tea-

spoon) and give this amount daily, always with 8 ounces of water.

Nutritional Supplements

Children's multivitamin—Provides a base of the essential vitamins and minerals. It is a good idea to make sure that your child is on a multivitamin for a few weeks leading up to the surgery.

Vitamin C—Supports tissue healing and has mild anti-inflammatory effects. The type with bioflavonoids is preferable. Dosage: the child's age in years times 50 milligrams, twice daily. Reduce the dosage if diarrhea occurs. Consider using a buffered vitamin C powder (nonacidic) or liquid vitamin C. Both work well for infants and children, and can be mixed in juice.

Probiotic—Choose a children's acidophilus supplement that also contains the good bacteria bifidus. It is especially important if antibiotics are given after the surgery. Give as directed on the container for 2 months.

Herbal Remedies

Echinacea and/or astragalus are good herbs to support the immune system and prevent infections associated with the surgery or hospital stay. Start giving these 1 week before and give for 2 weeks after surgery.

Homeopathy

Bach Flower Rescue Remedy—This is good to use before surgery if your child has a lot of anxiety. Give 2 drops as needed during the day to help reduce anxiety. It will not interfere with any medications.

Arnica montana 30C or 200C—Immediately after surgery, give a dose to speed the healing process and reduce pain. Give one 2-pellet dose of 200C, or if using the 30C potency, give a 2-pellet dose every 3 hours the first day.

Pick the one of the following remedies that best matches your child's symptoms. For the remedies below, unless otherwise indicated, give your child 2 pellets of a 30C potency three times daily. Improvements should be seen within 48 hours. If there is no improvement within 48 hours, try another remedy. After you first notice improvement, stop giving the remedy unless symptoms begin to return.

Note: Lower potencies (6X, 12X, 6C) may need to be given more often (four times daily).

Calendula—Give twice daily for 2 days to help with the healing of tissue that has stitches.

China officinalis—Used when there is a lot of blood lost from surgery and the child feels very weak.

Hypericum perforatum—Give if there is nerve damage or nerve pain, or for any surgery done where there is major trauma to nerve tissue (for instance, to the spine).

Nux vomica—Use if the child has nausea and vomiting and constipation that is associated with anesthetic use.

Phosphorus—Use if your child has had a severe reaction to an anesthetic.

Staphysagria—Give after abdominal surgery to promote healing and reduce pain.

■ ADVANCED PLAN

Nutritional Supplements

Zinc—Supports the immune system and enhances skin healing. Dosage: children 2 and younger, 5 milligrams; 2 and older, 10 to 15 milligrams. Use for 2 weeks and then stop.

Vitamin E—After surgery, give 100 international units per 50 pounds of body weight daily to help with tissue healing.

Note: Check with your doctor first to make sure that your child has not received any blood-thinning medications. Once the wound has completely healed, vitamin E can be applied topically to prevent scar tissue formation.

■ WHAT TO EXPECT

With these therapies, you should see a quicker healing time, and you lessen the chances of your child developing a secondary infection.

Sweating

Despite its reputation, sweating is usually healthy. When a child sweats excessively, it means that the body's temperature regulators are hard at work. This action of the sweat glands is designed to regulate the amount of water and minerals in the body and to rid the body of unwanted toxins. Sweat glands are located all over the body.

Normal perspiration happens when a child plays vigorously for a long time and races indoors with a sweaty but smiling face. Or when she spends some time outdoors on a hot, humid day. Or when she wears socks made of a synthetic material, such as polyester, acrylic, or nylon, which causes feet to sweat.

But sweating can occur for other reasons.

Emotional disorders can provoke excessive perspiration. Children who feel anxious or panicky or stressed often sweat profusely.

Certain illnesses can also unleash the sweat glands. A child with a fever due to the flu or a sore throat tends to sweat excessively once the fever drops. As the sweat evaporates on the skin, the body cools down. Sweating is also a common symptom of hypoglycemia (low blood sugar), bacterial pneumonia, and tuberculosis.

Serious physical conditions, such as heat exhaustion, can also cause profuse perspiration. Heat exhaustion is caused by the loss of fluids and salt through sweating and the failure to drink enough replacement fluids.

Some children are genetically inclined to sweat more easily than others.

The conventional approach is to look for an underlying infection or metabolic disorder and then institute appropriate therapy.

■ BASIC PLAN

Diet

Food sensitivities can aggravate excessive sweating in some children. (See "Food Allergies and Food Sensitivities" on page 298.) Spicy foods such as hot peppers and garlic may worsen excessive sweating as well.

Do not cut down on fluid intake for a child who sweats easily, as this could lead to dehydration.

Homeopathy

There are different remedies that can help balance out excessive sweating. Following are two of the common ones, but it is best to see a homeopathic practitioner for an individualized prescription. Unless otherwise indicated, give your child 2 pellets of a 30C potency twice daily. Improvements should be seen within 7 days. If there is no improvement within 7 days, try another remedy. After you first notice improvement, stop giving the remedy unless symptoms begin to return. *Note:* Lower potencies (6X, 12X, 6C) may need to be given more often (three times daily).

Calcarea carbonica—The typical Calcarea carbonica infant or child is chubby. She sweats easily on her head and feet. She wakes up with sweat on the back of her neck. Her hands and feet are cold and clammy.

Sulphur—For a child who sweats easily all over her body. She sticks her feet out of the covers at night or sleeps with no covers on. She has bad body odor. The child has a high thirst for cold drinks and may crave spicy foods.

■ WHAT TO EXPECT

Natural therapies can often help reduce excessive sweating within 4 to 6 weeks of treatment.

Swimmer's Ear

Medically called otitis externa, swimmer's ear occurs when excessive moisture gets trapped within the delicate lining of the ear canal.

Children tend to develop swimmer's ear during the hot, humid days of summer, especially if they spend a lot of hours in swimming pools, lakes, rivers, or oceans. Swimming in polluted waters can heighten a child's risk of developing this ear infection.

Usually, the first sign of a problem is an itchy feeling inside the ear canal. Unfortunately, vigorous scratching to relieve this itch often abrades the skin in the canal and causes a bacterial or fungal infection. Other symptoms associated with swimmer's ear include swelling of the ear canal, pain when tugging on the outside ear or when moving the jaw, greenish or yellowish discharge exiting the ear canal, and muffled hearing. Jiggling the child's ear causes a lot of pain.

Mild cases of swimmer's ear usually go away with proper treatment within 5 to 7 days. Left untreated, swimmer's ear can develop into a serious and painful infection. In rare cases, a child may develop malignant otitis externa, a serious condition characterized by reddish, swollen ear canal tissue that bleeds easily.

The conventional approach if the earlobe is infected is to give antibiotics, and cortisone eardrops may be prescribed.

■ BASIC PLAN

Herbal Remedy

Mullein—Place 1 or 2 drops in each ear before your child swims. Many people have found that this prevents swimmer's ear.

Homeopathy

Pick the following remedy that best matches your child's symptoms. Unless otherwise indicated, give your child 2 pellets of a 30C potency three times daily. Improvements should be seen within 48 hours. If there is no improvement within 48 hours, try another remedy. After you first notice improvement, stop giving the remedy unless symptoms begin to return.

Note: Lower potencies (6X, 12X, 6C) may need to be given more often (four times daily).

Belladonna—The ear pain and a fever come on quickly. The ear is very red.

Hepar sulphuris—The earlobe is very sensitive to touch and cold. The child is very irritable.

■ ADVANCED PLAN

Herbal Remedy

Echinacea—Taken internally for immune support for 5 days.

■ WHAT TO EXPECT

Your child should have a decrease in susceptibility to swimmer's ear.

Swollen Glands or Nodes

In healthy children, the lymphatic system of glands and nodes works all over the body to produce antibodies needed to fend off invading viruses or bacteria.

These glands become swollen when their cells (called lymphocytes) must multiply quickly at a site of infection. Their rapid growth causes the glands to swell in size.

Swollen glands are signals that your child's immune system is on the job.

However, seek medical attention if the glands became red, painful, or large enough for you to see, especially if they are accompanied by a high fever. This can be a sign of a serious bacterial infection. Also, see your doctor if your child has chronically swollen glands.

The conventional approach is to let minor cases of swollen glands run their course. Pain relievers such as acetaminophen may be given if the child has discomfort. Antibiotics are given if there is an underlying bacterial infection.

Caution: Do not give your child aspirin for swollen glands, because if he has a viral infection, there is the chance of him developing a serious condition known as Reye's syndrome.

■ BASIC PLAN

Diet

Follow a whole-foods diet (see "Diet" on page 4). Quality protein sources are important, such as fish, legumes, nuts, and lean poultry. Decrease the consumption of sugars and soft drinks, which leach minerals out of the body and have a suppressive effect on the immune system. Artificial sweeteners and preservatives should be avoided.

Foods that contain essential fatty acids are important for immune system health. Fish such as salmon, halibut, trout, and mackerel are good sources. Fresh fish two or three times weekly is recommended. Flaxseeds are an excellent source of the important alpha linolenic acid (ALA). They can be ground up and sprinkled on salads or added to healthy protein, fruit, or vegetable shakes. Grind 1 teaspoon per 50 pounds of body weight (children weighing 30 to 50 pounds may also use 1 teaspoon) and give this amount daily, always with 8 ounces of water.

Breastfeeding is important for a healthy immune system. What a breastfeeding mother eats is important, too. If she eats foods to which her baby is sensitive, these can be passed on through the breast milk, possibly leading to immune problems. For a bottlefed baby who has a weak immune system, switch to a hypoallergenic formula.

Food sensitivities can lead to a weakened immune system. (See "Food Allergies and Food Sensitivities" on page 298 on how to identify and treat this problem.)

Adequate fluid intake is important. Make sure that your child consumes water throughout the day.

Nutritional Supplements

Children's multivitamin—Provides a base of the essential vitamins and minerals.

Vitamin C—Supports the immune system. Dosage: the child's age in years times 50 milligrams, twice daily. Reduce the dosage if diarrhea occurs. Consider using a buffered vitamin C powder (nonacidic) or liquid vitamin C. Both work well for infants and children, and can be mixed in juice.

Herbal Remedies

Immune-enhancing herbs such as **echinacea**, **larix**, **astragalus**, and **reishi** can be used to strengthen a weakened immune system. Give one or a combination of these herbs daily for 10 days, for extra immune support. If the glands are still swollen, see your doctor.

Homeopathy

Pick the following remedy that best matches your child's symptoms. Unless otherwise indicated, give your child 2 pellets of a 30C potency twice daily. (For infants, crush the pellets into powder and mix it with water.) Improvements should be seen within 48 hours. If there is no improvement within 48 hours, try another remedy. After you first notice improvement, stop giving the remedy unless symptoms begin to return.

Note: Lower potencies (6X, 12X, 6C) may need to be given more often (three times daily).

Bromium—For stony hard, swollen lymph nodes of the neck. Tends to be worse on the left side.

Calcarea carbonica—The infant or child has chronic swelling of the neck lymph nodes. The child tends to be plump and sweats easily on the back of his neck.

Hepar sulphuris—For swollen lymph nodes that are very tender to the touch. Symptoms come on after exposure to cold weather.

Mercurius solubilis or vivus—For swollen lymph nodes (especially on the neck) along with bad breath, increased salivation, coated tongue, body odor, and sensitivity to hot and cold.

Phytolacca—For lymph node swelling of the neck area along with tonsil or throat infection. Tends to be worse on the right side.

Silica—For chronic swelling of the lymph nodes. The child gets infections easily.

Constitutional Hydrotherapy

This improves immune power. (See Hydrotherapy for Children on page 115 for directions.) Do daily.

■ ADVANCED PLAN

Nutritional Supplement

Children's whole-food supplement—Choose one that contains a blend of vegetables and fruits. Available in capsule or powder form. Give as directed on the container.

Herbal Remedies

Herbs such as **New Jersey tea** (*Ceanothus americanus*) and **burdock root** can be combined with **echinacea** to improve lymphatic flow and detoxification. Give for up to 10 days.

Aromatherapy

German chamomile—Add to a carrier oil and massage it into the lymph nodes in the direction of the heart. If the child is taking a homeopathic remedy, use aromatherapy at a different time.

Acupressure

Gently press the following acupressure points with a thumb for 10 to 15 seconds. Perform on both sides of the body and repeat three times each day.

Large Intestine 4—Located in the webbing between the thumb and index finger.

Stomach 36—Located four finger-widths below the kneecap and one finger-width toward the outside of the leg (outside of the shinbone on the muscle).

■ WHAT TO EXPECT

Many cases of swollen glands resolve on their own. Natural therapy optimizes the immune response to an infection, and swollen lymph nodes often resolve within 5 to 7 days.

Teeth Grinding

Teeth grinding, or bruxism, is a common condition that occurs when a child is asleep. This involuntary habit occasionally happens during waking hours. Muscles on both sides of the face contract, causing the top and bottom teeth to slide back and forth across each other in a gnashing motion.

About half of all children grind their teeth at some point, and fortunately, most outgrow this habit. Because this gnashing usually occurs during sleeping, it may not be detected until a regular dental checkup.

A child may wake up with a headache or a painful, achy face. Prolonged teeth grinding can wear down teeth, cause gums to recede, and erode jawbone joints. It can also develop into a more painful jaw condition known as temporomandibular joint disorder (TMD).

Stress and anxiety—or unconscious efforts to correct a faulty bite—can trigger teeth grinding. A child who grinds her teeth at night is often doing so as a subconscious response to fears, anxieties, and other upsetting emotions. In rarer cases, hypoglycemia or mercury leakage from dental fillings may provoke teeth grinding.

Teeth grinding can also be an underlying symptom of a worm infection such as pinworms.

A pediatric dentist can evaluate your child's teeth to see if there is any structural cause of the teeth grinding.

■ BASIC PLAN

Diet

Some cases of teeth grinding may be due to a child's food sensitivities. (See "Food Allergies and Food Sensitivities" on page 298 for more information.)

Increased food sources of calcium and magnesium are advised, as a deficiency of these minerals may aggravate teeth grinding. (See Vitamins and Minerals for Children on page 79 for foods that contain these minerals.)

Nutritional Supplement

Calcium and magnesium—Relaxes the muscles and nervous system. Give 500 milligrams of calcium and 250 to 500 milligrams of magnesium daily. Best taken with the evening meal. Available in liquid form. Almost always bought in a formula, but can be given separately.

Herbal Remedy

Passionflower—Promotes relaxation. Give before bedtime.

Aromatherapy

Lavender—Promotes relaxation. Add 2 or 3 drops to a vaporizer and allow the fragrance to fill the room, or add to a bath before bedtime.

Homeopathy

Bach Flower Rescue Remedy—For teeth grinding that is related to stress and anxiety. Give 2 drops before bedtime.

Kali phosphoricum 6X and Magnesia phosphorica 6X—This combination helps to reduce muscle tightness and relax the nerves. Give 2 pellets of each remedy twice daily, alternating remedies for a total of 4 doses.

Specific remedies can be prescribed for teeth grinding. See a homeopathic practitioner for an individualized remedy.

■ ADVANCED PLAN

Nutritional Supplement

Children's multivitamin—Provides a base of the essential vitamins and minerals needed for proper development. Sometimes, nutritional deficiencies can lead to teeth grinding.

■ WHAT TO EXPECT

There should be a reduction in teeth grinding over 4 to 6 weeks.

Teething

During the first few months, mouthwise, a baby is all gums. Family photos sport those wonderful toothless grins. The first tooth pokes through as early as 3 months or as late as 12 months. The rate is heavily influenced by heredity.

Usually, the front teeth on the top and bottom appear first, followed by molars. New teeth arrive monthly. By age 2 or 2½, most babies have all of their 20 temporary teeth (called deciduous teeth).

Teething is the term used to describe this uncomfortable time, when teeth push through the gums. Some babies drool excessively and want to chew and suck on everything. Their cheeks may become red and chapped due to the frequent removal of drooling on sensitive skin. As a tooth emerges up and out of the gums, the tissue surrounding the site can become inflamed and painful. It is not uncommon for babies to be up every night crying in pain, especially when the first few teeth emerge, until they can adjust to the pain and discomfort.

Other signs of teething include a low-grade temperature, fussiness, diarrhea, and a refusal to eat. Teething puts stress on a baby's body, so be aware that during this time, a baby is vulnerable to illnesses (especially diarrhea) and fevers. A child may be more susceptible to colds and ear infections during periods of teething.

By the time a child reaches age 6 or 7, these baby teeth start to be replaced by permanent teeth. Fortunately, the emerging permanent teeth do not create the pain and irritation commonly associated with baby teeth.

The conventional treatment is the use of pain relievers such as infants' acetaminophen and a topical anesthetic teething gel that relieves gum pain. Let your child chew or suck on your finger or a cool washcloth. A teething ring can also work well. Do not freeze the teething ring, to avoid frostbite of your child's gums. Instead, leave it in the refrigerator.

■ BASIC PLAN

Homeopathy

We have found that nothing works as well as homeopathy for teething, and in most cases, it is the only treatment that needs to be used. Most homeopathic companies have combination formulas that contain the most common remedies for teething. They relieve the pain and moodiness that accompany teething without any side effects. They are available at most health food stores and pharmacies.

Another option is to pick the one of the following remedies that best matches your child's symptoms. For the remedies below, unless otherwise indicated, give your child 2 pellets of a 30C potency three times daily. (Crush the pellets into powder and mix it with water, or put the powder in the child's mouth.) Improvements should be seen within 24 hours. If there is no improvement within 24 hours, try another remedy. After you first notice improvement, stop giving the remedy unless symptoms begin to return.

Note: Lower potencies (6X, 12X, 6C) may

Case History

Recently, our neighbor asked us what she should do with her 8-month-old boy, who was in some serious pain from teething. Normally, he was a very happy-go-lucky child. But since the teething had begun 5 days earlier, he had been irritable and crying a lot, with a runny nose and alternating bouts of constipation and diarrhea. We gave him one dose of Chamomilla. Within 15 minutes, he calmed down and stopped crying. His mother told us later that after he received this remedy, his teething symptoms disappeared. Parents report to us all the time that homeopathic remedies for teething "work like a miracle." We have noticed that many babies' and mothers' magazines now advertise homeopathic remedies for teething. This is great—we cannot think of a quicker, safer way to relieve teething.

need to be given more often (four times daily).

Belladonna—For teething where the cheek (especially the right side) gets very red. The child spikes a fever with the teething. The teething is better with pressure.

Calcarea carbonica—The child tends to be large and flabby and has chronic teething problems. This is a plump baby who sweats easily on the back of his head.

Calcarea phosphorica 6X or 30C—A

good remedy when the child is late teething or when other remedies do not help. The child is irritable and discontented.

Chamomilla—This is the most common remedy used for teething. The child is very irritable and very sensitive to pain. It is hard to console him; he wants something and then refuses it when you give it to him. He throws tantrums, screaming and kicking. Carrying and rocking the child provides temporary relief. One cheek may be pale and the other red. Diarrhea (which may be green) accompanies the teething. The child is better with something cold in his mouth, such as a cold teething ring or cloth. Ear infection accompanies the teething.

Coffea cruda—The child is very restless and does not sleep while teething.

Ferrum phosphoricum 6X or 30C—The child's cheeks are red, and he has a fever, but he does not seem to have high levels of pain from teething. Can be used as a preventive remedy during teething spells.

Magnesia phosphorica 6X or 30C—For teething that is better with warmth, such as a warm cloth in the mouth.

Podophyllum—The teething is better when the child is biting things. Green diarrhea accompanies the teething.

Silica 6X or 30C—For a thin child who is slow to teethe and who has susceptibility to tooth decay or abscesses.

■ ADVANCED PLAN

Herbal Remedy

White willow—Has properties similar to aspirin that help to relieve pain. Five to 10 drops two or three times daily may be helpful.

Caution: Do not use white willow if your child is feverish or has a virus.

Acupressure

Large Intestine 4—Located in the webbing between the thumb and index finger. Relieves tooth pain. Gently press the acupressure point with a thumb for 10 to 15 seconds. Perform on both sides of the body and repeat three times each day.

■ WHAT TO EXPECT

Homeopathic remedies usually provide relief within 5 to 30 minutes.

Temporomandibular Joint Disorder (TMD)

This painful condition is an umbrella term for a collection of medical and dental problems that affect the hinged jaw joint and surrounding facial muscles.

When conditions are optimal, the hinged jaw joint, called the temporomandibular joint, is covered with slick cartilage and a thin film of joint fluid. A protective disk within the joint keeps bones from rubbing against each other.

A child with TMD experiences pain when chewing, as well as a clicking or grating sound that comes from moving her jawbone joint to yawn, speak, or eat. In some instances, the jaw's mobility may be compromised, or it may lock when she attempts to open or close her mouth. The inability to fully open the jaw joint can also cause a child's face to look asymmetric. Some children suffer facial pain, frequent headaches, and spasms in the chewing muscles that attach to the bone around the joint.

Stress is often a big factor in TMD. But poor posture, teeth grinding, and keeping one's mouth open for prolonged periods of time can also lead to TMD. Muscle tension in and around the jaw—due to emotional or physical reasons—causes the teeth to clench and grind. Poor dental work and jaw biomechanics can cause a child's bite to be off, contributing to TMD. The alignment of the skull bones and neck vertebrae can also contribute to TMD.

Some infants have TMD problems if there was a lot of jaw and head trauma during delivery. These babies will tend to have a harder time breastfeeding.

The conventional approach to TMD is first to determine whether there is a structural defect or injury that is causing the TMD, and then to prescribe the appropriate therapy (such as dental work, physiotherapy, or surgery). Pain-relieving and muscle-relaxing medications may be prescribed for acute flare-ups.

■ BASIC PLAN

Diet

Your TMD specialist may recommend a temporary liquid or semiliquid diet for times of flare-up so that your child does not have to chew. If this is the case, make sure to use the nutritional supplements listed in this chapter.

Nutritional Supplements

Calcium and magnesium—Relaxes tense muscles surrounding TMD. Take 500 milligrams of calcium and 250 milligrams of magnesium daily.

Homeopathy

Pick the following remedy that best matches your child's symptoms. Unless otherwise indicated, give your child 2 pellets of a 30C potency two times daily. (For infants, crush the pellets into powder and mix it with water.) Improvements should be seen within 7 days. If there is no improvement within 7 days, try another remedy. After you first notice improvement, stop giving the remedy unless symptoms begin to return.

Note: Lower potencies (6X, 12X, 6C) may need to be given more often (three times daily).

Ignatia—Good for TMD that is due to emotional stress. Especially indicated for left-sided jaw pain.

Kali phosphoricum 6X and Magnesia phosphorica 6X—This combination is helpful to relax the jaw muscles. They can be taken on a long-term basis. Give 2 pellets of each remedy twice daily, alternating remedies for a total of 4 doses.

Acupressure

Consult with a practitioner for a specific treatment.

Other Recommendations

Chiropractic, osteopathic, or craniosacral therapy can help to treat the underlying musculoskeletal imbalances that can be causing TMD. Physiotherapy and massage can also be very helpful to relax the nerves and muscles that are tensed in a child with TMD. (See the Natural Health Care Modalities and Resource Guide on page 499 for more on these therapies.)

■ WHAT TO EXPECT

You should notice a reduction in TMD symptoms within 2 to 4 weeks.

Thrush

Thrush is a superficial mouth infection caused by the *Candida albicans* fungus. It affects the lips, the insides of the cheeks, the tongue, and the palate. It can also surface as diaper rash or a vaginal yeast infection. Thrush tends to thrive in warm, moist places such as inside the mouth and vagina and in the diaper area.

Newborns and babies under 6 months of age are most susceptible to thrush. However, anyone who has a weakened immune system or who is chronically ill or malnourished can develop this infection. New mothers who breastfeed their babies may develop thrush on their nipples, which may become puffy, dry, red, itchy, and flaky.

At first, thrush begins as white, flaky, moist patches covering all or a portion of the tongue and gums, the insides of the cheeks, and sometimes, the lips. Although these patches can be scraped off, they leave inflamed

red surfaces that bleed easily. A baby with thrush may lose his appetite. The affected area may itch or develop irritable sores. Don't confuse milk spots in the mouth with thrush. Milk spots are simply dribbles of milk from feeding; they can be easily wiped off, while thrush cannot.

Since yeast can be passed back and forth from the mother's nipple to the child and vice versa, it is good to treat both the breastfeeding mother and her child.

Thrush is often caused by antibiotics (which destroy the mouth's population of good bacteria), infectious mononucleosis, or viral upper respiratory infections.

Consult your doctor if your baby has a fever, cough, or upset stomach in addition to the mouth infection. These are signs that your baby's immune system may be weak or overworked.

The conventional approach is to use a topical antifungal medication.

■ BASIC PLAN

Diet

If you are breastfeeding, do not stop. The immune factors in breast milk will support your baby's immune system to help him fight the fungal infection.

A breastfeeding mother should eat yogurt with live cultures (this should be sugarless, so use the plain variety rather than the flavored) to increase her levels of good bacteria. She should also avoid sugar products, which feed the yeast.

Nutritional Supplements

Probiotic—Choose a powdered children's acidophilus supplement that also contains the good bacteria bifidus. It is especially important for infants who have been on antibiotics. With a washed-off finger, place a fingertip-full in the infant's mouth twice daily until the infection is gone. It is also a good idea to apply children's probiotic powder to the mother's nipple before breastfeeding.

The breastfeeding mother should take an adults' probiotic supplement for at least 1 month as well.

Homeopathy

Pick the following remedy that best matches your child's symptoms. Unless otherwise indicated, give your child 2 pellets of a 30C potency twice daily. (For infants, crush the pellets into powder and mix it with water.) Improvements should be seen within 4 days. If there is no improvement within 4 days, try another remedy. After you first notice improvement, stop giving the remedy unless symptoms begin to return.

Note: Lower potencies (6X, 12X, 6C) may need to be given more often (three times daily).

Borax—Specific for white patches of thrush in the mouth. The first remedy to try.

Hydrastis—For a yellow-streaked tongue and yellow mucus in the mouth.

Other Recommendations

If the baby is using a pacifier or a rubber nipple, make sure to boil these items for 15 minutes daily to kill any lingering yeast.

■ WHAT TO EXPECT

You should see marked improvement within 7 days of natural therapy.

Tonsillitis

The tonsils—two groups of tissue on either side of the pharynx, in the back of the throat—are important in the body's immune system. They help guard the body against invasive germs. When the tonsils become infected by bacteria or a virus, the condition is known as tonsillitis.

The symptoms of viral tonsillitis begin gradually over 1 or 2 days. A child often has a fever, queasiness, and a loss of appetite. Sometimes, there is also a sore throat, a cough, swollen and painful glands on the sides of the neck, and red or irritated tonsils.

Tonsillitis caused by a virus lasts about 24 hours and usually not more than 5 days.

Bacterial tonsillitis is almost always caused by streptococcus bacteria (strep throat). A child can have a sore throat, pain when swallowing, a headache, abdominal pain, and a fever as high at 104°F. Other symptoms include a middle ear infection, sinusitis, and sores around the tonsils.

Doctors used to remove the tonsils (a tonsillectomy) when chronic tonsillitis occurred. Today, it is recognized that the tonsils are part of the lymphatic system and serve as part of the immune system. They are typically not removed unless they are enlarged to the point that they interfere with breathing.

The conventional treatment for bacterial tonsillitis (and usually for viral tonsillitis as well) is antibiotics and a pain-relieving medication such as acetaminophen.

Caution: Do not give your child aspirin for tonsillitis. Aspirin can lead to Reye's syndrome in children with viral infections.

■ BASIC PLAN

Diet

Avoid refined sugars, which suppress the immune system. Food sources to avoid include sugar, soft drinks, and highly processed foods. In addition, avoid dairy products (which are usually the biggest culprit) and fast foods, which are harmful to the immune system.

Frozen fruit juice pops can help give temporary relief of sore throats but should be used sparingly, as their sugar content can suppress immune function.

Encourage lots of liquids to moisten your child's throat. Soups, broths, and herbal teas are excellent.

Nutritional Supplement

Vitamin C—Supports the immune system and has mild anti-inflammatory effects. The type with bioflavonoids is preferable. Dosage: the child's age in years times 50 milligrams, twice daily. Reduce the dosage if diarrhea occurs. Consider using a buffered vitamin C powder (nonacidic) or liquid vitamin C. Both work well for infants and children, and can be mixed in juice.

Herbal Remedies

Echinacea and goldenseal combination—Stimulates the immune system and fights infections. Goldenseal is specific for mucous membrane infections such as bacterial tonsillitis. The liquid form is preferred for sore throats, as direct contact stimulates the lymphatic part of the immune system in the throat.

Licorice root—Soothing to the throat and has immune-enhancing properties.

Homeopathy

Pick the following remedy that best matches your child's symptoms. Unless otherwise indicated, give your child 2 pellets of a 30C potency three times daily. Improvements should be seen within 48 hours. If there is no improvement within 48 hours, try another remedy. After you first notice improvement, stop giving the remedy unless symptoms begin to return.

Note: Lower potencies (6X, 12X, 6C) may need to be given more often (four times daily).

Apis mellifica—For a red, inflamed throat that feels better with cold drinks and worse with warm drinks. The child may describe the pain as stinging or burning. The tonsils and uvula (the tissue in the middle of the throat that hangs down) are swollen and bright red. Generally, this is right-sided tonsillitis.

Arsenicum album—For burning pain in the throat that is relieved by warm drinks or warm food and worsened with cold drinks or cold food. Pain is often worse on the right side, and the child sips water frequently throughout the day. He is restless, and his symptoms are worse from 12:00 to 2:00 A.M.

Belladonna—The most common remedy for strep throat. There is high fever and burning pain. Tonsils and throat are a bright or scarlet red color. This is more often right-sided tonsillitis.

Ferrum phosphoricum—The child has tonsillitis and a sore throat and fever but does not act or feel really sick.

Lachesis—For left-sided, sore tonsillitis. There is a tickling pain that is better when swallowing food and worse with empty swallowing. The child does not want anything to touch his throat.

Lycopodium—For right-sided tonsillitis that feels better with warm drinks.

Mercurius solubilis or vivus—The throat looks red and raw, with a lot of burning. The child salivates a lot (even though his throat is dry) and has bad breath. He is feverish. The glands are often swollen around the neck. Symptoms are worse at night.

Phytolacca—The pain radiates from the throat to the ears (particularly the right ear) when swallowing. The child may have pain at the root of his tongue. His throat feels better with cold drinks and worse with warm ones.

Streptococcinum—Helps the immune system fight a strep infection of the tonsils more effectively. Can also be given preventively when a child is exposed to someone with strep throat

Hydrotherapy

Alternate hot cloths (2 minutes) and cold cloths (3 minutes) over the throat to help reduce congestion and inflammation. Repeat this alternation twice daily.

■ ADVANCED PLAN

Nutritional Supplements

Vitamin A—Supports the immune system. Daily dosage: infants under 1 year, 1,875 international units (IU); children 1 to 3, 2,000 IU; kids 4 to 6, 2,500 IU; kids 7 to 10, 3,500 IU; males 11 and older, 5,000 IU; females 11 and older, 4,000 IU.

Note: These dosages are for short-term use, up to 10 days. Higher dosages may be used only under a doctor's supervision. Available in liquid drops.

Zinc—Supports the immune system. Dosage: children 2 and younger, 5 milligrams; 2 and older, 10 to 15 milligrams. Use for 2 weeks and then stop.

Herbal Remedies

Propolis—Destroys bacteria and viruses on contact. Best used as a spray or tincture on the tonsils and throat area.

Lomatium root—A strong antiviral herb that supports the immune system.

Slippery elm lozenges are very soothing to the throat. Most children over age 5 are able to suck on them without choking.

Garlic as a food or supplement is effective to treat bacterial sore throats.

■ WHAT TO EXPECT

You should notice improvement within 3 days of natural therapy. Natural therapies are also advised if antibiotics are prescribed by your child's doctor, to resolve the infection more quickly and for quicker relief of symptoms.

Toothaches and Tooth Decay

Although young children naturally lose their baby teeth, they are at risk for toothaches and tooth decay if they do not receive proper and regular dental care and eat healthful, fortifying foods.

Toddlers whose teeth are not brushed daily are prone to having their baby teeth fall out prematurely or decay. Either of these consequences can lead to damage or poor placement of permanent teeth.

A persistent toothache usually signals a cavity or an abscessed tooth. The pus from an abscess will either stay under the tooth or emerge to the surface. The surrounding gum becomes inflamed and painful. The abscess can burst and cause blood poisoning.

Tooth decay, known to dentists as dental caries, occurs when the outer covering of a tooth (called enamel) and the body of the tooth (called dentin) gradually disintegrate, often due to acidic erosion. Bacterial plaque slowly eats away at the enamel and dentin until it reaches the pulp, the source of sensitive nerve fibers and nourishment for the tooth.

The main causes of tooth decay are gum diseases. Topping this list are gingivitis, inflammation of gums, periodontitis, tissue inflamma-tion, and jaw bone erosion. Poor dental hygiene can contribute to these diseases. So can poor diet selection. A diet dominated by foods containing refined sugars and starches (including fruit), carbonated sodas, and sources of acid (such as chewable vitamin C tablets) can cause the loss of calcium from tooth enamel in a child.

The conventional approach is for a dentist to evaluate the cause of the toothache and/or tooth decay by visual examination and x-ray. The dentist will likely remove the decayed material and refill the cleaned area with a filling to stop further decay. If there is more serious decay, then an internal part of the tooth (the pulp) may be removed and restored with a metal crown. Also, a root canal or removal of the tooth may be recommended for serious decay.

■ BASIC PLAN

Diet

To reduce your child's susceptibility to tooth decay, greatly reduce the amount of sugars in her diet. This includes soft drinks, candy, and refined carbohydrates. Fruit juices should be used in moderation and always diluted with water. Alkaline foods that are rich in minerals that buffer the saliva include vegetables and whole grains.

Have your child drink water and swish it in her mouth after meals to rinse out bacteria and sugars.

Breastfed infants may have fewer tooth problems. Whether your baby is breastfed or not, do not let her sleep with a bottle of juice or milk. Bacteria build up more quickly with these fluids in the mouth.

Nutritional Supplements

Calcium and magnesium—For children 2 and older, give 500 milligrams of calcium and 250 to 500 milligrams of magnesium to support proper bone health.

Herbal Remedy

For ages 3 and up, a mouth rinse containing **myrrh** (5 drops) combined with either **Oregon grape** or **goldenseal** (5 drops) in an ounce of water helps to cleanse the mouth and reduce gingivitis. Have your child gargle this and spit out twice daily.

Homeopathy

Pick the following remedy that best matches your child's symptoms. Unless otherwise indicated, give your child 2 pellets of a 30C potency every 15 minutes to 1 hour for up to three doses. (For infants, crush the pellets into powder and mix it with water.) If there is no improvement within 2 hours, try another remedy. After you first notice improvement, stop giving the remedy unless symptoms begin to return.

Note: Lower potencies (6X, 12X, 6C) can be given at the same frequency.

Belladonna—For quick onset of tooth pain. The gums are swollen, the cheeks are flushed, and the pain is better with warm applications. Tooth pain is better with pressure.

Chamomilla—This is the most common remedy used for tooth pain. The child is very irritable and very sensitive to pain. It is hard to console her; she wants something and then refuses it when you give it to her. One cheek may be pale and the other red. The child is better with something cold in her mouth (for example, a cold teething ring or cloth).

Coffea cruda—The child is restless and cannot sleep from the pain. Cold water provides some relief, while warm drinks or food make the pain worse.

Hepar sulphuris—The pain is worsened by touch and cold air, water, or food. The child is very irritable.

Hypericum perforatum—For tooth pain as a result of trauma (such as a hit in the teeth, or dental work) where there is shooting nerve pains.

Kreosotum—This is the main remedy for decaying teeth. The child also may have inflamed gums that are spongy and bleed easily.

Mercurius solubilis or vivus—For pain in the teeth. Symptoms are worse at night. The child salivates excessively. Infection may be involved. Other indications include bad breath and decaying teeth.

Plantago major—For toothache on the left side of the mouth. Severe, piercing tooth pain is worse from cold or touch.

Silica—Gum boils or abscesses develop slowly and heal slowly. Gums are sensitive to cold. Teeth are very brittle and crumble easily.

Note: If your child requires surgery for decaying teeth, the following remedies can be helpful:

Aconitum napellus or Bach Flower Rescue Remedy—Give to a child who is fearful and anxious about seeing the dentist. The Rescue Remedy dosage is 2 drops.

Arnica montana—Give immediately after the surgery to reduce pain, inflammation, and bleeding.

Staphysagria—Use after Arnica montana for the residual pain from a tooth extraction.

Acupressure

Large Intestine 4—Located in the webbing between the thumb and the index finger. Helps to relieve tooth pain. Gently press the acupressure point with a thumb for 10 to 15 seconds. Perform on both sides of the body and repeat three times each day.

■ ADVANCED PLAN

Nutritional Supplements

Coenzyme Q$_{10}$—One of the best supplements if your child has chronic gingivitis. An average child's dosage is 10 to 20 milligrams. It's a good idea to work with a doctor when using this supplement.

Vitamin C—Supports tooth and gum health. The type with bioflavonoids is preferable. Dosage: the child's age in years times 50 milligrams, once daily. Give for at least 6 weeks. Reduce the dosage if diarrhea occurs. Consider using a buffered vitamin C powder (nonacidic) or liquid vitamin C. Both work well for infants and children, and can be mixed in juice.

■ WHAT TO EXPECT

Consult with a dentist to find the cause of the tooth pain or tooth decay. Natural therapies in this chapter can help reduce tooth pain within minutes to hours.

Underweight

Although parents should be concerned about their children becoming overweight or obese, equal attention should be given to ensure that children are not underweight for their age and height.

A child is classified as underweight when she ranks in the lower fifth percentile on standardized height and weight charts for children of her same age.

There are many reasons why a child may be underweight. She may not eat enough food to provide her body with an adequate supply of calories and nutrients. She may eat the wrong foods, such as junk foods and snacks that are high in calories but low in nutritional value. Malabsorption can be at the root of an underweight child's problem. Or she may be undernourished. All of these food-related causes can not only affect a child's weight and growth rate but can also leave her feeling constantly dizzy, tired, and weak.

Nutritional deficiencies such as anemia due to low iron can lead to poor growth and development.

Underweight may also be associated with a medical condition. Intestinal parasites, cystic fibrosis, celiac disease, heart problems, and a malfunctioning thyroid can also contribute to the inability to gain weight.

Finally, emotional issues can cause a child to be underweight. High-stress situations such as a death in the family, parents going through a divorce, peer pressure at school, or moving can make a child depressed, anxious, or withdrawn. These emotions can cause a child to lose her appetite.

Two weight-related problems that typically strike teenagers are anorexia nervosa and bulimia nervosa. With anorexia nervosa, the child is afraid of gaining weight and consumes inadequate amounts of food. Besides looking thin, the teen may have constipation, no menstrual cycle, intolerance to cold, fatigue, or excess energy. Bulimia nervosa occurs when there is binge eating followed by purging (such as vomiting, use of laxatives and/or diuretics, fasting, and/or excess exercise). The teen's teeth may change appearance and look ragged if there is self-induced vomiting.

The conventional approach to underweight is to find out if there is an underlying illness causing the child's low weight. A thorough history and lab tests will be used to identify any disease or imbalance causing the inability to gain weight. Children with severe weight loss may need to be hospitalized. Both anorexia nervosa and bulimia nervosa require medical and psychological help.

■ BASIC PLAN

Treatment depends on the reason why the child's weight is too low. Underlying illnesses or imbalances need to be diagnosed.

Diet

Your child may benefit from smaller, more frequent meals during the day to increase the overall calorie consumption in a day. A balance of quality carbohydrates (complex carbohydrates), protein, and fats is required for normal weight gain. Meals should be prepared at home as opposed to fast foods. Essential fatty acids are important for development and growth. Between meals, high-calorie protein and carbohydrate shakes can help ensure that your child consumes enough calories daily. (See "Diet" on page 4 for more details on a healthful whole-foods diet.) We also advise that you get specific diet recommendations from a naturopathic doctor or nutritionist.

Infants who are bottlefed may develop and gain weight better on a different formula. (See "What If You Are Not Breastfeeding?" on page 131 for more information on infant formulas.)

Nutritional Supplements

A whole-food supplement that contains protein, carbohydrates, vegetables, and fruits is a healthful way for your child to take in more nutrients and calories. Use under the supervision of a doctor or natural health care practitioner.

Children's multivitamin—Provides a base of the essential vitamins and minerals necessary for proper growth.

Homeopathy

Work with a homeopath to get a specific remedy for your child. Homeopathy can be quite effective for helping the body to assimilate foods more efficiently and for balancing the body's metabolism.

■ ADVANCED PLAN

Nutritional Supplements

Microbial-derived enzymes—Helpful if there are absorption problems. Give a digestive complex with meals as directed on the container or by a health professional.

Essential fatty acid complex—Supplies the good fats the body needs for proper growth and development. Choose a children's blend that contains omega-3 and omega-6 fatty acids, and follow the directions on the container. Or give fish oil or flaxseed oil at the following daily dosages. Fish oil: 1 gram per 50 pounds of body weight. Flaxseed oil: children 2 and under, 1 teaspoon; kids 3 to 6, 2 teaspoons; kids 7 and older, 2 to 3 teaspoons (reduce the dosage if diarrhea occurs).

■ WHAT TO EXPECT

With many cases of underweight, your child's weight should increase over 2 to 3 months. Work with a holistic doctor to have your child monitored and incorporate the natural therapies in this chapter. Anorexia nervosa and bulimia nervosa require many months to years of help from a mental health professional; each case is different.

Urinary Tract Infection

Urinary tract infections occur in any or all of the parts of the body that produce, store, or eliminate urine. These parts include the urethra, ureters, kidneys, and bladder.

Commonly called UTI, this condition can be hard to detect in babies and children because the symptoms are often subtle.

The condition offers few signs other than fever, frequent urination, or painful urination. A child's urine may be cloudy, smelly, or bloody. Night waking is a common symptom in babies with urinary tract infections. Sometimes, stomachaches or lower back pain accompany a UTI.

Girls are more at risk of developing urinary tract infections than boys. This is due to body structure. In girls, the urethra (the small tube that drains urine from the bladder and out the body) is located closer to the rectum. Bacteria from the lower intestine or vagina can easily reach the urethra and get into the bladder.

Urinary tract infections are usually caused by intestinal bacteria (especially *E. coli*) but can also develop due to viral infections. The infection can be contained within the lower areas of the urinary tract that include the bladder and urethra. A bladder infection is referred to as cystitis, and a urethra infection is called urethritis.

UTI may also be caused by sensitivities to chemicals in bubble baths or scents and dyes in toilet tissue. Malnutrition and constipation can also make a child more susceptible to urinary tract infections.

Contact your doctor if you suspect that your child has a urinary tract infection. Prompt treatment is required to prevent the infection from traveling to the kidneys, which is much more serious.

The conventional approach is to treat the infection with antibiotics and give pain-relieving medications such as acetaminophen.

■ BASIC PLAN

Diet

Fluid intake should be increased to help flush out a bacterial infection. Unsweetened cranberry juice is excellent; studies show that it prevents bacteria from adhering to the bladder wall. Have your child drink 8 to 16 ounces of cranberry juice throughout the day and for 5 days after the infection has cleared. The taste may be too strong for younger kids and should be diluted with water. Cranberry juice extract tablets are also available. Purified water should also be increased to six 6-ounce glasses of water daily. Avoid sugar products of any kind, as they can lower immunity. Fruit juices other than cranberry should be limited, and if used should be highly diluted—4 parts water to 1 part juice.

Chronic bladder or urinary tract infections can be the result of food sensitivities. Common ones for this condition include citrus fruit, milk, and sugar. (See "Food Allergies and Food Sensitivities" on page 298.)

Nutritional Supplement

Vitamin C—Supports the immune system. Dosage: the child's age in years times 50 milligrams, twice daily. Reduce the dosage if diarrhea occurs. Consider using a buffered vitamin C powder (nonacidic) or liquid vitamin C. Both work well for infants and children, and can be mixed in juice.

Herbal Remedies

Echinacea and goldenseal—This combination supports the immune system to get over an infection. Useful for either bacterial or viral infections of the urinary tract.

Uva-ursi—One of the best herbs to fight infections of the urinary tract.

Horsetail—An antiseptic herb for the urinary tract.

Marshmallow root—Soothing to the bladder and urinary tract.

It would be best to purchase a formula that contains all of the herbs above. But you could purchase each separately and give them throughout the day, using the following recipe for kids 3 and older (kids under 3 should use herb dosage based on weight): echinacea and goldenseal combination, 15 drops; uva-ursi or horsetail, 10 drops; and marshmallow root, 10 drops. Add the mixture to water or diluted juice (preferably cranberry) and serve. Give this remedy every 2 to 3 hours throughout the day. Continue giving the remedy until 1 week after the infection seems to have cleared.

Note: For children who are old enough to swallow capsules, these herbs can be purchased in capsule form and taken throughout the day as well.

Homeopathy

Pick the following remedy that best matches your child's symptoms. Unless otherwise indicated, give your child 2 pellets of a 30C potency every 3 hours for up to three doses. (For infants, crush the pellets into powder and mix it with water.) If there is no improvement

Vital Fact

Approximately 3 percent of girls and 1 percent of boys have an urinary tract infection by age 11.

within 9 hours, try another remedy. After you first notice improvement, stop giving the remedy unless symptoms begin to return.

Note: Lower potencies (6X, 12X, 6C) may need to be given more often (four times daily).

Aconitum napellus—For the very first symptoms of an urinary tract infection. The child may be spiking a fever and crying and/or screaming from the pain.

Apis mellifica—For stinging and burning pain with urination. The child feels better in a cold bath as opposed to a warm bath. Also helpful when the child is not able to urinate with the bladder infection.

Cantharis—The most common remedy for bladder infections. If it is hard to tell which homeopathic remedy to use, start with Cantharis and see if it is helpful. Symptoms include burning and cutting pains with urination, and a sense of urgency to urinate. Only small amounts of urine may come out at first when the child tries to empty her bladder. Blood may be present.

Mercurius corrosivus—For hot and burning urination. The urine may contain blood and pus, and has an offensive odor. The child has great burning pains.

Sarsaparilla—For burning pain that occurs at the end of urination.

Constitutional Hydrotherapy

This stimulates the immune system. (See Hydrotherapy for Children on page 115 for details.)

■ ADVANCED PLAN

Nutritional Supplements

Zinc—Supports the immune system. Dosage: children 2 and younger, 5 milligrams; 2 and older, 10 to 15 milligrams. Use for 2 weeks and then stop.

Vitamin A—Supports the immune system. Daily dosage: infants under 1 year, 1,875 international units (IU); children 1 to 3, 2,000 IU; kids 4 to 6, 2,500 IU; kids 7 to 10, 3,500 IU; males 11 and older, 5,000 IU; females 11 and older, 4,000 IU.

Note: These dosages are for short-term use, up to 10 days. Higher dosages may be used only under a doctor's supervision. Available in liquid drops.

Thymus glandular extract—Give one to two 250-milligram tablets or capsules daily.

Probiotic—Choose a children's formula that contains acidophilus and bifidus. In cases where antibiotics have been used, make sure to supplement with children's acidophilus for a minimum of 2 months to replace good bacteria. Give as directed on the container.

Cranberry extract—Inhibits bacteria from attaching to the bladder wall. Give 10 milligrams per pound of body weight daily in tablet or capsule form. Helpful to prevent chronic bladder infections.

Herbal Remedies
Chinese herbal therapy from a practitioner of oriental medicine can be helpful.

■ WHAT TO EXPECT
Your child will most likely be prescribed antibiotics. It is recommended to also use the natural therapies in this chapter as complementary treatment to fight the infection, to help your child recover more quickly, and to reduce discomfort. Chronic urinary tract infections are best prevented with natural therapies as reviewed in this chapter.

Vaccination Side Effects

Statistically speaking, most vaccinations do not cause acute illness or systemic damage in children. However, it has been suggested that many physicians do not correlate the advent of a disease with that of a vaccine being given. Also, the potential for side effects that occur over time has not been well-studied.

A normal reaction to a vaccine is pain, redness, and slight swelling at the area of the skin where the vaccine was injected. A mild fever, slight irritability, and fatigue for 1 to 2 days is not uncommon either. Signs of a more serious reaction include a high fever (higher than 102°F), inconsolable screaming, seizure, ana-

phylaxis (trouble breathing), and personality changes. These require immediate emergency attention. If your child has had one of these reactions, consider it a warning. Strongly consider discontinuing the series of vaccinations for the particular vaccine for which there was a reaction.

Suspected long-term vaccination side effects include arthritis, asthma, autism, attention deficit disorder, Crohn's disease, juvenile diabetes, middle ear infections, seizures, and other chronic conditions. More research needs to be done with regard to the potential side effects of vaccines.

As a matter of prevention, a child should not be given a vaccination if he has been sick in the last 48 hours (with a cold, the flu, fever, or another illness). Let the physician administering the vaccine show you the container, so you can verify that the right vaccine(s) are being given. Record the lot and batch number of the vaccine. If your child experiences an adverse reaction to a vaccine, make sure that your doctor writes this down in your child's chart and reports the reaction to the U.S. Centers for Disease Control and Prevention. (See "Vaccine Reporting" on page 506.) This way, you have legal documentation to verify the adverse reaction. Do not allow your child to receive another dose of the vaccine to which he reacted. Get as much information as possible from your pediatrician, from other health professionals, and from informational resources before deciding on whether to vaccinate.

The conventional approach is to use medicines such as acetaminophen to reduce pain and fever. Some physicians will discontinue giving another shot of the vaccine for which there was an adverse reaction.

■ BASIC PLAN

Diet

If your child has had an adverse reaction, reduce or cut out all sugars—they suppress the immune system.

Nutritional Supplement

Vitamin C—Supports the immune system and has mild anti-inflammatory effects. The type with bioflavonoids is preferable. Dosage: the child's age in years times 100 milligrams, twice daily. For prevention, start the vitamin C 1 week before the vaccination and continue for at least 1 week after. Reduce the dosage if diarrhea occurs. Consider using a buffered vitamin C powder (nonacidic) or liquid vitamin C. Both work well for infants and children, and can be mixed in juice.

Herbal Remedies

Echinacea—Supports the immune system. Use preventively by giving for 1 week before the vaccination and up to 1 week after. Nonalcoholic, glycerin-based products are available.

Larix is another good option for immune support. It mixes well in a formula or juice.

Homeopathy

Pick the following remedy that best matches your child's symptoms. Unless otherwise indicated, give your child 2 pellets of a 30C po-

tency twice daily. Improvements should be seen within 2 days. If there is no improvement within 2 days, try another remedy. After you first notice improvement, stop giving the remedy unless symptoms begin to return.

Note: Lower potencies (6X, 12X, 6C) may need to be given more often (three times daily).

Ledum—Give immediately after a vaccine shot to prevent tissue swelling as well as complications.

Silica—The most common remedy for a weakened immune system after a vaccine. The child may get colds, sore throats, and other infections very easily. The glands are always enlarged. An infant may have failure to thrive after the vaccine or have trouble putting on weight. A child may be slow mentally and may have development problems. He tires easily. This remedy may need to be taken for 2 weeks or longer for benefits to be noticed. Consult with a practitioner trained in homeopathy.

Carcinosin—An acute remedy for high fevers and sleeplessness after a vaccination.

Thuja occidentalis—For asthma and skin eruptions that occur after a vaccination.

DPT—A homeopathic combination of diphtheria, pertussis, and tetanus. Used for adverse reactions to the DPT vaccine. This remedy may need to be taken for 2 weeks or longer for benefits to be noticed. Consult with a practitioner trained in homeopathy.

Constitutional Hydrotherapy

This supports the immune system and aids in detoxification. (See Hydrotherapy for Children on page 115 for details.)

Other Recommendations

Craniosacral therapy may be helpful in cases where there has been neurological damage. See "Craniosacral Therapy" on page 503 for more information.

■ WHAT TO EXPECT

Natural therapy can help treat secondary infections and symptoms such as swelling that result from vaccines. More serious reactions may be helped with specific homeopathic and/or craniosacral therapy.

Vaginitis

Vaginitis is a term used to describe a host of conditions that cause inflammation of the sensitive walls of the vagina. Yeast, bacteria, or protozoa cause vaginitis. Prolonged use of antibiotics can also change the vaginal environment by destroying the beneficial bacteria and make a girl more vulnerable to infection.

Girls with this condition experience itchiness, burning, pain, and tenderness during urination. Some develop a white, curdlike vaginal discharge that resembles cottage cheese.

The most common culprit in vaginitis is a yeast infection known medically as *Candida albicans*. Symptoms include vaginal itch, possibly vaginal soreness, cottage cheese–like vaginal discharge, and a burning discomfort around the vaginal opening.

Other types of vaginitis include:

Bacterial vaginosis: The symptoms of this bacterial infection can include an abnormal grayish white vaginal discharge and foul-smelling vaginal odor.

Trichomonas vaginitis: Not a problem in children except for sexually active teens, this sexually transmitted disease is caused by a one-celled microorganism called *Trichomonas vaginalis*. Symptoms include a foul-smelling, yellowish-green vaginal discharge and itching. Symptoms worsen during menstruation.

Mild vaginal discharge in young girls can also be caused by sensitivity to underwear material. Wearing cotton panties and using non-perfumed toilet paper can help avoid this problem.

Baby girls may have a vaginal discharge for a few days after birth, which is common and nothing to worry about.

Repeated antibiotic use can make a girl susceptible to vaginitis, as the beneficial flora of the vagina are depleted.

Consult with your physician if your child has vaginal discharge, irritation, or pain. Chronic vaginitis can be a sign of an underlying condition such as diabetes. Also, chronic vaginitis can be caused by sexual abuse.

Conventional treatment focuses on the use of antifungal creams or vaginal suppositories for the treatment of yeast-related vaginitis.

■ BASIC PLAN

Diet

Sugars are notorious for feeding yeast. Refined carbohydrates and other simple sugars should be eliminated or greatly reduced in the child's diet. Yogurt that contains acidophilus with live cultures (and that doesn't contain sugar) is excellent for a girl to eat to increase the amount of good bacteria in her body.

Food sensitivities can be related to chronic cases of vaginitis and should be treated. (See "Food Allergies and Food Sensitivities" on page 298.)

Nutritional Supplement

An acidophilus supplement is useful for vaginitis. These good bacteria maintain an acidic environment in the vagina and also produce hydrogen peroxide, which kills yeast and bacteria. Inserting a capsule of acidophilus in the vagina each night and covering it with a pad can be very helpful. This may need to be done for a few days or a few weeks depending on the case. Also, the acidophilus supplement should be taken orally as well. We recommend that these treatments be done only with the guidance of a doctor.

Herbal Remedy

Echinacea—Give two or three times daily for immune support.

Homeopathy

See a practitioner for an individualized remedy. Or pick the one of the following remedies that best matches your child's symptoms. For the remedies that follow, unless otherwise indicated, give your child 2 pellets of a 30C potency three times daily. Improvements should be seen within 24 hours. If there is no improvement within 24 hours, try another remedy. After you first notice improvement, stop giving the remedy unless symptoms begin to return.

Note: Lower potencies (6X, 12X, 6C) may

need to be given more often (four times daily).

Kreosotum—For tremendous vaginal itching and putrid odor.

Pulsatilla—For yellow or creamy discharge. The problem feels worse in a bath or in a warm stuffy room. The child is very weepy and clingy.

Sepia—For thin, burning, white or yellow discharge. The child is irritable.

■ ADVANCED PLAN

Nutritional Supplements

Children's multivitamin—Provides a base of the essential vitamins and minerals for immune support.

Vitamin C—Supports the immune system and has mild anti-inflammatory effects. The type with bioflavonoids is preferable. Dosage: the child's age in years times 50 milligrams, twice daily. Reduce the dosage if diarrhea occurs. Consider using a buffered vitamin C powder (nonacidic) or liquid vitamin C. Both work well for infants and children, and can be mixed in juice.

■ WHAT TO EXPECT

You should see improvement in 2 to 3 days. Doctor supervision is required.

Warts

These harmless, small, bumpy mounds of overgrown skin usually appear on fingers, hands, knees, elbows, or toes. Warts are usually brown or flesh-colored and have rough, dry surfaces.

Although anyone at any age can develop warts, they seem to strike more often during childhood and adolescence. They tend to recur and spread.

Warts are caused by a host of viruses and can be spread to other parts of the body or other people through direct contact. Experts have identified at least 70 different types of the human papillomavirus (HPV) known to infect the skin and leave warts.

A few of the more dominant types of warts are listed here.

Common warts: This type tends to surface on the skin of the hands and fingers. These warts usually don't hurt and are caused by HPV types 2 and 4.

Plantar warts: This type usually appears on the soles of the feet and tends to grow down into the skin instead of creating mounds. Caused by HPV type 1, plantar warts are painful and attack blood vessels embedded deep in the skin.

Plane warts: These are small, flat, flesh-colored warts that grow in clusters.

Venereal warts: This type (known medically as *condylomas acuminata,* or genital warts) affects the genital and anus areas. These moist, fleshy mounds of skin have surfaces that resemble cauliflower. At least four different types of HPV cause this type of wart, which is spread through sexual contact. This can be a sign of sexual abuse in children.

Childhood warts often disappear over time without treatment.

The conventional treatment for warts is a topically applied acid (salicylic acid) to slowly peel away the skin. Also, cryosurgery involves freezing the wart with liquid nitrogen, which destroys the wart cells. The last resort is to surgically remove a wart. This may be done for stubborn plantar warts that cause foot pain while a child is walking or standing.

Note: Venereal warts need to be treated by a doctor.

■ BASIC PLAN

Diet
Avoid simple sugars, which can reduce the effectiveness of the immune system against the virus that is causing your child's warts.

A whole-foods diet is recommended. (See "Diet" on page 4 for more information).

Nutritional Supplement
Children's multivitamin—For immune support. Choose one that contains selenium, which inhibits viruses from replicating.

Herbal Remedies
Antiviral herbs such as **echinacea** and **lomatium** can be effective in stimulating the immune response against the virus causing the wart growth.

Thuja—One or 2 drops of the tincture or oil can be applied to the wart daily (with a cotton swab) for 2 to 3 weeks. Thuja is believed to have a direct antiviral effect.

Banana peel—Tape the inside of a fresh piece of banana peel to a plantar wart with adhesive tape every day for 2 to 4 weeks. It contains a substance that kills warts.

Homeopathy

Pick the following remedy that best matches your child's symptoms. Unless otherwise indicated, give your child 2 pellets of a 30C potency two times daily for 2 weeks, then stop giving the remedy. Wait and see if the warts improve over the next 2 weeks. If there is no improvement, try a different remedy.

Note: Lower potencies (6X, 12X, 6C) may need to be given more often (three times daily).

Antimonium crudum—For hard, flat warts. These are often located on the tips of the fingers or toes (plantar warts) and under or around the nails.

Causticum—For large, fleshy, soft warts that bleed easily. Often located on the hands especially around the fingernails, and on the arms and face.

Dulcamara—For large, smooth warts found on the back of the hand or on the palm.

Nitric acid—For cauliflower-looking warts that bleed easily and are painful. Often found on or near the genital area, mouth, and anus.

Note: Genital warts should be treated by a doctor.

Thuja occidentalis—For large crops of warts (usually large warts) that tend to come back after being burned off or surgically removed. For warts that have formed since vaccination.

■ ADVANCED PLAN

Aromatherapy

Lemon and tea tree oil—Place 1 drop of each on a cotton swab and dab it onto the wart(s). Cover with an adhesive bandage. Repeat daily for 2 to 3 weeks. Use under the supervision of a doctor.

■ WHAT TO EXPECT

The warts should disappear within 1 to 2 months. If there is no improvement, change to a different treatment, or consult with a natural health care practitioner such as a naturopathic doctor.

Part 3

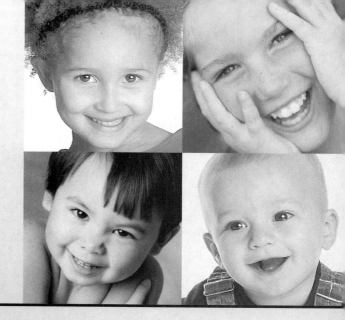

vital resources

chapter 10

emergency information

I. Cardiopulmonary Resuscitation (CPR)

This section provides a review of the lifesaving techniques of mouth-to-mouth and CPR, which all parents should know. We strongly recommend getting formal emergency training from a local hospital or Red Cross or from another certified professional.

If your child shows any of the following signs, he may need either mouth-to-mouth resuscitation or CPR:

- Unresponsive, does not appear to be breathing
- Extreme difficulty breathing (could be from an obstruction in the respiratory tract)
- Blue lips associated with respiratory distress
- Rapid or labored breathing (for example, grunting)
- Severe wheezing
- Drooling, or difficulty swallowing
- Extreme paleness

If your child has any of these signs, call for emergency help and begin the steps that follow.

Evaluate the child's condition. Is the child conscious? Try to wake him by shouting or tapping him. Check to see if the child is breathing by placing your ear directly over his mouth.

- If the child is not breathing but his heart is still beating, position him on his back and do the following:

1. Clear his mouth. Look for any gum or foreign body. If you can see an object, remove it with your fingers. If any liquid is in his mouth, remove it by tilting his head to the side.

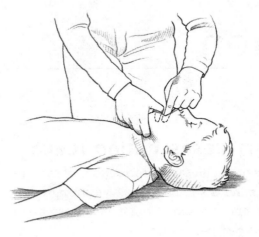

Gripping your child's jaw, sweep your finger inside his mouth to remove any foreign materials.

2. Open the child's airway by tilting his head back so that his nose is in the air. Lift his chin up with one hand while pushing down on his forehead with the other hand. In some cases, this opening of the airway will allow the child to breathe.

To open your child's airway, gently tilt back his head by pressing on his forehead and lifting his chin; make sure his mouth is open.

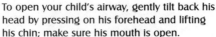
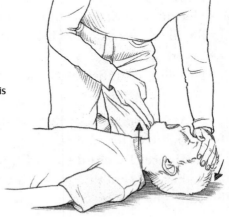

3. If the child is still not breathing and does not appear to be choking, then give mouth-to-mouth resuscitation. Pinch the child's

nostrils closed with one hand and seal the child's mouth with yours. (For infants and small children, you can seal both the child's nostrils and mouth with your mouth.) Give two rescue breaths, blowing air forcefully enough into the child's lungs until you see the chest rise slightly. Then, remove your mouth, and if the child does not start breathing, give another breath. Continue at approximately 20 breaths per minute (one breath every 3 seconds). Continue at this rate until the child is breathing on his own.

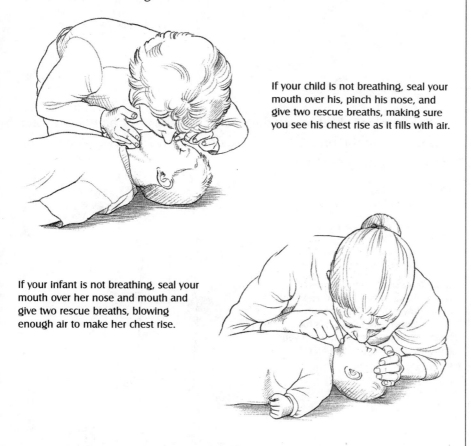

If your child is not breathing, seal your mouth over his, pinch his nose, and give two rescue breaths, making sure you see his chest rise as it fills with air.

If your infant is not breathing, seal your mouth over her nose and mouth and give two rescue breaths, blowing enough air to make her chest rise.

- If the child is not breathing and also has no pulse that can be felt, you must begin chest compressions:

  1. Place the child on a firm surface. For an infant, place two or three fingers on the breastbone, one finger-width (an adult's finger-width)

below the nipple line. Press down ½ to 1 inch, at a rate of about 100 times per minute. Make sure not to apply too much pressure.

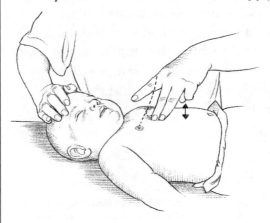

Before beginning chest compressions on your infant, imagine a line between the nipples, then place two fingers on her breastbone, one finger-width below that line.

For an older child, place the heel of one of your hands over the lower third of the breastbone. Press down 1 to 1½ inches at a rate of 80 to 100 times per minute.

To perform chest compressions on your child, place the heel of one hand on the lower third of his breastbone while gently pressing back his forehead with your other hand. Keep your arm straight, and your shoulder directly over your hand.

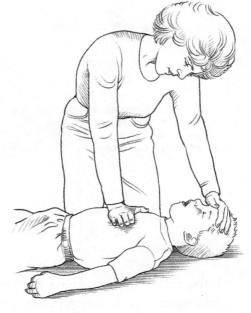

2. After five compressions, give the child one breath. Continue repeating five compressions to one breath until you feel a pulse.

II. Choking

Choking is the most common cause of accidental death in children under age 1. Food is the item most commonly involved. Choking becomes life-threatening when a child swallows an object that blocks air from getting to the lungs. This prevents your child from being able to talk or make normal sounds. Her face may turn bright red or blue due to the lack of oxygen.

You must take immediate action in this situation with the proper response as described below. The technique to be used depends on the age of the child and her symptoms.

Coughing but Able to Breathe and Talk

For Children of All Ages

Coughing is an automatic response for expelling an object from the throat. If your child is able to breathe and talk, give her verbal assurance that everything is okay, and let her cough. Do not try to remove the object with your fingers, which could make the situation worse. If necessary, take your child to an emergency room or call 911 if the object cannot be expelled.

Cannot Breathe and Is Turning Blue

Children Under 1 Year Old

Immediate first-aid is required. Be gentle, so as to not damage the baby's internal organs.

1. Place the infant facedown on your forearm, in a head-down position (her head in your hand). Hold her jaw with your hand from underneath, keeping her head and neck stabilized. Rest your forearm firmly against your upper thigh for support.

If the baby is large, then you may want to lay the baby facedown over your lap; she should be firmly supported with her head lower than her trunk.

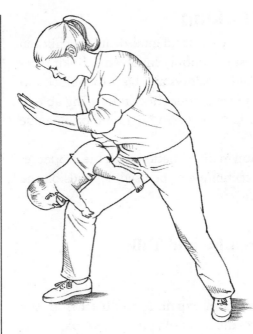

Before performing back blows on your infant, be sure she is stabilized by resting her facedown on your forearm and supporting your arm on your upper thigh. Gently hold her jaw in your hand.

2. Give four back blows rapidly with the heel of your hand between the baby's shoulder blades.

Give four rapid back blows between your baby's shoulder blades, using the heel of your hand.

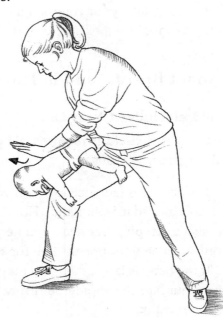

3. If the baby still cannot breathe, turn her onto her back on a firm surface. Give four rapid chest thrusts over the breastbone, using only two fingers.

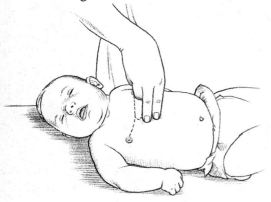

If your baby still is not breathing, place her on a firm surface and give four chest thrusts with two fingers placed on her breastbone, one finger-width below the nipple line.

4. If the baby is still not breathing, open the airway by tilting her head and chin back, and attempt to see if there is a foreign body. Do not try to pull anything out unless you can see it. If you can see it, then sweep it out with your finger.

5. If the baby does not start breathing, then give her two breaths by mouth-to-mouth, or mouth-to-nose (see page 469).

6. Keep repeating steps 1 to 5 as you or someone else calls for emergency help.

Children Over 1 Year Old

1. Apply a series of up to 10 abdominal thrusts (the Heimlich maneuver) as described below until the foreign object comes out.

- If the child is small, place him on his back. An older, larger child can be treated while standing, sitting, or lying down.
- Kneel at the child's feet if he is on the floor; stand at his feet if he is on a table.
- Place the heel of one hand in the center of his body between the navel and the rib cage, your second hand on top of your first.
- Press into the abdomen with a rapid inward and upward thrust. This must be done gently with a small child.

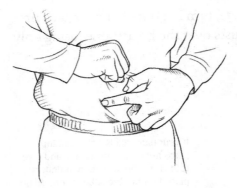

To perform the Heimlich maneuver, place the thumb-side of one fist above your child's belly button.

Either kneeling or standing behind your child to provide support, wrap your other hand over your fist and give rapid inward and upward thrusts.

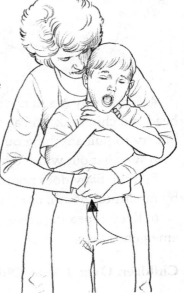

2. If the object has not been expelled with the Heimlich maneuver, open the child's mouth and tilt his head back. If you can see the object, try to sweep it out with your finger. If you cannot see the object, do not attempt to sweep it out.

3. If your child does not start breathing, give mouth-to-mouth resuscitation. If the child still is not breathing, repeat a series of up to 10 abdominal thrusts.

4. Repeat steps 1 to 3 as you or someone else calls for emergency help.

III. Poisoning

There are a number of ways that poisoning can occur. It can occur because of a dangerous mixture of medications, from overdose, from swallowing dangerous household chemicals or insecticides, or from ingesting poisonous plants, food, or nicotine.

A child's reactions can vary depending on the type and amount of toxins ingested—possibly with emergency and fatal outcomes. Reactions can include inflammation or burning around the lips, if the substance was taken orally; difficulty swallowing; nausea; sudden behavior changes; extreme thirst; breathing difficulties; unconsciousness; headaches; convulsions; vomiting; and death.

Improper use of medications, such as overdosing or mixing one medication with another without a doctor's recommendation, can trigger an adverse reaction. Many prescription medications can have negative effects when combined with others. Also, some people unknowingly harbor allergies to medications, which could lead to poisonous predicaments.

Because they are curious, children are vulnerable to household chemicals, detergents, and cleaners that are poorly capped and stored. Their immediate response could include vomiting or gagging. Also, children may accidentally lick, chew, or swallow poisonous plants or nicotine patches. This could induce symptoms that range from dizziness or transitory distress to diarrhea, vomiting, gagging, or difficulty breathing.

Another more common form of poisoning comes from the ingestion of tainted food that was improperly cleaned, cooked, or refrigerated. Such foods can contain dangerous bacteria and contaminants that create a feeling of pain, bloating, and nausea for 3 to 6 hours after consumption, as well as diarrhea, stomach cramps, and vomiting.

Vital Fact

Millions of poisoning exposures occur each year in the United States, resulting in nearly 900,000 visits to emergency departments. About 90 percent of poisonings happen in the home, and more than half of them involve children under age 6.

Preventing Poisoning

With poisoning, prevention is the key. Following are recommendations from the American Association of Poison Control Centers that can help you protect children from poisons:

- Post the telephone number for your poison control center near your phone, in a place where all family members would be able to find it quickly in an emergency.
- Remove all nonessential drugs and household products from your home. Discard them according to the manufacturer's instructions.
- If you have small children, avoid keeping highly toxic products, such as drain cleaners, in the home, garage, or shed, or any other place that children can access.
- Buy medicines and household products in child-resistant packaging and be sure that caps are always on tight. Do not remove child safety caps. Avoid keeping medicines, vitamins, or household products in anything but their original packaging.
- Store all of your medicines and household products in a locked closet or cabinet—including products and medicines with child-resistant containers.
- Crawl around your house, including inside your closets, to inspect it from a child's point of view. You'll likely find a poisoning hazard you hadn't noticed before.
- Never refer to medicine or vitamins as "candy."
- Make sure that visiting grandparents, family friends, or other caregivers keep their medications away from children. For example, if Grandma keeps pills in her purse, make sure that the purse is out of your children's reach.
- Keep a bottle of syrup of ipecac in your home—it can be used to induce vomiting. (*Note:* This is not the same as the homeopathic Ipecacuanha.) Use syrup of ipecac only when the poison control center tells you to.
- Avoid products such as cough syrup or mouthwash that contain alcohol. These are hazardous for young children. Look for alcohol-free alternatives.
- Keep cosmetics and beauty products out of children's reach. Remember that hair permanents and relaxers are toxins as well.

The most serious case of food poisoning, particularly with improperly canned foods and seafood, is a potentially fatal form known as botulism. Generally, the longer it takes for the symptoms of food poisoning to appear, the more serious the poisoning.

Carbon Monoxide Poisoning

Carbon monoxide (CO) is an invisible, odorless, poisonous gas that can also cause sickness and death. The incomplete burning of fuels such as natural gas, oil, kerosene, coal, and wood produces carbon monoxide. Also, fuel-burning appliances that are not working properly or that are installed incorrectly can produce fatal concentrations of carbon monoxide in your home. Other hazards include burning charcoal indoors and running a car in the garage, both of which can lead to dangerous levels of CO in your home.

The following are some simple tips from the U.S. Centers for Disease Control and Prevention to prevent carbon monoxide poisoning:

- Install carbon monoxide alarms near bedrooms and on each floor of your home. If your alarm sounds, the U.S. Consumer Product Safety Commission suggests that you press the reset button, call emergency services (911 or your local fire department), and immediately move to fresh air (either outdoors or near an open door or window). If you learn that fuel-burning appliances were the most likely cause of the poisoning, have a serviceperson check them for malfunction before turning them back on. Refer to the instructions on your CO alarm for more specific information about what to do if your alarm goes off.
- Symptoms of CO poisoning are similar to the flu, only without a fever (headache, fatigue, nausea, dizziness, shortness of breath). If you experience any of these symptoms, get fresh air immediately and contact a physician for proper diagnosis. Also, open windows and doors, turn off combustion appliances, contact emergency services, and take the steps listed above to ensure your home's safety.
- To keep carbon monoxide from collecting in your home, make sure that any fuel-burning equipment, such as a furnace, stove, or heater, works properly, and never use charcoal or other grills indoors or in the garage. Do not leave your car's engine running while it's in the garage, and consider putting weather stripping

Vital Fact

Among children ages 5 and under, 60 percent of poisoning exposures are to non-pharmaceutical products such as cosmetics, cleaning substances, plants, foreign bodies and toys, pesticides, art supplies, and alcohol. The remaining 40 percent of exposures are to pharmaceuticals.

around the door between the garage and the house if they're connected.

Iron Poisoning from Supplements or Medicines

From 1986 through 1997, more than 218,000 children ages 5 and under ingested iron preparations. Forty-six died. Again, make sure that medicines and supplements are out of the reach of children.

Lead Poisoning

The ingestion of dust from deteriorating lead-based paint is the most common cause of lead poisoning among children. Currently, more than 80 percent of public and privately owned housing units built before 1980 contain some lead-based paint. (See "Environment" on page 25 for more information on the environment and children's health.)

Treatments for Poisoning

Immediate treatment by a doctor or in an emergency room can help prevent serious damage. Work with a doctor to incorporate these natural therapies, which aid detoxification and prevent liver damage.

Acute poisoning (internal)—If you suspect that your child has ingested a poison, first get the poisonous substance away from your child. If there is still some in her mouth, have her spit it out into a bowl, so that you have the substance if a doctor needs to examine it. Next, check your child for these signs:

- Severe throat pain or discomfort
- Excessive drooling
- Trouble breathing
- Convulsions
- Drowsiness

If your child has any of these signs, call an ambulance or get to an emergency room immediately. If there is no sign of these serious symptoms, call your local poison control center. The number is usually listed on the inside cover of your phone book, but it's best to have it on a sheet near your phone for emergency use. If you cannot find the number, call 911 and ask for poison control. You can also call your pediatrician. Do not make your child vomit unless instructed to do so by the poison control center or your doctor.

Poison on the skin—If a chemical is spilled on your child, remove his clothes and rinse the skin with lukewarm water for 15 minutes. Then call the poison control center for further advice. Do not apply any topical treatment unless instructed to do so.

Poison in the eye—Immediately flush your child's eye with lukewarm water. Aim for the inner corner of the eye. You may need another adult to help you hold the child. Flush for 15 minutes and call the poison control center for further directions.

Nutritional Supplements

Charcoal capsules—Help to absorb toxins. Use as directed by your doctor.

Probiotic—A children's acidophilus supplement that contains bifidus can be helpful to recover from the effects of poisoning, especially food poisoning. Give as directed on the container.

Alpha lipoic acid—Protects the liver cells from being damaged by drugs and other toxins. Give as directed by a doctor.

Herbal Remedies

Milk thistle and **dandelion root** can be used to help the liver and body recover from various types of poisoning. Give for 6 to 8 weeks after the poisoning incident. Use under the guidance of a nutrition-oriented doctor.

Homeopathy

The following remedies are *not* to be used to replace the advice or prescription of a doctor to treat a case of poisoning. Rather, they can be used in a complementary manner to help ease symptoms and to quicken the recovery process.

Arsenicum album—For the effects of poisoning that cause vomiting and diarrhea, or just diarrhea by itself. Give the child 2 pellets of a 30C potency three times daily, for 2 days.

Nux vomica—Helps the child to recover from the effects of poisoning from foods or medications. Symptoms of nausea and vomiting are indications for this remedy. Give the child 2 pellets of a 30C potency twice daily, for 2 days.

your child's natural medicine kit

We recommend that all parents and caregivers have a children's natural medicine kit at home or when traveling. You can design a kit containing all of the medicine listed below or select the ones that you feel would be most needed, based on your child's health history. A fish tackle box makes a great storage container for these items.

Herbal Remedies

- Aloe vera gel or cream for burns or dry skin
- Calendula succus or tincture for cuts and scrapes
- Echinacea (liquid or capsules) for infections
- Echinacea and goldenseal combination (liquid or capsules) for infections
- Ginger root (liquid or capsules) for digestive upset or nausea

Homeopathic Remedies

Homeopathic first-aid kits are available through some practitioners, by mail order, or at health food stores. (See "Homeopathy" on page 504 for ways to find a practitioner near you.) You can also compose your own kit containing the remedies shown on page 482.

Nutritional Supplements

It's a good idea to keep vitamin C with bioflavonoids and vitamin A drops on hand. Both supplements support the immune system.

Homeopathic Remedies for First-Aid

Remedy	Uses
Aconitum napellus	Fever, infection
Apis mellifica	Bee sting
Arnica montana	Trauma, bruising
Arsenicum	Food poisoning
Belladonna	Fever, infection
Cantharis	Burns
Chamomilla	Teething, ear infection
Ferrum phosphoricum	Fever
Gelsemium	Flu
Hypericum perforatum	Nerve trauma
Ledum	Puncture wounds
Lycopodium	Gas and bloating
Magnesia phosphorica	Muscle cramps
Nux vomica	Indigestion, food poisoning
Pulsatilla	Infections, earaches
Rhus toxicodendron	Sprains and strains
Sulphur	Skin rashes
Bach Flower Rescue Remedy	Emotional upset

Other Medicine Kit Essentials

- Elastic bandages (such as Ace)
- Adhesive bandages (such as Band-Aid)
- Bulb syringe
- Hot water bottle
- Scissors and tweezers
- Sterile gauze pads and adhesive tape
- Syrup of ipecac (used under the direction of a physician for certain types of poisoning to induce vomiting; do not confuse with homeopathic Ipecacuanha)
- Thermometer

chapter 12

vaccinations

Making an informed decision as to whether to vaccinate your child is one of the more important decisions you will make as a parent. Each vaccine has its own risks and benefits, and each parent needs to make an educated decision about which vaccines their child will receive. As the decision maker for your child, you must understand each disease and decide if the risks from the vaccine outweigh the risks from catching the disease. We cannot go into full detail in this section, so please research this information before you take your child to the doctor for shots. There are many books, magazine articles, and Web sites that contain positive and negative information regarding vaccinations. As the decision maker for your child, you need the most accurate information available. Both pro and con vaccine positions contain scare tactics that support their opinion. It is important that you determine which information is fact and which information is exaggerated opinion.

Before your child receives any vaccinations, your physician should give you a sheet of paper that explains the vaccination and its possible risks. If your physician does not offer this information, then you need to ask for it. This source of educated material should not be your only source of vaccine information. Deciding whether or not to vaccinate can take weeks or months for some parents.

Keep in mind that each state (including provinces in Canada) allows reasons to be exempt from vaccines. These exemptions include philosophical, medical, and religious reasons. The parents are allowed to excuse their children from vaccines and, by law, their children can still attend school and related functions (state laws vary). It is very important to find a pediatrician who respects your decision. Shopping around for a pediatrician is more important than shopping around for a car! It may take weeks or months to find a pediatrician with whom you feel comfortable. We recommend that you start looking for a pediatrician and researching vaccine information when you are pregnant.

The U.S. Centers for Disease Control and Prevention, or CDC, is one source of public information about vaccinations. Your doctor should also report any adverse vaccine reactions to the Vaccine Adverse Event Reporting System (VAERS) immediately. You, the parent, can also report any adverse reaction to the U.S. Department of Health and Human Services' Vaccine Adverse Event Reporting System. (See "Vaccine Reporting" on page 506 for contact information.)

Current Pediatric Vaccination Schedule (United States, 2001)

This schedule comes from the American Academy of Pediatrics. It is updated frequently. For the most recent information, visit the Academy's Web site at www.aap.org.

Hepatitis B: Three doses, with a fourth dose given only if necessary (this is determined by your physician). All children and adolescents through 18 years of age who have not been immunized can be given the series at any time.

Diphtheria, tetanus, and pertussis (DTP, DTaP): These three are usually given together, with the acellular pertussis (aP) replacing the whole cell pertussis vaccine. There are five required doses in this series. For children who cannot tolerate the acellular pertussis portion of this vaccine, the DT (diphtheria, tetanus) vaccine is available. Boosters for tetanus and diphtheria are recommended every 10 years.

Haemophilus influenzae type b: There are three *Haemophilus influenzae* type b conjugate vaccines licensed for use. Depending upon which vaccine is used, two to four doses are required.

Polio: To eliminate the risk of vaccine-associated paralytic polio, it is now recommended that the inactivated polio vaccine be used for routine childhood polio vaccination in the United States. Four doses of this vaccination are required. The oral polio (if available) is only to be used under special circumstances—for instance, in unvaccinated children who will be traveling in less than 1 month to an area where polio is common.

Measles, mumps, and rubella (MMR): These three are usually given together, and two doses are required.

Varicella (chicken pox): One or two doses are required for this vaccine.

Hepatitis A: This vaccine is recommended in selected areas. Your local public health center can give you information on requirements.

Pneumococcal conjugate vaccine (PCV): Sold under the brand name Prevnar, this newest vaccine of the bunch is recommended for all children 2 to 23 months old. Four doses are required.

Hepatitis B

Currently, the U.S. Centers for Disease Control, the American Academy of Pediatrics, and the Canadian Paediatric Society recommend that all infants receive vaccination against hepatitis B, a disease affecting the liver. Hepatitis B can be transmitted through sharing of needles (drug use), through sexual intercourse, and through exposure to blood or blood products. We have strong reservations about the routine vaccination of infants and children with hepatitis B. Considering the route of transmission of this disease and the risk factors associated with the vaccine, we only recommend that high-risk infants and children be vaccinated (for example, those whose mothers are hepatitis-B positive).

Contraindications

Absolute: Do not give further injections to patients who develop symptoms of severe hypersensitivity after an injection of hepatitis B vaccine.

Relative: Patients with a history of allergic reaction to common baker's yeast may react adversely to the vaccine. Defer vaccination if the patient has a moderate or severe active infection.

Adverse Reactions

Complaints include those at the injection site (17 to 22 percent) and systemic complaints (those that affect the whole body; 14 to 15 percent). They may include pain, tenderness, itching, induration (a smooth, hardened, slightly elevated area of tissue), redness, bruising, swelling, warmth, and nodules (a knot or swelling in the injection area).

Systemic reactions include fatigue, weakness, headache, fever over 100°F, malaise, nausea, diarrhea, dizziness, sore throat, upper respiratory tract infection, abnormal liver function, a decrease in blood platelets, eczema, bruising, and abnormally fast heartbeat or palpitations. Erythema multiforme (Stevens-Johnson syndrome) is another possible reaction; it includes a rash with dark red patches, usually on the arms and legs, that goes away after a while without itching or burning.

Reactions following less than 1 percent of injections include sweating, achiness, chills, tingling, hypertension (elevated blood pressure), loss of appetite, abdominal pain or cramps, constipation, flushing, vomiting, paresthesia (abnormal sensations such as burning or prickling), rash, hair loss, angioedema, hives, joint pain, arthritis, muscle pain, back pain, enlarged lymph nodes, hypotension (lowered blood pressure), and bronchial spasm that leads to difficulty breathing.

Anaphylaxis is a rare but serious reaction: It begins with unease, agitation, and sometimes flushing and may progress to irregular heartbeat, tingling limbs, itching, and throbbing in the ears before turning into hives, swelling, difficulty breathing, shock, and possibly death if emergency assistance is not available.

Another rare reaction is *Guillain-Barré syndrome,* an inflammation of the nerves with progressive muscle weakness in the arms and legs, which may lead to paralysis. Guillain-Barré syndrome usually occurs after an infectious disease, and the person usually recovers completely.

As with any medicine, there is a very small risk that serious problems, even death, could occur after getting a vaccine.

Booster Doses and Immunity

The duration of protection from hepatitis B is undetermined, but it apparently lasts more than 5 to 7 years in most healthy recipients. Seventy to 80 percent of recipients are protected after the second dose, and more than 95 percent are protected after the third dose.

Diphtheria

This vaccine is usually given as one injection with tetanus and pertussis. There are two different forms of the diphtheria vaccine, one for children under 7 years old and one for anyone over 7 years old.

This vaccine is not to be used for the treatment of diphtheria.

Contraindications

Anyone under 6 weeks of age or over 7 years of age should not be given the diphtheria vaccine for pediatric use. People 7 or older should be given the adult diphtheria toxoid.

Any acute infection with fever is a reason to defer administration of routine boosters.

Adverse Reactions

Redness, tenderness, and induration may occur surrounding the injection site. In addition, fever, malaise, generalized aches and pains, flushing, hives or itching, increased heartbeat, and low blood pressure

Vital Fact

Between 1990 and March 1999, more than 24,000 reports of possible adverse reactions to the hepatitis B vaccine were registered with the FDA's Vaccine Adverse Event Reporting System. These include a significant number of severe injuries and death. Preliminary evidence indicates that some people might be genetically disposed to an adverse autoimmune or neurological response to the recombinant hepatitis B vaccine. The French and Canadian governments are funding research on hepatitis B vaccine adverse-events reports. In France, the hepatitis B vaccine was taken off the market in 1998.

may occur. These reactions are more likely to occur in people who have received an unusually large number of booster doses. Keep in mind that postvaccine neurological disorders have followed injection of almost all vaccines, including the diptheria vaccine. However, this is uncommon.

Booster Doses and Immunity

The duration of this vaccine is usually 5 to 10 years. Therefore, it is recommended that the diphtheria vaccine be readministered every 5 to 10 years (this is usually given in conjunction with the tetanus vaccine). Immunity to diphtheria usually develops a few weeks after the second dose, and complete immunity develops after completing the entire series. The immunization with diphtheria reduces the incidence of the disease by more than 95 percent in people who have been vaccinated.

Tetanus

This vaccine is usually given as one injection that includes diphtheria and acellular pertussis for children under 7. For people over 7 years of age, there is a separate diphtheria and tetanus vaccination for adults. The tetanus vaccine is also available by itself and, if it is desired, the patient should inform his physician of wanting this vaccine by itself so that it can be ordered.

The tetanus vaccine should not be used for the treatment of tetanus.

Contraindications

Any patient with a history of neurological symptoms following administration of the tetanus vaccine should not receive more tetanus vaccine doses.

If a person is hypersensitive to aluminum (which is part of the routinely used tetanus vaccine), the fluid tetanus toxoid, a different tetanus vaccine, should be used for vaccination.

In addition, if a person has an acute infection and/or a fever, routine vaccination should be deferred.

The FDA recommends that elective tetanus vaccination be deferred during any outbreak of polio. Injections are a cause of provocative polio.

The safety of the tetanus vaccine is known for children as young as 2 months.

Adverse Reactions

Redness and induration around the injection site are common. A nodule or bump may also be present for a couple of days. Abscesses and atrophy of the skin layer may also occur (surrounding the injection site). In people who have received multiple booster shots, adverse reactions can occur 2 to 12 hours after injection. These include redness, swelling, itchiness, enlarged lymph glands, and induration around the site. Occasionally, pain and tenderness can occur.

Systemic reactions following tetanus injections include low-grade fever, chills, fatigue, generalized aches and pains, headaches, hives, itchiness, increased heart rate, anaphylaxis, hypotension, and neurological complications. There can also be a hypersensitivity to the protein of the tetanus organism itself. The cause of this is unknown. In some people, there is an interaction between the tetanus vaccine and high levels of preexisting antibody from prior tetanus vaccines (booster doses). This is the most common cause of arthritis-like responses. People with this problem should not be given even emergency doses of tetanus vaccine more than every 10 years.

Booster Doses and Immunity

Booster doses of tetanus vaccine should be given at 10-year intervals throughout life. The onset of protection occurs after the primary immunizing series (3 doses) and continues as long as the booster doses are given. If a wound occurs that requires the protection of the tetanus vaccine and the person has not received the primary tetanus vaccine series, then protection from tetanus can be achieved through the tetanus immune globulin shot.

Pertussis

This vaccine is usually given with tetanus and diphtheria (known as the DTP shot). There is a whole cell pertussis vaccine (DTwP) and an acellular pertussis vaccine (DTaP). Recently, the recommendation has been to use only the acellular pertussis vaccine because the incidence of side effects is less than with the whole cell pertussis vaccination.

This vaccine should not be given for the treatment of pertussis.

Contraindications

The pertussis vaccine should not be given to children who have recovered from pertussis. In addition, it should not be given to anyone who has a history of serious adverse reactions to a previous dose of a pertussis vaccine. These reactions include an immediate anaphylactic reaction, or encephalopathy occurring within 7 days following the injection. Symptoms of encephalopathy may include major alterations in consciousness, unresponsiveness, and generalized or focal seizures that persist for more than a few hours. A person may fail to recover from encephalopathy within 24 hours.

Data are unavailable as to the use of the acellular pertussis vaccine in children who cannot be given the whole cell pertussis vaccine. Therefore, until data are available, all the contraindications for the whole cell pertussis vaccine are to be adopted as contraindications for the acellular pertussis vaccine.

The pertussis-containing vaccine should not be given to children under 6 weeks old or to people over 7 years old.

Precautions

The following instances warrant careful consideration as to whether the child should receive additional doses of the pertussis-containing DTwP or DTaP injection:

- Temperature over 105°F within 48 hours of receiving the pertussis-containing vaccine (and no other cause can be found as to why the child has this fever)

- Collapse or shocklike state within 48 hours of the injection
- Persistent, inconsolable crying that lasts more than 3 hours, occurring within 48 hours of the injection
- Convulsions with or without fever within 3 days of the injection
- Occurrence of any type of neurological symptom or sign (including one or more convulsions) following injection. This is a contraindication to further use of the pertussis vaccine, whether whole cell or acellular.
- Any evolving or changing disorder that involves the central nervous system, even if a seizure does not occur, contraindicates using the pertussis vaccine (whole cell or acellular).
- DTaP should be given with caution to children who have blood coagulation disorders that would contraindicate any injection.
- With children for whom the pertussis component of the vaccine is contraindicated, the DT shot (diphtheria and tetanus toxoids for pediatric use) should be used instead.

Vital Fact

Studies suggest that infants and children with a history of convulsions in first-degree family members (parents or siblings) have an increased risk of neurological events linked to the pertussis vaccine, compared with those who have no such history. Some experts feel that these studies may be flawed by selection bias or genetic confounding.

Adverse Reactions

Pain, redness, and nodule development can occur at the injection site. Rarely, an abscess may develop. Fevers that range from 101° to 104.7°F are considered mild reactions to the pertussis-containing vaccine. Within 12 hours of vaccination, irritability, malaise, sleepiness, and vomiting may occur and persist for 1 to 7 days.

Several types of reactions have occurred after the pertussis vaccine (by itself) and the DTP shot. Most of these reactions are due to the pertussis component of the vaccine. Reactions that contraindicate further vaccination with pertussis include convulsions, encephalopathy, neurological disease, collapse, shock, and altered consciousness.

Booster Doses and Immunity

Three doses of pertussis vaccine produce a 50 to 95 percent reduction in the incidence of the disease. The vaccination is effective for more than 4 to 6 years.

Haemophilus influenzae Type b

There are various forms of this vaccine. The vaccine leads to active immunity against diseases caused by *Haemophilus influenzae* type b bacteria. Groups with increased susceptibility to this disease include children in day care, people with low socioeconomic status, and African-Americans (especially those lacking a specific immune globulin). In addition, Caucasians lacking a specific immune globulin, Native Americans, and individuals with sickle cell disease are also considered high-risk.

Contraindications

Patients who are hypersensitive to any component of this vaccine should not receive it. Patients who have an illness or acute infection have reason to delay this vaccination until they are better.

Those with a mild illness can be given this vaccine.

Adverse Reactions

A fever over 101°F occurred at least once in 2 percent of recipients during clinical trials. Redness, swelling, and tenderness are additional reactions seen after given this vaccine. Irritability, restless sleep, diarrhea, vomiting, loss of appetite, rash, hives, thrombocytopenia, convulsions, and renal failure or Guillain-Barré Syndrome are all post-vaccine reactions that may or may not be due to the vaccine.

Booster Doses and Immunity

Booster doses after 15 months of age are not currently recommended. Roughly a 45 to 88 percent reduction of disease incidence among children 18 to 24 months of age or older has been demonstrated. Since there are many different forms of this vaccine, the efficacy range varies. Protection lasts several years.

Inactivated Polio Vaccine

This vaccine is the preferred method of protecting against polio. Immunization of children is recommended. Immunization of adults living within the continental United States is not usually necessary because of the low probability of exposure to the disease.

Contraindications

Patients with a history of hypersensitivity to any component of this vaccine should not receive it.

If anaphylaxis occurs within 24 hours of this injection, no further injections of polio should be given. Immunization should be delayed during an acute illness.

Adverse Reactions

Redness, induration, and pain at the injection site may occur. Temperatures over 102°F have been reported in 38 percent of patients.

Booster Doses and Immunity

A total of three or four doses is necessary to complete the series (this depends on the age of the patient). It is possible to develop 97.5 to 100 percent protection after two doses. Protection lasts many years.

Measles, Mumps, and Rubella
(Live Vaccine)

Also known as MMR, this vaccine actively immunizes against all three illnesses.

Contraindications

The following people should not be given this vaccine:

- Pregnant patients
- Patients who are hypersensitive to any of its components (including eggs, if there has been an anaphylactic reaction)
- Patients receiving immunosuppressive therapy

Vital Study

Doctors and researchers are concerned about the rise of autism, childhood diabetes, asthma, learning disabilities, and other chronic conditions of childhood and their possible association with the increase in childhood vaccinations. You can find studies and ongoing research information on the Internet and in many natural or health magazines.

- Patients with blood disorders
- Patients with primary or acquired immunodeficiency
- Patients with any febrile illness or infection
- Patients with active and untreated tuberculosis

Adverse Reactions

Short-term burning or stinging can occur at the injection site. Local pain, induration, and redness can occur at the injection site. In addition, symptoms of the same kind following natural measles or rubella infection can occur. These include mild gland swelling, hives, rash, fatigue, sore throat, fever, headache, nausea, vomiting, diarrhea, joint pain, nerve inflammation, and arthritis. Fevers ranging from 101° to 103°F can appear 5 to 12 days after vaccination.

Guillain-Barré syndrome has been reported after immunization with rubella-containing vaccines.

Encephalitis and other nervous system reactions have also occurred very rarely in people given this vaccine. Rarely, vaccine recipients have reported chronic joint symptoms after this injection.

Booster Doses and Immunity

In most states, one booster dose is recommended to ensure protection against these diseases. Disease is usually reduced by 95 percent. Protection lasts 11 or more years.

Interesting Opinions

Due to the possible association between autism and the MMR vaccine, we recommend our patients get these vaccines separately and spaced apart. Talk with your physician if you want him to order the single measles, mumps, and rubella vaccines. They are available.

Varicella (Live Vaccine)

This vaccine is given to protect people from chicken pox. There are not enough data to state whether there is protection against the *complications* of chicken pox (for example encephalitis, hepatitis, and pneumonia) in children who have had the vaccine and contract the disease anyway.

Contraindications

The following people should not be given this vaccine:

- Those with hypersensitivity to any part of the vaccine, including gelatin
- Those with a history of anaphylactic reaction to neomycin
- Patients with certain blood disorders
- Patients receiving immunosuppressive therapy
- Those with active, untreated tuberculosis
- Pregnant women
- Those with any febrile respiratory illness or other active illness

Adverse Reactions

In clinical trials involving children, the following occurred: pain and soreness at the injection site, swelling, redness, rash, and itchiness, as well as induration, stiffness, and fever above 102°F. Rashes included injection rashes (peaking after 8 to 19 days) and general rashes (peaking after 5 to 26 days). Allergic responses, general illness, and encephalitis have also been reported.

Booster Doses and Immunity

Booster doses are not currently recommended. This vaccine provides 70 to 90 percent protection against infection for up to 10 years.

Interesting Opinions

Many natural health care providers worry that vaccinating children against chicken pox might lead to these kids getting chicken pox as adults, which can be serious.

Vital Facts

- On July 16, 1999, the U.S. Centers for Disease Control and Prevention (CDC) recommended phaseout of the rotavirus vaccine following reports of intussusception (bowel obstruction) after vaccination.
- The CDC's Advisory Committee on Immunization Practices has recommended changing the American policy for poliovirus vaccination. The change states that four doses of the inactivated polio vaccine as of January 1, 2000, are to replace the oral polio vaccine (a live vaccine). The American Academy of Pediatrics has agreed to discourage the use of the oral polio vaccine, to reduce the small risk of vaccine-associated paralytic polio, which can occur using the live, oral vaccine.
- In 1986, the National Childhood Vaccine Injury Act was created by the U.S. Congress to allow parents to seek compensation for children adversely affected by vaccines.
- In 1999, the FDA instructed vaccine manufacturers to cease making vaccines with thimerosal, a mercury preservative. The hepatitis B vaccine is the first vaccine available that is thimerosal-free. A list of thimerosal-containing vaccines can be found at www.vaccinesafety. edu.

Hepatitis A

This vaccine is used to induce active immunity against hepatitis A.

The CDC's Advisory Committee on Immunization Practices (ACIP) recommends vaccination of children in states, counties, and communities with baseline hepatitis A infection rates of 20 or more cases per 100,000 people per year. These states include Arizona, Alaska, Oregon, New Mexico, Utah, Washington, Oklahoma, South Dakota, Idaho, Nevada, and California.

In addition, there is further suggestion to consider vaccinating children in areas with hepatitis A incidence between 10 and 20 cases per 100,000 people per year. These states include Missouri, Texas, Colorado, Arkansas, Montana, and Wyoming.

Contraindications

Patients who are hypersensitive to any component of the vaccine or who have had a hypersensitivity reaction to the hepatitis A vaccine in the past should not receive it. The vaccination should be delayed in patients with any illness or active infection.

Adverse Reactions

Pain, tenderness, warmth, redness, and swelling at the injection site have been seen after this vaccination, as have fever (over 102°F), headache, abdominal pain, sore throat, bruising, upper respiratory infection, cough, diarrhea, vomiting, and laboratory abnormalities.

Booster Doses and Immunity

If persistent protection is desired, a booster dose is recommended 6 to 18 months after the initial dose. The disease rate of prevention is around 94 percent after the vaccine is administered. Protective antibody levels develop within 1 month after vaccination and should last at least 6 months.

Pneumococcal Conjugate Vaccine (PCV)

Also known by the brand name Prevnar, this vaccine is marketed to induce immunity in infants and toddlers against disease (such as meningitis) caused by *Streptococcus pneumoniae*. The ACIP recommends that all children up to 23 months be vaccinated. Older children (up to 59 months) may also be vaccinated, depending upon risk factors. Some doctors may recommend this vaccine for older children with recurrent ear infections, though it has not been approved for this use.

Contraindications

Patients with severe hypersensitivity to any component of the vaccine, including the diphtheria toxoid, should not receive it.

Temporarily defer vaccination if the child has an active infection.

The safety of this vaccine for children less than 6 weeks old has not been established. Immune response has not been studied in premature infants.

Adverse Reactions

In prelicensure trials, the most frequently reported events were injection site reactions, fever over 100°F, irritability, drowsiness, restless sleep, decreased appetite, vomiting, diarrhea, rash, and hives. More serious reactions such as seizures and anaphylaxis are rare.

Booster Doses and Immunity

No boosters are currently recommended. Immunity increases with successive doses. It is not determined how long immunity lasts.

Depending upon the age of the recipient, one to four doses are required.

Booster Doses and Immunity

Pneumococcal Conjugate Vaccine (PCV)

natural health care modalities and resource guide

13

Acupuncture/Acupressure

These therapies are based on the ancient Chinese medicinal concept that the body contains 12 main channels of acupuncture/acupressure points. Through these channels run the life-giving energy known as *qi*. Disease arises when one or more of these channels (meridians) are blocked. Through the use of needles (acupuncture), or by pressing on specific points (acupressure), one can reestablish energy flow and balance in the body. There are hundreds of acupuncture/acupressure points. Since acupressure does not involve the use of needles, it is the preferred treatment for children. Practitioners of oriental medicine use acupuncture and acupressure in their practices.

American Oriental Bodywork Therapy Association
1010 Haddonfield-Berlin Road, Suite 408
Voorhees, NJ 08043
(856) 782-1616

American Association of Oriental Medicine
433 Front Street
Catasauqua, PA 18032
(610) 266-1433
www.aaom.org

Aromatherapy

Essential oils from plants, leaves, bark, roots, seeds, and flowers are used to treat a wide range of conditions.

National Association for Holistic Aromatherapy
4509 Interlake Avenue North #233
Seattle, WA 98103-6773
(888) ASK-NAHA
(206) 547-2164
www.naha.org

Biofeedback

Biofeedback is information supplied instantaneously about an individual's own physiological processes. Data concerning a person's cardiovascular activity (blood pressure and heart rate), temperature, brain waves, or muscle tension are monitored electronically and returned, or "fed back," to that person by a gauge on a meter, a light, or a sound. It has been shown that an individual can be taught to use biofeedback to learn how to voluntarily control the body's reactions to stress or related events. An individual learns through biofeedback training to detect his physical reactions (inside-the-skin events) and establish control over them. An example would be a child with anxiety who learns to calm his nervous system with the use of biofeedback. Clinical psychologists, counselors, and some health practitioners use biofeedback in their practices.

Biofeedback Certification Institute of America
10200 West 44th Avenue, Suite 310
Wheat Ridge, CO 80033
(303) 420-2902
www.bcia.org

Breastfeeding

Following are a list of organizations that have local chapters that provide breastfeeding moms with support. In addition, information is available through the following organizations regarding pumping breast milk, storing it, and proper breastfeeding techniques. Your local hospital should also have information regarding breastfeeding support, feeding techniques, and storage information.

Healthy Children 2000
Center for Breastfeeding
8 Jan Sebastian Way #13
Sandwich, MA 02563-2359
(508) 888-8044
www.aboutus.com/a100/hc2000/index.htm

International Childbirth Education Association, Inc.
PO Box 20048
Minneapolis, MN 55420
(952) 854-8660
www.icea.org

Lact-Aid International, Inc.
PO Box 1066
Athens, TN 37371-1066
(423) 744-9090
www.lact-aid.com

International Lactation Consultant Association
1500 Sunday Drive, Suite 102
Raleigh, NC 27607
(919) 787-5181
www.ilca.org

La Leche League International
1440 North Meacham Road
Schaumburg, IL 60168-4079
(800) LA-LECHE (also check your local phone book)
www.lalecheleague.org

Nursing Mothers Counsel
PO Box 50063
Palo Alto, CA 94303
(650) 599-3669 (national referral line)
www.nursingmothers.org

Wellstart International Corporate Headquarters
4062 First Avenue
San Diego, CA 92103
(619) 295-5192

Chelation Therapy

Chelation therapy is the use of certain agents or nutrients that help pull toxic substances out of the body (for instance, heavy metals such as lead). This can be done in intravenous form with chelating agents such as ethylenediaminetetraacetic acid (EDTA), or, less commonly, with oral agents (such as certain vitamins). Medical doctors and some naturopathic doctors use chelation therapy.

American College for Advancement in Medicine
23121 Verdugo Drive, Suite 204
Laguna Hills, CA 92653
www.acam.org

Chiropractic

This is a system of healing based on the premise that poor spinal health (subluxations) leads to improper nerve flow and disease. Through specific adjustments of the spine and extremities, one can restore spinal health and normal body function. Doctors of chiropractic are trained as primary health care physicians.

American Chiropractic Association
1701 Clarendon Boulevard
Arlington, VA 22209
(800) 986-4636
www.amerchiro.org

Craniosacral Therapy

Craniosacral therapy is a gentle, noninvasive type of bodywork. The craniosacral system consists of the membranes and fluid that surround and support the brain and spinal cord. It extends from the bones of the head (the cranium) down to the bones at the base of the spine (the sacrum). The fluid within the membranes is continuously draining and refilling. The filling and draining creates gentle, rhythmic, expanding and contracting movements that can be felt and monitored by a craniosacral therapist. The therapist then applies gentle manipulations to correct imbalances and reestablish proper fluid movement. Specific training is required to become a craniosacral therapist.

The Upledger Institute, Inc.
11211 Prosperity Farms Road, Suite D-325
Palm Beach Gardens, FL 33410
(800) 233-5880
www.upledger.com

Guided Imagery

This is the use of imaging techniques in one's mind to enhance health and well-being. Studies have shown a benefit to the immune system. For example, many children with cancer are taught to visualize their immune cells becoming active and fighting cancer cells. Clinical psychologists, counselors, naturopathic and medical doctors, and various other health practitioners use guided imagery.

The Academy for Guided Imagery
PO Box 2070
Mill Valley, CA 94942
(800) 726-2070
www.healthy.net/agi

Herbal Medicine

Herbal medicine is the therapeutic use of plant extracts for the prevention and treatment of illness. Herbalists and naturopathic doctors are trained extensively in therapeutic uses of herbs as medicine.

American Botanical Council
PO Box 144345
Austin, TX 78714-4345
(512) 926-4900
www.herbalgram.org

Herb Research Foundation
1007 Pearl Street, Suite 200
Boulder, CO 80302
(303) 449-2265
www.herbs.org

Homeopathy

Homeopathy is based on the premise that "like cures like." Homeo-pathic remedies are highly diluted medicines that stimulate the healing powers of the body. Homeopaths or homeopathic doctors have had extensive training in a certified program.

National Center for Homeopathy
801 North Fairfax Street, Suite 306
Alexandria, VA 22314
(703) 548-7790
www.homeopathic.org

Homeopathic Academy of Naturopathic Physicians
12132 Southeast Foster Place
Portland, OR 97266
(503) 761-3298

Massage

Massage is the therapeutic use of external pressure applied to the skin and muscles of the body.

American Massage Therapy Association
820 Davis Street, Suite 100
Evanston, IL 60201-4444
(847) 864-0123
www.amtamassage.org

Naturopathy

This is a system of natural medicine that focuses on working with the healing systems of the body. Naturopathic doctors are trained as primary health care providers. As general practitioners, they work to prevent and restore health using clinical nutrition, herbal medicine, homeopathy, physical medicine, counseling, hydrotherapy, and other forms of natural healing.

The American Association of Naturopathic Physicians
8201 Greensboro Drive, Suite 300
McLean, VA 22102
(703) 610-9037
www.naturopathic.org

Canadian Naturopathic Association
1255 Sheppard Avenue East
Toronto, Ontario, M2K 1E2
Canada
(416) 496-8633

Osteopathy

Osteopathy is a system of medicine based on the premise that the structure (the spine and extremities) is related to the internal health of the body. Osteopathic doctors may use spinal manipulation to treat patients. They are also trained in drugs and surgery and practice as primary doctors.

American Osteopathic Association
142 East Ontario Street
Chicago, IL 60611-2818
(800) 621-1773
www.am-osteo-assn.org

Parasitology Testing

Testing for intestinal parasites is generally done using a stool sample. Your doctor can order a specialized kit from a lab that does comprehensive parasitology testing. We have listed one major lab for your convenience.

Great Smokies Diagnostic Laboratory
63 Zillicoa Street
Asheville, NC 28801
(800) 522-4762
www.gsdl.com

Physiotherapy

Physiotherapy is the use of external therapies to prevent and treat health conditions: the use of heat, cold, light, and physical and mechanical means to enhance healing within the body. Physiotherapists are trained health care specialists in the use of physiotherapy.

American Physical Therapy Association
1111 North Fairfax Street
Alexandria, VA 22314-1488
(800) 999-2782
www.apta.org

Vaccine Reporting

To report an adverse reaction to a vaccine, contact the Vaccine Adverse Event Reporting System (VAERS).

VAERS
(800) 822-7967
(847) 434-4000 (American Academy of Pediatrics)
www.aap.org

Centers for Disease Control and Prevention (CDC)
1600 Clifton Road
Atlanta, GA 30333
(800) 311-3435
www.cdc.gov

VOC Information

If you're concerned about exposing your child to volatile organic compounds (VOCs), which can cause health problems such as asthma, allergies, headaches, fatigue, and possibly even cancer, these companies can provide more information.

Scientific Certification Systems
1939 Harrison Street, Suite 400
Oakland, CA 94612
(510) 832-1415
www.scs1.com
(Certifies cleaners based on their biodegradability, toxicity, and VOC content)

Northwest Coalition for Alternatives to Pesticides
PO Box 1393
Eugene, OR 97440-1393
(514) 344-5044
www.pesticide.org
(Offers fact sheets on the dangers of pesticides and alternatives for specific pest problems)

American Formulating and Manufacturing
3251 Third Avenue
San Diego, CA 92103
(619) 239-0321
(Offers low-VOC paints, stains, sealants, carpet cleaner, and flooring adhesive)

Benjamin Moore and Company
51 Chestnut Ridge Road
Montvale, NJ 07645
(800) 826-2623
www.benjaminmoore.com
(Offers VOC-free paint and some low-VOC Crayola brand paints)

Environmental Construction Outfitters (ECO) of New York
(800) 238-5008
www.environproducts.com
(Offers no-VOC paints, flooring, carpets, and low-pollutant wallpaper)

references

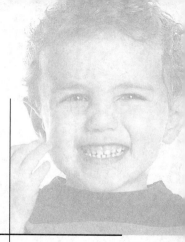

Following is a list of recommended reading on children's health and natural medicine. For a complete listing of *Your Vital Child* references and other recommended reading, visit our Web site at www.thenaturalphysician.com.

Childhood Illness and the Allergy Connection by Zoltan Rona, M.D.

The Baby Book by William Sears, M.D.,
and Martha Sears, R.N.

Encyclopedia of Natural Medicine by Michael Murray, N.D.,
and Joseph Pizzorno, N.D.

The Family Nutrition Book by William Sears, M.D.,
and Martha Sears, R.N.

Healing the Hyperactive Brain by Michael Lyon, M.D.

How to Raise a Healthy Child by Lendon Smith, M.D.

The Infant Survival Guide by Lendon Smith, M.D.

The Natural Physician's Healing Therapies
by Mark Stengler, N.D.

Prescription for Nutritional Healing by Phyllis Balch, C.N.C.,
and James Balch, M.D.

index

Underscored page references indicate boxed text. **Boldface** references indicate illustrations.

E